'This book demonstrates the continuing development and creativity of the discipline rooted in Freud's work. It offers expert coverage of the proliferation of psychoanalytic ideas providing an excellent introduction to the discipline. It is brought together and integrated with great care to make a clear statement about the continuing relevance of our discipline.'

Peter Fonagy *is professor of Contemporary Psychoanalysis and Developmental Science, University College London*

'Huppertz has put together an extraordinary volume that covers the development of psychoanalytic theory and practice from Freud's talking cure through modern relational perspectives. A particular strength of the volume is that it traces the evolution of psychoanalysis from a one-person to a two-person sensibility. This makes it an invaluable volume for teaching and learning about psychoanalytic thinking.'

Peter Buirski *is dean emeritus at the Graduate School of Professional Psychology, University of Denver*

'Huppertz demonstrates his masterful understanding of the study of the human mind as a dynamic science in which fundamentals are fluid to interpretational biases, cultural beliefs, and other influential circumstances. Assumptions, confounding of opposition between psychoanalytic schools and diversified cultural influences, are powerless against the symphony of insight given by the prominent psychoanalytic professionals featured here.'

Susan P. Sherkow *is a training analyst and instructor at the Berkshire Psychoanalytic Institute*

'Huppertz has done a great service by bringing together this extraordinary volume that provides clear and compelling glimpses into the assumptions of many schools of psychoanalytic thought. Written by esteemed experts, this eminently readable volume captures the vitality of the global psychoanalytic community.'

Kerry J. Sulkowicz *is president of the American Psychoanalytic Association*

Underlying Assumptions in Psychoanalytic Schools

This book offers a comparative study of the major schools of psychoanalysis by exploring their historical development, their differences and similarities, and the underlying assumptions made by each.

Encompassing the expertise of colleagues from different schools of psychoanalytic thought, each chapter explores a particular perspective, defining specific theoretical assumptions, theories of etiology, and implications for technique, as well as providing each author's view on the historical development of key psychoanalytic concepts.

With contributions from leading authors in the field, and covering both historical and international schools, the book provides an enlightening account that will prove essential to psychoanalytic practitioners and students of psychoanalysis and the history of medicine.

Bernd Huppertz is a physician in private practice. He is a psychotherapist (child, adolescent, adult, and group), a psychiatrist, a neurologist, and, formerly, a brain researcher. In 2002, he qualified to teach further education in psychiatry and psychotherapy (lecturer, teaching therapist, and supervisor) (Brandenburg Medical Association). He is also a part-time medical director of non-profit outpatient counseling/rehabilitation centers for addicted patients. He is a research associate of the American Psychoanalytic Association (APsaA), a member of the Association for Child Psychoanalysis (ACP), a member of the American Psychological Association (APA) (Division 39), a fellow of the International College of Psychosomatic Medicine (ICPM), and the founder of the Institute for Comparative Psychotherapy. He has published in the fields of psychiatry, psychoanalysis, psychotherapy, and psychosomatic medicine and is the editor of *Psychotherapy in the Wake of War: Discovering Multiple Psychoanalytic Traditions* and of *Approaches to Psychic Trauma: Theory and Practice.*

Underlying Assumptions in Psychoanalytic Schools

A Comparative Perspective

Edited by Bernd Huppertz

Routledge
Taylor & Francis Group
LONDON AND NEW YORK

Designed cover image: Staircase Berggasse 19, Vienna, photographed by the editor.

First published 2023
by Routledge
4 Park Square, Milton Park, Abingdon, Oxon OX14 4RN

and by Routledge
605 Third Avenue, New York, NY 10158

Routledge is an imprint of the Taylor & Francis Group, an informa business

British Library Cataloguing-in-Publication Data
A catalogue record for this book is available from the British Library

ISBN: 978-0-367-46255-0 (hbk)
ISBN: 978-0-367-46256-7 (pbk)
ISBN: 978-1-003-02776-8 (ebk)

DOI: 10.4324/9781003027768

Typeset in Times New Roman
by MPS Limited, Dehradun

Dedicated to Elisabeth Spillius, Anne-Marie Sandler, Joseph Lichtenberg, Anne Alvarez, Robert Hinshelwood, and Neil Skolnick: without their support this book would not be possible.

Contents

Contributors

Miri Abramis is a faculty, fellow, training and supervising analyst at the William Alanson White Institute in New York City, US. She teaches courses on applications of child development research to adult treatment and the work of Edgar Levenson. She is also the director of the WAWI Intensive Psychoanalytic Psychotherapy Program (IPPP). She is an associate editor of *Contemporary Psychoanalysis*. Dr. Abramis is in private practice in Manhattan, specializing in psychoanalysis, and psychotherapy with individuals and couples. She supervises widely.

Ann Addison is a lecturer at Essex University, UK, and a training analyst of the Society of Analytical Psychology, with a private practice in Central London for the treatment of adult patients. She has published papers on Jung and Bion in *The Journal of Analytical Psychology* and the *International Journal of Jungian Studies* and her book, *Jung's Psychoid Concept Contextualised*, published by Routledge, covers her research on Jung.

Samuel Arbiser is a full member, with the didactic role, of the Buenos Aires Psychoanalytic Association, a lecturer at the APdeBA Mental Health University Institute (IUSAM), a former member of the Committee of Publications of the IPA, author of *El Grupo Interno—Psiquis y Cultura (The Internal Group—Psyche and Culture)*, co-editor of *On Freud's "Inhibitions, Symptoms & Anxiety,"* and author of numerous articles in Spanish, English, French, Italian, German, and Portuguese for several psychoanalytic journals.

Orit Badouk Epstein is a UKCP attachment-based psychoanalytic psychotherapist, a training supervisor, and a training therapist. She trained at the Bowlby Centre, London, where she is the editor of the journal *Attachment: New Directions in Psychotherapy and Relational Psychoanalysis*. She has a private practice and has a particular interest in working with individuals who suffered extreme abuse. She specializes in attachment and trauma and regularly lectures, teaches, and writes articles and book chapters. She is the editor of various books, the most recent being *Shame Matters* published by Routledge, in 2021.

Joshua R. Burg is a licensed psychologist located in Denver, Colorado, US. He is an elected council representative of the International Association for Psychoanalytic Self Psychology (IAPSP) and chair of the Students & Candidates/Website & Social Media committees. He focuses his professional time on providing individual psychotherapy, teaching, and supervising students. Josh remains passionate about the psychoanalytic practice and often pursues continued training in self-psychology, intersubjective systems theory, and other contemporary relational approaches to psychodynamic practice.

Graham S. Clarke is a visiting fellow in the Department of Psychosocial and Psychoanalytic Studies, University of Essex, UK. He is the author of *Personal Relations Theory: Fairbairn, Macmurray and Suttie* (2006) and *Thinking Through Fairbairn* (2018). He was lead editor of *Fairbairn and the Object Relations Tradition* (2014) with David Scharff.

Les Fleischer is an associate professor at Lakehead University Orillia, Faculty of Health and Behavioural Sciences, and is on faculty at the Toronto Institute of Psychoanalysis. He is a psychoanalyst in private practice. He has published papers on psychoanalytic theory, castration depression, body image, unconscious fantasies, the superego, psychoanalytic education, and the education of mental health professionals. Additional research interests include classical theory, modern ego psychology, dreams, anxiety, mood disorders, and character disorders.

Tomasz Fortuna has been trained as a psychoanalyst at the Institute of Psychoanalysis in London, UK. He is a member of the British Psychoanalytical Society and the Hanna Segal Institute for Psychoanalytic Studies. He is a visiting professor at the Department of Psychiatry of Universiti Putra Malaysia. He worked as a psychiatrist in the NHS for 16 years and is now at the Portman Clinic and in private psychoanalytic practice. He teaches and supervises at the Tavistock and Portman Clinics, the Institute of Psychoanalysis, and abroad. His professional interests include the relationship between psychoanalysis and the arts, and the understanding of severe emotional disturbance and criminal behavior. He has published several articles and chapters and co-authored *Melanie Klein: The Basics.*

Roger Frie is a professor of education, at Simon Fraser University; an affiliate professor of psychiatry, at the University of British Columbia, Canada; and a faculty and supervisor at William Alanson White Institute in New York. He has published ten books and is co-editor, most recently, of *Culture, Politics and Race in the Making of Interpersonal Psychoanalysis* (Routledge, 2022). He is a former co-editor of *Psychoanalysis, Self and*

Context and an Editorial Board member of *Contemporary Psychoanalysis* and *Psychoanalytic Psychology.*

Alexandra Harrison is a practicing child and adult psychiatrist and psychoanalyst in Cambridge, Massachusetts, US, with a special interest in children ages 0–5 years old and children on the autistic spectrum. She is a part-time assistant professor at Harvard Medical School at the Cambridge Health Alliance and president of a nonprofit, Supporting Child Caregivers. She is a training and supervising analyst in adult, child, and adolescent psychoanalysis at the Boston Psychoanalytic Society and Institute and a member of HMS (CHA) and SCC.

Leon Hoffman is a psychiatrist and child and adolescent psychiatrist; training and supervising analyst in adult, child, and adolescent analysis, co-director, Pacella Research Center at NYPSI (New York Psychoanalytic Society and Institute); faculty, Icahn School of Medicine at Mount Sinai; chief psychiatrist/psychoanalyst, West End Day School in New York City, US. Most notably, he is the author of *Manual for Regulation-Focused Psychotherapy for Children (RFP-C) with Externalizing Behaviors: A Psychodynamic Approach*, co-written with Timothy Rice and Tracy Prout.

John Keene is a training and supervising analyst of the British Psychoanalytical Society, UK. He teaches and supervises across the world and is the co-editor of *Independent Psychoanalysis Today* (2012) with Paul Williams and Sira Dermen. He also works with groups and institutions and is the author of "Unconscious Obstacles to Caring for the Planet: Facing up to Human Nature" (2012).

Amanda Kottler is a clinical psychologist practicing as a psychoanalytic psychotherapist in Cape Town, South Africa. She is a founding and faculty member of the Cape Town Psychoanalytic Self Psychology Group and an emeritus council member of the International Association of Self Psychology. She has previously held a post as a senior lecturer at the University of Cape Town but now works full-time in private practice, teaching occasionally. She has published in South Africa, the UK, and the USA, and co-edited two previous books. She is a co-author of *Kohut's Twinship across Cultures: The Psychology of Being Human*, published by Routledge in 2015.

Patrick Landman is a psychoanalyst, child psychiatrist, and lawyer. He was president of the association Espace Analytique founded by the famous child psychoanalyst Maud Mannoni. He has worked on the transmission of psychoanalysis and as a child psychiatrist on the demutualization of autistic children.

Francois Louw is a chartered clinical psychologist (British Psychological Society), psychoanalyst (British Psychoanalytical Society), and psychosomatician

(IPSO P. Marty), UK. He is the Psychological Therapies Lead for Pain Management Services of the Royal Free London NHS Foundation Trust. Furthermore, he works in private practice in London, teaches various courses at the Institute of Psychoanalysis, and is a visiting lecturer on the Tavistock Adult Psychotherapy course and University College London's MSc in Theoretical Psychoanalytic Studies.

Iréne Matthis is a professor of psychoanalysis and an associate professor of clinical neuroscience, at Umeå University, Sweden. Now retired, she has been a training analyst for the Swedish Psychoanalytic Association (IPA). She is one of the founders, in 2000, of the International NeuroPsychoanalysis Society and was editor of the regional bulletin *Journal Neuropsychoanalysis* for the first 8 years. She has published more than ten books and many articles on psychoanalysis, women's issues, psychosomatics, and neuropsychoanalysis. In 1968, she was one of the founders of Group 8, the Swedish Women Liberation Movement.

Isabelle Meier is a graduate of the C.G. Jung Institute Zürich (1996) and maintains a private practice in Zürich, Switzerland. She received her doctorate in psychology from the University of Zurich, as well as her degree in history and philosophy. She is a training analyst and supervisor of the C.G. Jung-Institut, Zürich, and of ISAPZURICH. Isabelle has authored several publications in German, and English. Her special area of interest lies in the links of imagination, complexes, and archetypes.

Judit Mészáros is a habil. professor honoris causa—Eötvös Loránd University, Budapest. Mészáros is a training and supervising analyst of the Hungarian Psychoanalytical Society (affiliated with the IPA); and a staff member at the European Psychotherapy Training Institute, Budapest. She has written scores of papers and book chapters, edited or authored books, curated exhibitions of the "Budapest School of Psychoanalysis" in London and Budapest, and was an expert consultant for a Ferenczi film (Hungarian TV). Her latest book: *Ferenczi and Beyond. Exile of the Budapest School and Solidarity in the Psychoanalytic Movement during the Nazi Years*, Karnac, 2014. She is the president of the Sándor Ferenczi Society, an Executive Board member of the International Sándor Ferenczi Network, and a psychoanalyst/psychotherapist in private practice.

Alejandra Perez is a psychoanalyst in private practice, a member of the British Psychoanalytic Society, and a parent-infant psychotherapist at the Anna Freud National Centre for Children and Families (AFNCCF). She is also the programme director of the MSc Early Child Development and Clinical Applications at University College London/AFNCCF and gives talks in the UK and internationally on clinical work with parents and infants, psychoanalysis, psychic development, and parenting. She is currently head of Longitudinal Experiences and Adjustments in Parenthood Study

(LEAPS) which explores the parent-child relationship and parents' experiences in the early years.

Neil Skolnick is a faculty member, supervisor, and past co-director of the Relational Track at the NYU Postdoctoral Program in Psychoanalysis. Additionally, he is a faculty member and supervisor at the National Training Program (NTP) of the National Institute for the Psychotherapies (NIP), the Institute for the Psychoanalytic Study of Subjectivity (IPSS), and the Westchester Center for the Study of Psychoanalysis and Psychotherapy. His most recent book, published by Routledge in 2020, is *Relational Psychoanalysis and Temporality: Time Out of Mind.* He has authored numerous journal articles and book chapters, and edited two books: with Susan Warshaw (1992), *Relational Perspectives in Psychoanalysis,* and with David Scharff (1998), *Fairbairn: Then and Now.* He maintains a private practice in Manhattan, US, where he also supervises and conducts study groups.

Allen Siegel is a psychoanalytically trained psychiatrist with 50 years of experience in treating, teaching, and writing about psychoanalytic treatment from a self-psychological perspective. He is the author of the well-received book *Heinz Kohut and the Psychology of the Self.* He is the American Director of the Anatolian Association of Psychanalytic Psychotherapies and a founding member of the International Association for Psychoanalytic Self Psychology. He also teaches self-psychology internationally.

Frank Summers is a clinical psychologist, psychoanalyst, a professor of clinical psychiatry and the behavioral sciences, at Feinberg School of Medicine, Northwestern University, and a supervising and training analyst at the Chicago Psychoanalytic Institute and the Chicago Center for Psychoanalysis. Author of four books on psychoanalytic theory from an object relations perspective, including *The Psychoanalytic Vision,* winner of the Gradiva Award in 2013, Dr. Summers maintains a private practice of psychoanalysis and psychoanalytic therapy in Chicago, Illinois, US.

Frances Thomson-Salo is an affiliate researcher, at Murdoch Children's Research Institute, is a training adult and child psychoanalyst, and has worked in private practice and teaching hospitals in London and Australia as an infant mental health consultant. She is a member of the British Psychoanalytical Society and the Australian Psychoanalytical Society. As an associate professor, at the Department of Psychiatry, University of Melbourne, she taught the Masters of Mental Health Sciences for 20 years, specializing in infant mental health, and her books include *Engaging Infants: Embodied Communication in Short-Term Infant-Parent Therapy* (2018) and *Infant Observation: Creating*

Transformative Relationships (2014). She is an Editorial Board member of *The International Journal of Psychoanalysis* and chaired committees on Women and Psychoanalysis, and Sexual and Gender Diversity Studies of the International Psychoanalytic Association.

Koichi Togashi is a faculty and training and supervising analyst at Training and Research in Intersubjective Self Psychology, New York; a professor at Konan University, Kobe, Japan; and is in private practice in Hiroshima & Kobe, Japan. He is a council member of the International Association for Psychoanalytic Self Psychology. He is an editor of *Psychoanalytic Inquiry*, and an international editor of *Psychoanalysis, Self and Context*. He is also a member of the Executive Board of the Japan Psychoanalytical Association, and an editor of *The Japanese Journal of Psycho-Analysis*. He has published numerous books and articles in the US, Japan, and Taiwan. His latest book, *The Psychoanalytic Zero: Decolonizing Study of Therapeutic Dialogues*, won the 2020 Gradiva Award for Best Book.

Ed Tronick is a university distinguished professor in the Developmental Brain Sciences Program of the University of Massachusetts Boston and a research associate at the Harvard Medical School. He is the faculty chief of the Infant Parent Mental Health Post Graduate Certificate Program at the University of Massachusetts Boston in the US.

Massimo Vigna-Taglianti is a child neuropsychiatrist. He is a full member of the International Psychoanalytical Association and of the Italian Psychoanalytical Society, of which he was scientific chair from 2017 to 2021; he is a training and supervising analyst, and an expert in the analysis of children and adolescents. He is also an adjunct professor of child and adult psychiatry at Aosta University. For 20 years, his theoretical-clinical interest and his publications in various Italian and foreign journals and books concerned research in psychoanalysis and the area of pre-verbal trauma and transference phenomena, with particular reference to role-reversal and the importance of the transformative functions performed by action, play, and dream in the analytic process.

Foreword

Every time a new book is published it feels like a celebration. It is the outcome of an intense work of writing, and compilation—in this case—and it is the result of a painstaking task of editing. It is also a beginning, since the volume has become public it can be read and thus begins its own path, its journey, and becomes independent from the authors.

In this very interesting and appealing book, Bernd Huppertz presents 29 chapters written by different authors that carry the common thread of a question: what are the underlying assumptions in the different theoretical schools of psychoanalysis? These schools were, of course, born after Freud's fundamental and revolutionary contributions to the foundation of psychoanalysis. Freud's main contributions and the authors who followed him have had an enormous impact on our culture, influencing many fields such as mental health, pediatrics, law, and education, among others. I find a remarkable significance in this book as it creates a current mapping of the psychoanalytic schools and these perspectives are presented by authors that are, in fact, renowned in their own field. As a conclusion, in the final chapters we are offered an interesting comparative overview and some thoughtful considerations by the editor.

It is always a stimulating exercise and a needed task to examine and sometimes question the axioms (as they are called in mathematics) that sustain our psychoanalytic model, hence our practice. These underlying assumptions call for definitions and explanations that give our practice a meaningful theoretical basis, and it is also imperative to take into account the unconscious or implicit dimensions of the model of the mind that each analyst works with.

If psychoanalytic theory relies on our clinical work, then our practice and the current social and cultural realities work as a compass and, in turn, they sometimes demand modifications, adaptations, and revisions of our models of the mind. So, it is impossible not to take into account the culture in which we practice psychoanalysis.

This book also illustrates how each culture provides a different point of view and how each author provides another perspective, because as Huppertz says, behind each model of the mind there are authors that carry specific sensitivities to diverse aspects of a theory, in this way there are multiple versions of the different theories of the mind, that enrich them.

Coming from Argentina, I have to say that it makes me very proud to see *a* chapter about Argentine psychoanalysis, as they have made invaluable contributions to our discipline. And, importantly, this book also brings the Asian psychoanalytic perspective that has been on a path of significant development for so long.

Finally, I believe that this book will become a must-read because it offers an updated map of the current ideas coming from an international psychoanalytical community.

Virginia Ungar
IPA former President
2017–2021

Acknowledgments

First, I would like to express my gratitude to Bob Hinshelwood whose wealth of knowledge and deeply thoughtful comments provided the motivation for this book. Our telemeetings and discussions during its development and completion over a period of years will remain unforgettable for me: it was an exciting journey of discovery as we followed up leads, moves, and eventual new movements over the decades.

I would also like to thank Anne Alvarez for her encouragement and enthusiastic support, our lively discussions, and her help with editing issues.

Further, I have to thank Seth Aronson, Kathrin Asper, Tessa Baradon, Tony Bass, Mark J. Blechner, Peter Buirski, Margaret Crastnopol, David L. Downing, Joseph Fernando, Denis Flynn, Aikaterin Fotopoulou, Glen Gabbard, Penelope Garvey, Adrienne Harris, Andre Haynal, Ruth Imber, Theodore Jacobs, Marinella Lia, Nancy McWilliams, Mariângela Mendes de Almeida, Joan Raphael-Leff, Andrew Samuels, David Scharff, Joan Schachter, Joyce Slochower, Mark Solms, Alain Vanier and especially Sheila Hafter Gray for their support. Special thanks go to Sibylle Schacke.

I thank Taylor Frecker for her assistance with the grammar, proofreading, and formatting. My special thanks go to Alexis O'Brien, Susannah Frearson, Russell George, and Katie Randall from Routledge.

Special thanks to the contributors to this difficult project, for their willingness, support, and hard work.

In addition to this I would like to thank the following people for their helpful advice:

Jan Abram, Salman Akhtar, Maxine Anderson, David Armstrong, Anna Balas, Giovanni Battista Foresti, Francis Baudry, Ariane Bazan, Beatrice Beebe, Ricardo Bernardi, Christopher Bonovitz, Claudia Lucia Borensztejn, Sandra Buechler, Fredric Busch, Lesley Caldwell, Dana Charatan, Richard D. Chessick, Nancy Julia Chodorow, Marco Conci, Coline Covington, Elizabeth Danto, Sophie de Mijolla-Mellor, Jack Drescher, Judith Dupont, Judith Edwards, Gerard Fromm, Szönyi Gábor, Viviane Green, Jay

Greenberg, Rafael Groisman, Anne Harrison, Anton Hart, Irwin Hirsch, Jeremy Holmes, Douglas H. Ingram, Verena Kast, Gil Katz, Helena Klímová, Gregorio Kohon, Anton Kris, Thomas Kohut, Emily Kuriloff, Marie Christine Laznik, Susan Loden, George J. Makari, Norka Malberg, Jill Miller, Jane Milton, Juliet Mitchell, Marina Mojovic, Donna Orange, Anna Ornstein, Michael Parsons, Gerald Perman, Nydia and Alberto Pieczansky, Liana Pinto Chaves, Alfred Ribi, Helen Taylor Robinson, Eduardo Russo, Edgard Sanchez, Jill Scharff, Joy Schaverien, Tamar Schonfield, Joseph Schwartz, Andreas Schweizer, Caroline Sehon, Jonathan Shedler, Susan P. Sherkow, Jonathan Sklar, Alan Slomowitz, Donnel Stern, Anna Streeruwitz, Adrian Sutton, Jane Tillman, Mary Trowell, Steven Tublin, Mary Twyman, Martha Vennersten, Vamik D. Volkan, Monica Vorchheimer, Sherwood Waldron Jr., Douglas F. Watt, Mitchell Wilson, Jessica Yakeley, Margaret R. Zellner, and Samuel Zysman.

Introduction

Bernd Huppertz

Early in my professional life, I was confused by the contrast between the relative agreement among thinkers in the medical field and the differences between the various psychoanalytic schools and perspectives. What were the reasons for so many psychoanalytic approaches? I wanted to clarify this for myself, so I started studying some of these perspectives and traveled to London every month for nearly two decades. At that time, it was the center of European psychoanalysis and the city of Sigmund and Anna Freud, Melanie Klein, Wilfred R. Bion, Donald W. Winnicott, John Bowlby, and others.

During this period of my life, on a Saturday in 2006, I walked through an exhibition called "Constable: The Great Landscapes" at the Tate Britain Gallery in London. I saw that Constable had painted many mills, some several times, in winter, in the summer, from the side, back, in a different light, day, and night. It was always another painting, another perspective, and another view. That is, things were changing not only through the perspective, but also through the context, the changing environments such as time of day, day of the week, the season of the year, or year of the decade. In this sense, Constable could be seen to be conducting a great experiment using the type of chronobiological clock used in laboratory research. He invited the eye to look ever more closely at the object.

From this day on, I could better understand what Bion meant by the terms vertices, transformations, and the invariant. He wrote, "Significance therefore varies according to the point of view (or vertex) with which they are associated. Vertices may have as their approximate realizations various recognized disciplines such as religion, mathematics, physics, music, painting, and other arts" (1970, p. 21). Bion argued that a psychoanalyst transforms the facts he describes "by regarding them in a particular way. My description is therefore a transformation, analogous to the artist's painting that is a product of the particular artist's approach" (1965, p. 10). He saw the work of a psychoanalyst lying "between the point where a man receives sense impressions and the point where he gives expression to the transformation that has taken place" (1965, p. 46).

DOI: 10.4324/9781003027768-1

It is as a result of these experiences and readings that I have been driven to offer this comparative study of the major schools of psychoanalytic thought.

A Short Overview of the History of Psychoanalysis

(1) Sigmund Freud was the founder and developer of the psychoanalytic theory of the mind and of its treatment methodology. He and his followers succeeded in creating a powerfully cohesive and persuasive group to spread his ideas. After an initial phase, however, colleagues and pupils of Freud began to develop their own differing perspectives and ways of thinking. Then, so-called deviant theories (Guttman, 1985) followed, with the schisms of Alfred Adler (later the Adlerians) on one side and of Carl Gustav Jung (later the Jungians) on the other side (Freud, 1914).

Influenced by Abraham (1924), a gradual and slow move toward an object-relations perspective was begun. On the other side, a conflict emerged between Freud and Ferenzci about the importance of the issue of trauma. Later, other trajectories were pursued. In the beginning these schools were always strongly connected with a founder.

Then, developed in the following decades, (2) Anna Freud, Ego-Psychology, and finally the contemporary UK Freudians.

After a short time of consolidation, newer schools began to emphasize additional features in psychological development with (3) Melanie Klein, Kleinians, and post-Kleinians (drives as object-seeking). The controversial discussions (King & Steiner, 1991) between the Anna Freud group and the Melanie Klein group led to the development of a third group, the British Independents (Kohon, 1986, 2017) or the so-called Middle group. To this Middle group also belonged (4) Fairbairn, (5) Winnicott and the Winnicottians as part of the independents (though originally Kleinian), and other British Independents such as Balint and Bowlby. This group has sometimes also been referred to as the British object relations school (with different perspectives on each other as well). The group placed more emphasis than the Kleinians on the role of external objects.

(6) Bion (at first a Kleinian until 1959 and his paper "Attacks on Linking" then later perhaps post-Kleinian) struck off in a new direction in his attempt to study processes of thinking and the way in which emotion not only underlaid such processes but was central to them. (In the US many analysts have emphasized another thread in Bion's thinking, that is, the distinction between the omnipotent process of knowing what is in someone else's mind versus the slow process of *getting to* know, with the implication of the fundamental unknowability of another's mind (O)).

(7) At the same time Bowlby developed his own form of departure from the classical psychoanalytic emphasis on the internal world, by stressing the importance of processes of actual attachment between mother and infant.

Other new schools developed in Europe and the US: in France, (8) Lacan (until 1953 Kleinian), and the Lacanians under the influence of structuralism. In the US, (9) in the New York Psychoanalytic Society (founded 1911) and the New York Psychoanalytic Institute (founded 1930) the US Freudian school, and together with the emigrées from Nazi Europe, North American ego psychology was developed. This (10) North American ego psychology splintered into various approaches, from modern conflict theory to modern ego psychology.

Another major shift involved the change from a "one-person psychology" to a "two-person psychology" (Ferenczi, Balint, and Sullivan). One-person psychology, a term at first used by John Rickman in 1957, is focusing clinically on the intrapsychic world of the individual, that is the internal world. The use of concepts of transference and countertransference marked something of an intrapsychic parallel of that which later was called a two-person psychology in the United States. While in Europe, object relationists tried to integrate internal and external, in the United States the two-person psychology became, clinically, a relationship-based approach, focusing more on the interpsychic interactions of real individuals. Gradually, Sándor Ferenczi (11) and the Budapest school of psychoanalysis (important in the early years of psychoanalysis) had been taken up again in the United States as offering a bridge between the one-person and the two-person psychologies; it left room for environmental influences. Furthermore, in the decades since the 1920s, an interpersonal approach (12)—the integration of Sullivan's "interpersonal psychiatry" into a branch of psychoanalysis—meant that interpersonal relations became important and gave rise to a two-person psychology.

Then in the 1930s, a new group, the Neo-Freudians (13) such as Fromm, Karen Horney, and Clara Thompson focused, far more than Freud, on social and cultural factors in human development.

In the 1950s, Self-psychology, Kohut, and Kohutians (14) began the focus on the "self" with a new appreciation and understanding of different types of narcissism and other new lines of development. Kohut's ideas were further developed in various ways by the post-Kohutians (15).

In the 1980s, in New York, relational psychoanalysis (16) was born. The integration of relational theories, which were elaborated by Greenberg and Mitchell (1983), focused on the importance of the relational dimension for human development.

A little later in the same decade (1980s) the term intersubjectivity (17) was coined by George Atwood and Robert Stolorow (1984) in California and was grounded in inter-subjective systems theory and the importance of affect. They looked at "defenses" such as narcissism and obsessionality and suggested it was important to identify when such processes were pre-stages of defense and therefore represented genuine developmental needs and not simple defenses against something else.

(18) Individual American object relations theorists, for example Kernberg, developed various theories which saw object relationships as constituting the basic unit of the human personality.

Looking at the development aspects of psychoanalysis we can differentiate two main centers of research, the UK and the US.

Parent-infant psychotherapy in the UK (19) arose from followers of Anna Freud and Melanie Klein using Esther Bick's infant observation and later infant research as bases.

Infant research-rooted therapies in the US (20), derived from the observations of the early baby watchers, led to more fully-fledged psychoanalytic theories enriched by a developmental thinking (Boston Study Group and others).

(21) Neuropsychoanalysis/psychodynamic neuroscience forges a link between the neurosciences and psychoanalysis.

Other, more geographically rooted psychoanalytic schools, are marked by a diversity of approaches as in (22) the Italian psychoanalytic schools with, for example, Ferro, Civitarese, Borgogno, and Bolognini; the (23) South American schools with people such as Bleger, Pichon-Riviere, Racker, and the Barangers; or (24) the Asian psychoanalytic schools which are also marked by regional and cultural differences of their psychoanalytic schools or institutes.

Other Schools

The Jungian school approach, the analytical psychology (traditional and contemporary) (25) is marked by its difference from the other more Freudian-oriented schools. There is a wider definition of the unconscious which includes the distinction between a personal and a collective unconscious. There is also more emphasis on the role of culture in the making of meaning.

The post-Jungian approach (26) is marked by various regional and culturally influenced approaches. Nowadays it returns to the period of Jung's Red Book.

The Differences Between the Various Schools of Thought

After editing two books about different approaches and uses of psychodynamic thinking, *Psychotherapy in the Wake of War* and *Approaches to Psychic Trauma: Theory and Practice*, I was asked what were the real differences between these schools. I think these schools emerged because psychoanalysts have different views about certain essentials and the labels of the schools give their members a group identity. To cite Eisold:

> And that identity, in turn, as Ellenberger (1970) has pointed out, is linked to a "school" in the sense of the ancient Greco-Roman philosophical schools. Analysts are Freudian or Kleinian or Sullivanian, etc. in much the same way that ancient philosophers were Epicurean or Stoic or Pythagorian. Internalizing their training as part of their identities ....
>
> (2018c, p. 91)

I remembered and became aware that I had always easily, in the beginning of creating this manuscript, found authors who wanted to write under a specific label. Most of my authors of the one-person psychology type wrote about an important founder of a school labeled by his name, whereas those of the two-person psychology type tended to think and work more along the lines of the ideas of the school as a whole. Mostly they both adapted the models to the changing social environment and made them functional in their own way for the current time. They used these models mostly as a personal model or as a tool, as Paul Denis maintained:

> Furthermore, behind each explicit psychoanalytic model there is an author, who has been particularly sensitive to an aspect of mental functioning and the process of psychoanalytic treatment. New models may correspond to a broadening of the author's field of vision, but other models can correspond to an author's restriction of the field of vision or failure to take into consideration fundamental factors of psychoanalytic understanding.
>
> (quoted in Fischbein, 2015)

Only sometimes did someone want to remain in the classical style and to write in the rules and terms of the founders. I recognized furthermore that between the so-called schools of thought are fluid transformations as in a rainbow. We shall discover many mutations and interpenetrations from one color to the next.

The development of the various schools of psychoanalysis and the evolution of psychoanalytical/psychodynamic theory and therapy resulted in tremendous changes. These extend from the "Metapsychology" (Freud) to a "Psychoanalytic Phenomenology" of a subjective representational world (Sandler & Rosenblatt, 1962) and to a methodological system of interpretative principles and the work of Atwood and Stolorow (1980) which involved adding a psychology of deficit to the psychology of conflict.

Wallerstein was very much in favor of pluralism under the umbrella of psychoanalysis. However, "Stepansky's (2009) concerns about how the term 'pluralism' is used in psychoanalysis remain valid: Theorists from different perspectives 'have evidenced little desire to engage in such effectful imaginative activity' (p. 249)" (i.e. pluralism) (Jurist, 2018, p. 17).

In terms of reaction to these various schools Ken Eisold thought "The problem was—and, I believe, still is—the splintering and fragmentation of the psychoanalytic community: split apart, psychoanalysts lost the capacity to talk across their differences" (Eisold, 2018d, p. 51).

Looking at reactions on this diversity of psychoanalytic perspectives we can find:

> Anne-Marie Sandler (1990) noted her shock at discovering her own prejudices: 'I found myself wanting to deride those methods, which were different from those I was accustomed to, and it took some time to overcome my culture shock and to accept, at an emotional level, the reality that there were outstanding analysts who have followed a different training route' (p. 49).
>
> (Eisold, 2018c, p. 85)

"The historical corollary of this intolerance is the remarkable history of schisms in psychoanalytic institutes, testifying to the difficulty of containing, much less accepting, theoretical differences within existing organizations" (Eisold, 2018c, p. 85).

"This inward focus has led to an extraordinary history of schisms and splits, the institutional effects of which still divide the analytic landscape and prevent its professional organizations from speaking with one voice" (Eisold, 2018b, p. 185).

The Science of Investigating Variations (In Psychoanalytic Schools and Perspectives)

With time, after Victoria Hamilton's research concerning "The analyst's preconscious" (1996) in various schools and perspectives, a science of investigating these variations in psychoanalytic schools and theories developed. The question of whether a translation and communication between psychoanalytic concepts and different linguistic cultures is, in general, possible (Tuckett et al., 2008) or only in some cases or for a part of the schools, remains open. So Fischbein thought, "in this babble of different versions the possibilities of misunderstanding or reductionism will remain" (2015). Another attempt at identification of the problem is Kenneth Eisold's (2018a) book about the history of theoretical conflicts in psychanalysis.

Dana Birksted-Breen edited the book *Translation/Transformation: 100 Years of the International Journal of Psychoanalysis* (2021) concerning the problems of translations, language, and cultures. In this context I can add my two comparative studies about different schools of thought, *Psychotherapy in the Wake of War: Discovering Multiple Psychoanalytic Traditions* (2013) and *Approaches to Psychic Trauma: Theory and Practice* (2019). Robert Hinshelwood (2008) tried to compare different psychoanalytic concepts in his

"Repression and Splitting: Towards a Method of Conceptual Comparison" based on an early paper in 1999 (British Psychoanalytical Society). Later he developed his own Hermeneutic Deductive System in his book *Research on the Couch* (2013).

Much debate has existed about whether psychoanalysis can be called a science (personal information). Freud thought psychoanalysis was "a natural science like any other" (Freud, 1938, p. 158). However, what is considered 'science' has changed since then. Carl Hempel (1942) based his argument on Viennese logical positivism to require all knowledge to conform to scientific materialist principles of logic without metaphysics. It was a view taken up by Braithwaite (1953, see also Malin, 2021), with some application to psychoanalysis and social science. Others (Grunbaum, 1984; Hook, 1959; Popper, 1959) debated whether psychoanalysis could qualify as a science according to these newer principles. Science now demands that we not only generalize from facts to create hypotheses and theories (a process of induction) but we must subject those theories to deductive testing as well. As Grunbaum indicated, the criteria of a deductive scientific system need to be fully met, and psychoanalysis is still regarded by many as dubious in that respect.

Central to the problem of a scientific psychoanalysis is the fact that it does not deal with physical matter. Rather it deals with felt experience. That experience is the patient's feelings, and for the analyst, the meaning is to be given to those feelings. Meanings and feelings are not quantifiable in any simple way, as the facts about material substances are. This inexactitude leads to the assumption that psychoanalytic facts are subjective and therefore slippery in the hands of those wishing to prove anything scientifically.

Hinshelwood (2013), in his *Research on the Couch* has sought a defense of psychoanalytic research and practice as a deductive system analogous to a scientific one. As a starting point, he takes Ezriel's (1956) account of the analytic setting as exactly comparable to an experimental one in other physical sciences. Ezriel was convinced that the analytic process is a linear one just like that process in a scientific experiment. An intervention is made that changes the data observed; in the analytic setting the intervention is made which changes the associations afterward. This is an identical process.

Ezriel described the change in the psychoanalytic data as a one that brings the unconscious anxiety and defense more toward a conscious awareness. As an example, he described an aggressive man, frightened of his aggression, who before complained of the government in Whitehall, and after the interpretation of his fear, complained of the clinic where Ezriel worked. This is a striking move, literally geographical. But mostly psychoanalytic change cannot be measured in space, time, and substance. They are changes in the awareness of anxiety.

Hinshelwood was concerned about the reliability of this kind of change, regarding it as a hermeneutic change, rather than a quantitative one. And it is therefore at risk of a considerable bias from the observing analyst's subjectivity, and not least his own allegiance to a particular metapsychology that could influence the perception of anxieties and defenses in his patient. As a result, Hinshelwood suggests a method of addressing, even harnessing the subjectivity of the analyst, and he quoted Heimann saying the analyst's countertransference is a tool for understanding the patient's transference. However, it is only part of a tool, since Heimann clearly said we must "check [the analyst's countertransference and] interpretations against the actual data of the analytic situation" (Heimann, 1960, 1989, Hinshelwood, 2012, 2015). This recommends a comparison of the actual material, the patient's free associations, against the feelings (countertransference) of the analyst. Using Ezriels' model and Heimann's recommendation, it is therefore possible to define the research data, before and after the interpretation, as the overlap between the associations and the countertransference in terms of anxiety and defenses.

Moreover, it is possible to predict the outcome of the interpretation, just as the scientist predicts the outcome of an experimental intervention. The prediction in a psychoanalysis is, in general, that following the interpretation the anxiety will be more apparent consciously and the defense is less strong—as with the man who moved his aggression nearer to the analyst, focusing on the clinic rather than the government. As with the predictions in physical science, they need to be strict as it is then possible to exclude false positives. Hinshelwood then gave some clinical examples.

The upshot of this hermeneutic deductive model is that meanings can take the place of quantitative measurements. The conditions in the linear process, before and after the intervention, are the meanings of the associations and the countertransference checked against each other which gives some considerable protection against bias. And moreover, the intervention itself is a meaning—the interpretation. The deduction is then this: If the change in the before and after associations is precisely in line with an opening up to the unconscious anxiety, then the meaningful interpretation is confirmed as valid; it is not falsified. It is a logic that can be used to compare two different sets of metapsychology. If they can each give a meaning to the pre-interpretive associations then the anxiety hidden there—shall we say Oedipal in one metapsychology and paranoid-schizoid in another—will predict different anxieties to be revealed. The comparison of the two theories will then rest on which anxiety in fact does come more to the fore after an interpretation of one or the other metapsychology. Thus comparing different theoretical metapsychologies becomes possible without the quantitative measurement of physical science.

When dealing with the question of the comparability of psychoanalytic terms of different psychoanalytic schools, I remembered the study of comparative literature on which I had once taken a course at the beginning of my studies. This discipline has a great similarity with the well-known psychoanalytic complex of topics. Veselovsky founded the subject of comparative literature with his fundamental work, which today could be defined as follows:

> the study of literature and cultural expression across linguistic, national, geographic, and disciplinary boundaries .... The characteristically intercultural and transnational field of comparative literature concerns itself with the relation between literature, broadly defined, and other spheres of human activity, including history, politics, philosophy, art, and science.
>
> ("Comparative Literature," 2021)

Still Goethe had already coined the term Weltliteratur (1827, October 12) in a letter to Sulpiz Boisserée ("Comparative Literature," 2021) (quoted in Strich, 1949: 349).

The questions of psychoanalysis are in parts similar to these of comparative literature. Both comparative approaches of literature and psychoanalysis terms can perhaps be summarized under the field of comparative studies or research:

> Comparative Studies encourages critical reflection about culture across boundaries of discipline, nation, and language. We attend to the dynamics of knowledge, power, and authority in a range of discourses and practices: social, religious, literary, aesthetic, technological, scientific, political, and institutional.
>
> (Department of Comparative Studies, n.d.)

The Underlying Assumptions and Their Main Topics

In order to differentiate the wide range of terms, conceptualizations, and models, sometimes with a variety of different meanings, I asked contributors to focus on the following main topics:

1 Underlying assumptions. These are defined as involving a willingness to accept something as true without question or proof. Basic assumptions usually involve a set of rules a person may hold about themselves, others, and the world. These rules are seen as unquestionably right. They may be used to identify the essential nature of a phenomenon as well as its causes and effects. For example, all criminals have faulty genes and are dangerous. Some basic assumptions are held consciously and others unconsciously.

   I have suggested the following differentiation:

   1.1 The main, general underlying assumptions of the perspective (Contributors were asked to choose one or as many as two, three, or four basic assumptions.)
   1.2 Specific theoretical assumptions (Contributors were asked to choose one or as many as two, three, or four assumptions for each category.)

I asked them to feel free to elaborate on the assumptions of their school so that the reader could become familiar with the ways in which the assumptions influenced the conceptualizations and practice.

1.2.1 Assumptions about the nature of psychic structure.
1.2.2 Assumptions about sources and nature of energy.
1.2.3 Assumptions about the nature of relationship.
1.2.4 Assumptions about developmental stages.
1.2.5 Assumptions about the body.
1.2.6 Assumptions about anxieties/instincts and defenses.

1.3 Assumptions concerning etiology.
1.4 Implications for technique, for example, different assumptions about the level of attention to transference, countertransference, developmental thinking, defense, relationships, field, self, internal objects, deficits, and trauma.

2 Subsequent development of the core concepts of the respective school, is described in terms that involve amplification, elaboration, and even deviation.

I have attached labels such as Freudian, post-Freudian, Kleinian, or post-Kleinian, to each contributor. All of these are in some ways spurious and artificial, especially because some of these contributors have changed their minds over time and may have extended the thinking of their schools or developed their own new schools. Psychoanalysis is continuously developing, psychoanalysts continue to learn from their patients, and the search for fuller theories and more adequate techniques goes on and influences contemporary psychoanalytic practice.

We should always examine new and old assumptions periodically and not take for granted that these assumptions correspond to reality. Rather, we need to understand that these are conceptualizations in the context of a specific period connected with analysts' and patients' specific experiences, which may or may not correspond to other realities.

Procedure

In summary, I asked colleagues from different schools to demonstrate in their chapter the underlying assumptions of their theory of the mind in a short overview focusing on the topics mentioned. This is followed by their thoughts on psychodynamic etiology and the respective implications for their technique and interventions. I asked for the rationale of their therapeutic thinking on the issues outlined above and also to give their view on the historical development of the core concepts. At the end of each chapter, a summary should be given in a schematic overview. Criteria for selecting these colleagues were, first, that they had published on a particular school of thought and second, that they were interested in going back to original sources and/or tracing the changes which led to the modern version.

The Summary and Overview (27) will give an overview of the results concerning the underlying assumptions of these schools of thought.

In the Epilogue (28), the editor describes his psychoanalytic journey from natural to social science.

Prospectus and Perspectives (29) will demonstrate the Motivational Systems Approach of Lichtenberg and the growing influence of systems theories on psychoanalysis.

References

Abraham, K. (1924). Versuch einer Entwicklungsgeschichte der Libido auf Grund der Psychoanalyse seelischer Störungen [A short history of the development of the libido. Selected papers on psychoanalysis]. *Neue Arbeiten zur ärztlichen Psychoanalyse, 3*, 7–99.

Atwood, G. E., & Stolorow, R. D. (1980). Psychoanalytic concepts and the representational world. *Psychoanalysis and Contemporary Thought, 3*(2), 267–290.

Atwood, G. E., & Stolorow, R. D. (1984). *Structures of subjectivity: Explorations in psychoanalytic phenomenology*. Routledge.

Bion, W. R. (1965). *Transformations: Change from learning to growth*. Tavistock.

Bion, W. R. (1970). *Attention and interpretation*. Tavistock.

Birksted-Breen, D. (Ed). (2021). *Translation/Transformation: 100 years of the International Journal of Psychoanalysis*. Routledge.

Braithwaite, R. B. (1953). *Scientific explanation: A study in the function of theory, probability and law in science*. Cambridge University Press.

Comparative literature. (2021, July 10). In *Wikipedia*. https://en.wikipedia.org/w/index.php?title=Comparative_literature&oldid=1044234855

Department of Comparative Studies. (n.d.). *Our mission*. The Ohio State University. Retrieved July 11, 2021 from https://comparativestudies.osu.edu/about-us/mission

Eisold, K. (2018a). *The organizational life of psychoanalysis: Conflicts, dilemmas, and the future of the profession*. Routledge.

Eisold, K. (2018b). Psychoanalysis as a profession: Past failures and future possibilities. In K. Eisold (Ed.), *The organizational life of psychoanalysis: Conflicts, dilemmas, and the future of the profession* (pp. 181–209). Routledge.

Eisold, K. (2018c). The intolerance of diversity in psychoanalytic institutes. In K. Eisold (Ed.), *The organizational life of psychoanalysis: Conflicts, dilemmas, and the future of the profession* (pp. 85–110). Routledge.

Eisold, K. (2018d). The splitting of the New York Psychoanalytic Society and the construction of psychoanalytic authority. In K. Eisold (Ed.), *The organizational life of psychoanalysis: Conflicts, dilemmas, and the future of the profession* (pp. 32–54). Routledge.

Ellenberger, Henri F. (1970). *The discovery of the unconscious: The history and evolution of dynamic psychiatry*. Basic Books.

Ezriel, H. (1956). Experimentation within the psychoanalytic session. *British Journal for the Philosophy of Science, 7*, 29–48.

Fischbein, S. V. (2015). Panel Report, IPA Congress Boston 2015: Is translation between psychoanalytic concepts possible? *International Journal of Psychoanalysis, 96*(6), 1671–1675.
Freud, S. (1914). On the history of the psycho-analytic movement. In J. Strachey (Ed. and Trans.), *The standard edition of the complete psychological works of Sigmund Freud* (Vol. 14, pp. 1–66). Hogarth Press.
Freud, S. (1938). An outline of psycho-analysis. In J. Strachey (Ed. and Trans.), *The standard edition of the complete works of Sigmund Freud* (Vol. 23, pp. 139–208). Hogarth Press.
Greenberg, J. R., & Mitchell, S. A. (1983). *Object relations in psychoanalytic theory*. Harvard University Press.
Grunbaum, A. (1984). *Foundations of psychoanalysis*. California University Press.
Guttman, S. A. (1985). The psychoanalytic point of view: Basic concepts and deviant theories. A brief communication. *International Journal of Psychoanalysis, 66*, 167–170.
Hamilton, V. (1996). *The analyst's preconscious*. Routledge.
Heimann, P. (1960). Counter-transference. *British Journal of Medical Psychology, 33*, 9–15.
Heimann, P. (1989). On counter-transference. In P. Heimann (Ed.), *About children and children-no-longer* (pp. 73–79). Routledge. (Original work published 1950).
Hempel, C. G. (1942). The function of general laws in history. *Journal of Philosophy, 39*, 35–48.
Hinshelwood, R. D. (2008). Repression and splitting: Towards a method of conceptual comparison. *International Journal of Psychoanalysis, 89*, 503–521.
Hinshelwood, R. D. (2012). On being objective about the subjective: Clinical aspects of intersubjectivity in contemporary psychoanalysis. *International Forum of Psychoanalysis, 21*, 136–145.
Hinshelwood, R. D. (2013). *Research on the couch: Single-case studies, subjectivity and psychoanalytic knowledge*. Routledge.
Hinshelwood, R. D. (2015). Alive moments: A personal reflection on what countertransference means. *Free Associations, 16*, 50–58.
Hook, S. (Ed.). (1959). *Psychoanalysis, scientific method, and philosophy*. New York University Press.
Huppertz, B. (Ed.). (2013). *Psychotherapy in the wake of war: Discovering multiple psychoanalytic traditions*. Aronson.
Huppertz, B. (Ed.). (2019). *Approaches to psychic trauma: Theory and practice*. Rowman and Littlefield.
Jurist, E. L. (2018). A defense of strong pluralism in psychoanalysis. Mentalizing the hermeneutic-science debate. In S. D. Axelrod, R. C. Naso, & L. M. Rosenberg (Eds.), *Progress in psychoanalysis. Envisioning the future of the profession* (pp. 17–35). Routledge.
King, P., & Steiner, R. (Eds.) (1991). *The Freud-Klein controversies 1941-45*. Routledge.
Kohon, G. (Ed.). (1986). *The British school of psychoanalysis: The independent tradition*. Yale University Press.
Kohon, G. (2017). *British Psychoanalysis: New perspectives in the Independent tradition*. New Library of Psychoanalysis.

Malin, B. (2021). R. B. Braithwaite's influence on Bion's epistemological contributions. *International Journal of Psychoanalysis* (in press).
Popper, K. (1959). *The logic of scientific discovery*. Hutchinson.
Sandler, A.-M. (1990). Comments on varieties of psychoanalytic training in Europe. In M. Meisels & E. Shapiro (Eds.), *Tradition and innovation in psychoanalytic education* (p. 472). Hillsdale Lawrence Erlbaum.
Sandler, J., & Rosenblatt, B. (1962). The concept of the representational world. *Psychoanalytic Study of the Child, 17*, 128–145.
Stepansky, P. (2009). *Psychanalysis at the margins*. Other Press.
Strich, F. (1949). *Goethe and world literature*. Routledge & K. Paul.
Tuckett, D., Basile, R., Birksted-Breen, D., Böhm, T., Denis, P., Ferro, A., Hinz, H., Jemstedt, A., Mariotti, P., & Schubert, J. (Eds.). (2008). *Psychoanalysis comparable & incomparable: The evolution of a method to describe and compare psychoanalytic approaches*. Routledge.

Chapter 1

Historical Introduction: The Beginnings of Psychoanalysis, Sigmund Freud, Metapsychology, Ego Psychoanalysis, the Developing Freudian School of Thought, and the Deviants

Bernd Huppertz

Note: Writing this historical chapter, I remembered a period more than three decades ago, when I took my psychoanalytic preliminary examination after finishing my medical studies. This was necessary in Germany in order to subsequently be able to carry out analytical treatments under supervision. At that time, the theories of Sigmund Freud were the main topic: there were only one or two small German-language paperbacks of about one hundred pages each about Melanie Klein.

...

In order to grasp the huge significance of Sigmund Freud, it is necessary to know a little about the strange ideas concerning the psyche in Freud's time. Freud's historical predecessors in the field of psychiatry and psychotherapy included names such as Franz Anton Mesmer (1734–1815) and his theory of animal magnetism, as well as Amand-Marie-Jacques de Chastenet, Marquis de Puységur (1751–1825), who had developed a new magnetism with "artificial somnambulism," which was later called "hypnosis" by the English surgeon Braid. This was followed by the school of Nancy with the further development of hypnosis and suggestion by Auguste Ambroise Liébeault (1823–1904) and Hippolyte Bernheim's (1840–1919) "Psychotherapeutics". There was also the school of the Salpêtrière with Jean Martin Charcot (1825–1893) and his students. Pierre Janet (1859–1947), who coined the term "sub-conscious," should be mentioned in particular.

After his neuroanatomical and neuropathological studies and his work on cocaine, the scientifically trained Freud developed an increasing interest in psychological processes and the existing ideas about suggestion and hypnotism. He studied for 4 months with Charcot in Paris 1885–1886 and worked then with Breuer in Vienna on hypnosis and hysteria from the 1880s. Together in 1895, they published the "Studies on Hysteria."

DOI: 10.4324/9781003027768-2

Despite everything new that Freud discovered, he remained integrated into his own historical context. Very much influenced by his teachers believing that psychology was a branch of philosophy and that science had to correspond to the scientific models of the time, he remained faithful to the mechanistic-energetic-positivistic thought structure of his time. However, during his life he often oscillated between an idealist (ideas) and an empirical (reality) position.

As a result of Freud's work, something like a Freudian school of thought developed over time, which became more and more widespread worldwide and developed into a movement via the Wednesday Society. In 1910, Freud gave it an international structure with the International Psychoanalytical Association and, in 1920, the International Journal of Psychoanalysis. Freud also found it necessary to separate himself from colleagues who developed or wanted to go their own ways, such as Adler, Jung, Stekel, and Ferenczi (Freud, 1914a).

The development of psychoanalysis from a historical point of view shows that the founders of various subsequent schools of thought had often found themselves in Freud's personal environment. Later, they were excluded as "dissenters" and often founded new schools of thought. Not only were the latter somehow connected to Freud, but they were often connected or influenced by their "analyses" and their analysts. The main centers of the psychoanalytic movement in Freud's time were Vienna, Budapest, Berlin, London, New York, and Moscow until about 1927.

The Development of Psychoanalysis by Sigmund Freud

In Breuer and Freud's "On The Psychical Mechanism of Hysterical Phenomena: Preliminary Communication from Studies on Hysteria" (1893), for the first time, the term repressions was specified as a defense against hidden painful meanings in the sense of anxiety-defense structures. Anxiety-generating thoughts and unacceptable ideas and feelings would be caused by inner-psychic conflicts and/or external stress. The uncathected psychic energy produces anxiety. The persons concerned would be unconsciously protected from these fears and/or conflicts by the so-called defense mechanism (for example, regression, reaction formation, or isolation) described by Freud. These would distort the stimuli from the id or unconsciously or consciously block them. Thus humans would be able to cope with anxiety-generating, stressful situations. In some cases, a defense, which should in normal life be a normal reaction to stress, may persist and produce symptoms in the sense of maladaptation which are pathological.

Neurosis Theory

Freud distinguished, on the one hand, an actual neurosis with origin in the present sexual life of the patients, which he again distinguished into neurasthenia and anxiety neurosis and on the other hand a psychoneurosis with origin in the previous developmental periods of infantile sexuality of the patients, which he again distinguished into hysteria and obsessive-compulsive neurosis.

Freud then designed a new concept that saw the origin of hysteria as well as other psychological complaints in the defense, the "forgetting" of embarrassing memories and ideas of sexual content.

In "The Interpretation of Dreams" (1900), in which Freud demonstrated a new technique, dream interpretation via free associations, he explained that the psyche with its different functions was driven by forces that would make up the dynamics of the personality. Freud used the term energy more in analogy to physical energy and Fechner's "psychophysics" to describe the intensity of psychic forces and psychic dynamics. This idea was closely related to the term cathexis. Changes in the cathexis of objects would be expressed as an expression of an energetic balance in terms such as consumption, displacement, mixing, and exchange (Freud, 1900).

Etiology

Freud distinguished two levels of mental life. The upper level formed the consciousness with its manifest expressions, the lower level the unconscious and its hidden manifestations. If these two levels should come into conflict with each other, symptoms would show up at the level of consciousness, and traumatic memories and relivings at the level of the unconscious.

A trauma, seen as excessive frustrations from undischarged energy-producing anxiety, would be held back with the help of the active force of repression in the unconscious, consuming psychological energy in the process. The symptom was seen as a kind of compromise between the trauma of puberty and/or childhood striving for consciousness versus repression. A disorder in one of the developmental phases of infantile sexuality would result in a persistence at the corresponding psychosexual organizational levels (partial infantilisms) and a corresponding psychopathology. Fixation or regression of the sex drive to the different stages of development (oral, anal, or phallic) could lead to a wide variety of psychological complaints and character development. Symptoms would be seen as a kind of compromise between the conscious traumas of puberty and/or childhood and repression. So that after puberty the genital aspirations may be disturbed.

Neurosis Therapy

How Freud treated his first patients is not known. Later he used a modified form of Breuer's cathartic treatment and a new method—analysis of dream symbols, using associations to dream symbols. However, dissatisfied with the existing concepts, he began looking for a new theoretical model in about 1895. It became a "Project for a Scientific Psychology," (1895/1950) a still quite artificial model.

From about 1900, Freud began to use the method of free association and rejected hypnosis. "Transference," the unconscious re-experience of events in the patient's life, became Freud's most effective therapeutic window. Freud saw his task as researching these unconscious processes and bringing them into consciousness by means of his therapeutic methods of free association and interpretation.

In Freud's "Papers on Technique," he developed his new approach: the method of free association. The patient should lie relaxed on a couch and say everything that comes to his mind, no matter what the content is. When the patient showed inhibitions and/or other difficulties, Freud called them "resistance." During the sessions, patients were seen to develop irrational feelings of love or hostility toward the therapist, which Freud called "transference." The analysis of resistance and transference became Freud's basic tool of therapy.

Basic Concepts of Psychoanalysis

Over the course of decades, Freud developed in different phases the theory and method, which he called psychoanalysis. "It is enough to say that psycho-analysis, in its character of the psychology of the deepest, unconscious mental acts, promises to become the link between Psychiatry and all of these other branches of mental science" (Freud, 1926b).

Metapsychology

The term metapsychology was first used by Freud in letters to Fliess in 1898. Later in a letter to Abraham he explained: "Metapsychology supposes models of the "psychic apparatus"—e.g., id, ego, super-ego; unconscious, preconscious, conscious; distribution of drive energy—at a high level of abstraction" (Freud, 1907).

Freud's metapsychology can be summarized as a system in which psychic processes should be described according to their dynamic, topographical, structural, economic, and developmental relationships. The term dynamic refers to psychic forces that are in conflict with each other; the topographical point of view means the distinction between the unconscious, the preconscious, and the conscious; the structural refers to the agencies/instances (id, ego, super-ego) involved in psychological processes; the economic one captures the regulation of psychic forces/energy, which are uncathected and produce anxiety through the pleasure-unpleasure principle, the search for pleasure and the avoidance of unpleasure; and the developmental in the sense of certain developmental and maturational steps. In Freud's "Papers on Metapsychology" he developed his thinking further, especially in his paper "The Unconscious" (Freud, 1915b).

The Unconscious

Freud proceeded from unconscious psychic processes, which manifest themselves especially in dreams, slips of the tongue, or failures and should influence consciousness to a different degree.

The Topographic Model

In the topographic model, Freud (1900) tried to divide psychic processes according to the degree of their consciousness and distinguished between a conscious, a preconscious, and an unconscious. He tried to classify them and summarize them in systems. Their relations with each other were seen as regulated by a censor. The system Cs (consciousness) was compared to a psychic space that was responsible for grasping stimuli of the inner and outer worlds. It was seen as a kind of sensory organ for the perception of psychic qualities. The system Pcs (preconscious) contained those psychic contents that were not present in the consciousness but could be retrieved by means of deliberate or sometimes unintentional attention orientation. The system Ucs (unconscious) consisted of psychic content which could not be raised into consciousness even by targeted concentration. There were various kinds of unconscious processes and Freud gave the most important theoretical place to the process of repression/suppression. This acted upon impulses and ideas regarded by the individual and/or culture as unpleasant, which had to be repelled or pushed into the Ucs. The therapeutic work taught Freud that the repressed contents could repeatedly gain access to the Cs in a distorted way (return of the repressed) (Freud, 1900).

Infantile Sexuality

In 1905, Freud published his "Three Essays on the Theory of Sexuality." Freud was certain that sexuality would exist from early childhood. The so-called psychosexual development runs along prevailing erogenous zones (oral mucosa, intestinal and genitourinary mucosa, genitals) an oral, anal (urogenital), and phallic-oedipal phase.

Freud's three phases and the resulting partial drives of childhood sexuality:

1 The oral phase, where the mouth became the erogenous zone and satisfaction would be obtained by sucking.
2 The anal phase, where the anus became the main erogenous zone and satisfaction would be obtained by retaining the stool.
3 The phallic phase, whereby the child in this phase would know only one genital organ, the male. It would only be able to distinguish between phallic and neutered, male and female.

During these phases, these so-called partial shoots would still be imperfectly united under the primacy of the genital organs.

The early mother-child relationship would lead to the Oedipus complex. Infantile-sexual claims would be made on the parents: out of love for the mother, the boy would compete with the father for the love of his mother and the daughter with the mother for the love of her father. These internalized infantile parental relationships—called Oedipus complex—would need to be overcome and dissolved. After abandoning these infantile claims, there would be internalization and identification with the parents.

These phases of autoeroticism would be followed by a period of latency. In puberty autoeroticism would pass to sexual objects and the partial shoots would unite under the primacy of the genital zone. Psychosexual differentiation between men and women would follow (Freud, 1905).

The Drive Theory

Freud hypothesized from 1905 via the existence of three phases of development an inconsistent, unfinished drive theory with the sex drives, the ego, and self-preservation drives. Later in 1920, he substituted the two dualistic primal drives (erotic) libido and (destructive) destrudo, life and death instincts.

Freud defined the drive as the mental representation of a continuously flowing, inner-somatic stimulus source, which would manifest itself in a so-called urge forward, which would find its mental expression in drive representations starting from the physical. These exciting processes in one's own body would be the source of the drive, whose drive aim would be the reduction of tension of this stimulus. The object of the shoots would be one's own body and its own body zones or an external object. These processes would occur again and again and be independent of conscious control. Freud called the drive energy itself libido (Freud, 1915a).

Freud later distinguished the drives in his paper "Beyond the Pleasure Principle" (1920) according to their functions on the one hand into erotic, libidinous and on the other hand into destructive, aggressive drives. He therefore took two dualistic primal instincts for granted: Eros (erotic libido) and Thanatos (destructive destrudo), life and death instinct. Both shoots should be able to occur individually, but often also together and mixed with each other.

Object and Object Relations

Freud's development of the term and the concept of object occurred in a variety of ways. It would range from an inner representation of an object to an external real object (person). Later he added the term and concept of object relation/object relationship. Initially, the term was used in the context of the drive theory where drives took precedence over the object from which they gain satisfaction. The first object of childlike infantile sexuality would be one's own body and the mother's breast (as a partial object). After weaning from the maternal breast, infantile sexuality would then move on to include the Oedipus complex. With repression comes latency. After puberty, genital sexuality would focus on an external object.

The Body

Freud was interested in the relation between body and mind for various reasons. The soma as the biological ground and the body as the mental representation of the soma was very important in Freud's thinking. Soma and body build during psychosexual development and are later the source of the drives (Freud, 1905).

The soma/body would play a big role in the development of the ego. The body ego would be formed from the physical sensations of the infant from early childhood. It would be a representation of the earliest experiences of the baby in the sense of a body-ego, the first manifestation of a developing ego.

Freud's term "somatic compliance" demonstrates the thought that somatic symptoms can be a product of psychic processes and result in symptoms of the body or of diseases.

The Structural Model of the Psyche

Freud's model of the psyche became the structural model consisting of the id, ego, and super-ego. Each structure had different tasks (Freud, 1923).

The id became the agency/instance that formed an unconscious structure that included drives, needs, and affects, especially the repressed material and later libido and detrudo (unconscious mind). It was to be determined by the instinctual pleasure principle (so-called primary process [unconscious]).

The ego became the structure that included perception, thinking, and memory (conscious mind). It should be the structure of everyday life, conscious thinking, and self-confidence. It should mediate between id, super-ego, and reality and be determined by the reality principle (secondary process [consciously]). The id should slowly develop as an early self from the body ego of early childhood.

The super-ego became the authority that included social norms, values, morality, conscience, and the ego ideal. It became the structure of internalized values.

Freud saw consciousness as a separate structure, which included external perception (seeing, hearing, feeling, etc.) as well as inner sensations. In this theory inner arousals were thought to leave no traces, but to fizzle out with the arrival of their consciousness.

Ego Psychoanalysis

The new theory of ego psychoanalysis began to develop in a number of different publications over 10 years. In his "On Narcissism: An Introduction" (1914b), Freud replaced the earlier distinction between non-sexual ego drives and sexual libido, two types of ego drives, libidinous and non-libidinous. With the beginning of the differentiation of the ego, the hitherto diffuse libido would concentrate on the ego. Freud called this primary narcissism. Part of the primary narcissism would be maintained in the subsequent phases, but the libido is largely directed at the mother and later turned toward other objects. Should the object libido later be withdrawn and directed at the ego, this was called secondary narcissism by Freud. In particular, in "Inhibitions, Symptoms and Anxiety" (1926a), Freud developed his thinking from metapsychology to an ego pathology.

After the conceptions of the psychoanalytic theory it began to spread to applications by Freud himself beyond the therapy, for example to fields such as religion, art, literature, sociology, and cultural history (for example Freud, 1921).

1. The Beginnings of Psychoanalysis—Freud and the Freudian School	
Main, general underlying assumptions	1 The Unconscious 2 Infantile Sexuality and Sexual Theory 3 Drive Theory (Libido and Destrudo) 4 Metapsychology (models of the "psychic apparatus," e.g., id, ego, super-ego; unconscious, preconscious, conscious)
Specific theoretical assumptions	
psychic structure	• Topographic model (conscious, preconscious, unconscious) • Relations with a censor • Structural model of the psyche—id (primary process, unconscious), ego (secondary process, conscious), and super-ego. • Disruption of the developmental phases of infantile sexuality (oral, anal, phallic-oedipal) could lead to partial infantilisms and corresponding psychopathology.
energy	The psyche is seen as driven by forces that form the dynamics of the mind. The term energy was used by Freud more in analogy to physical energy (Fechner) to describe the intensity of psychic forces. Changes in cathexis would build something like an energetic balance via processes such as consumption, displacement, mixing, or exchange.

(Continued)

relationships	The object enters first by being seen as a drive object which provides satisfaction (partial object; sexual object), then later seen in a fuller object relation.
developmental stages	Infantile sexuality: psychosexual development along erogenous zones (oral mucosa, intestinal and genitourinary mucosa, genitals) oral, (urogenital) and phallic-oedipal phase (latency, puberty, and genital sexuality)
body	• Soma and body source of the drives • Body first manifestation of the ego as body ego • Body is the mental representation of the soma
anxieties/instinct and defenses	Anxieties resulting from internal and outer conflicts and unacceptable ideas and feelings. Defense mechanisms would unconsciously protect against these fears and/or conflicts and anxieties.
Assumptions concerning etiology	Origin of neuroses in the defense, the "forgetting" of embarrassing memories, and ideas of sexual content. Symptom is seen as a kind of compromise between the trauma of puberty and/or childhood striving for consciousness and repression. Disturbance in a developmental phase of infantile sexuality could lead to persistence at the respective psychosexual organizational levels (partial infantilisms) with appropriate psychopathology (fixation; regression).
Implications for technique	Investigation of unconscious processes and bringing them into consciousness by means of free association and interpretation (therapeutic method) (resistance, transference, fixation, regression). Inner arousals are thought to fizzle out as a result of awareness by verbalizing anxieties and making them conscious and more tolerable.
Subsequent developments of the core concept	Many developments have added to or adapted the core concepts. Other schools of mind can be contrary or in antithesis to the Freudian core concepts, whereby the main divergences are toward (a) object-relations and (b) Lacanian symbolization.

References

Breuer, J., & Freud, S. (1893). On the psychical mechanism of hysterical phenomena: Preliminary communication from studies on hysteria. In J. Strachey (Ed. and Trans.), *The standard edition of the complete psychological works of Sigmund Freud* (Vol. 2, pp. 1–17). Hogarth Press.

Freud, S. (1900). The interpretation of dreams. In J. Strachey (Ed. and Trans.), *The standard edition of the complete psychological works of Sigmund Freud* (Vol. 4–5, pp. ix–627). Hogarth Press.

Freud, S. (1905). Three essays on the theory of sexuality. In J. Strachey (Ed. and Trans.), *The standard edition of the complete psychological works of Sigmund Freud* (Vol. 7, pp. 123–246). Hogarth Press.

Freud, S. (1907). Letter from Sigmund Freud to Karl Abraham, October 21, 1907. *The Complete Correspondence of Sigmund Freud and Karl Abraham 1907–1925, 52*, 11–12.

Freud, S. (1914a). On the history of the psycho-analytic movement. In J. Strachey (Ed. and Trans.), *The standard edition of the complete psychological works of Sigmund Freud* (Vol. 14, pp. 1–66). Hogarth Press.

Freud, S. (1914b). On narcissism: An introduction. In J. Strachey (Ed. and Trans.), *The standard edition of the complete psychological works of Sigmund Freud* (Vol. 14, pp. 67–102). Hogarth Press.

Freud, S. (1915a). Instincts and their vicissitudes. In J. Strachey (Ed. and Trans.), *The standard edition of the complete psychological works of Sigmund Freud* (Vol. 14, pp. 109–140). Hogarth Press.

Freud, S. (1915b). The unconscious. In J. Strachey (Ed. and Trans.), *The standard edition of the complete psychological works of Sigmund Freud* (Vol. 14, pp. 159–215). Hogarth Press.

Freud, S. (1920). Beyond the pleasure principle. In J. Strachey (Ed. and Trans.), *The standard edition of the complete psychological works of Sigmund Freud* (Vol. 18, pp. 1–64). Hogarth Press.

Freud, S. (1921). Group psychology and the analysis of the ego. In J. Strachey (Ed. and Trans.), *The standard edition of the complete psychological works of Sigmund Freud* (Vol. 18, pp. 65–144). Hogarth Press.

Freud, S. (1923). The ego and the id. In J. Strachey (Ed. and Trans.), *The standard edition of the complete psychological works of Sigmund Freud* (Vol. 19, pp. 1–66). Hogarth Press.

Freud, S. (1926a). Inhibitions, symptoms and anxiety. In J. Strachey (Ed. and Trans.), *The standard edition of the complete psychological works of Sigmund Freud* (Vol. 20, pp. 75–176). Hogarth Press.

Freud, S. (1926b). Psycho-analysis. In J. Strachey (Ed. and Trans.), *The standard edition of the complete psychological works of Sigmund Freud* (Vol. 20, pp. 259–270). Hogarth Press.

Freud, S. (1950). Project for a scientific psychology. In J. Strachey (Ed. and Trans.), *The standard edition of the complete psychological works of Sigmund Freud* (Vol. 1, pp. 281–391). Hogarth Press. (Original work published 1895).

Chapter 2

Contemporary UK Freudians

Francois Louw

Main, General Underlying Assumptions

The contemporary Freudian tradition (CFT) denotes a richly diverse group. The "Controversial Discussions" which occurred between 1942 and 1944 (King & Steiner, 1991) and the institutional compromise reached reverberated through successive generations and over time fostered an environment of mutual influence (Robinson, 2015; Sandler & Sandler, 1994). The work of Joseph and Anne-Marie Sandler on internal objects (Sandler & Sandler, 1998) is an example of productive cross-fertilization with Kleinian concepts. With respect to the independent tradition, Winnicott has been particularly influential among CFs.

The CFT includes analysts who identify more with classical Freudians, some influenced more by Anna Freud, and analysts who draw on traditions from other countries, most notably France and Italy. Robinson and Schachter (2020) suggest that the nature of the CFT is best approached via Wittgenstein's notion of "family resemblances" (p. 2). According to the authors, the CF family rests on Freud's metapsychological perspectives; dynamic, topographical, structural, economic, and developmental. They however point out that not all members think in economic terms and there is individual difference in emphasis as well (Robinson & Schachter, 2020). There is also agreement, that the dynamic unconscious can only be apprehended indirectly and partially through its derivatives (e.g., Perelberg, 2009; Yorke, 1988).

Specific Theoretical Assumptions

Assumptions about the Nature of Psychic Structure

The CFT assumes a broadly developmental perspective, embracing a complex notion of temporality within which a gradual process of psychic structuring takes place (Sandler & Schachter, 2014). Structuring involves interrelated drive and object-relations vicissitudes (Sandler & Sandler, 1998; Yorke, 1988).

DOI: 10.4324/9781003027768-3

The ego does not exist at birth and is at first a bodily ego (Freud, 1923), shaped by repeated experiences of physical contact with a mother or primary carer who responds to the infant's needs. Initially there is an absence of a continuous sense of self, with sporadic experiences of self and other, alternating with experiences of non-differentiation. Undifferentiated experiences gradually make way for differentiation between inside/outside, self/other, and phantasy/reality and give rise to the development of psychic structures (Sandler & Schachter, 2014). These maturational processes occur within the context of separating from the matrix of the early relationship with the mother (Kennedy et al., 1985; Sandler & Schachter, 2014).

The first basic structures are representations of objects and of self (Sandler & Sandler, 1998). Representations are shaped by drives, affects, defense, and phantasy. The Sandlers distinguished between internalization, identification, and introjection (Sandler, 1960; Sandler & Sandler, 1998). The process of internalization is an organizing activity whereby the gradual formation of representations creates a representational world (Sandler & Rosenblatt, 1962). Internalization forms the basis for all subsequent processes. Sandler (1960) distinguishes between primary and secondary types of identification; the former denotes a momentary fusion of self- and object representations that preserves their boundaries and separateness, whereas secondary identification refers to the alteration of the shape of the ego aimed at attaining similarity with an aspect of an object representation. Introjection pertains to the formation of super-ego and refers to the establishment of representations of parental authority as substitutes for "actual" parents (Sandler, 1960).

Both masculine and feminine (bisexual) identifications are formed. Psychic bisexuality is central to the Oedipus complex and its resolution, which leads to the consolidation of identity (Edgcumbe & Burgner, 1975; Perelberg, 2018). Oedipal resolution furthermore inaugurates repression which takes place *après-coup* and consolidates the structural division of the id, ego, and superego.

Assumptions about the Sources and Nature of Energy

Drives are seen as the prime motivational force. A dual conception of drives in conflict is shared. There is however no agreement upon Freud's (1920) final drive conception. Different elements of Freud's thinking about the nature of aggression and destructiveness are partly reflected in the range of views amongst CFs (Robinson & Schachter, 2020). Some use the concept of the death drive clinically to refer to a primary destructive force directed against internal objects. Others prefer Freud's conception of aggression as self-preservative, with some seeing self-preservative aggression as a defense against overwhelming helplessness. Many CFs view destructiveness as the outcome of a failure to sufficiently integrate aggressive and libidinal drives (Robinson & Schachter, 2020). The notion of a compulsion to repeat, because the death drive is beyond representation, is also of importance to many CFs (Perelberg, 2018).

The existence of the drives can be inferred only through their representatives; ideation and affect. Some CFs, influenced by Anna Freud (1993) and Joseph Sandler (e.g., Sandler & Sandler, 1998) accord affect a more primary role in their understanding of unconscious motivation. The Sandlers argued that from "a clinical point of view, anxiety, or any unpleasant affect, can be an extremely powerful motivation for an unconscious wish, at times even more powerful than the instinctual drives themselves" (p. 287).

Assumptions about the Nature of Relationship

Relationships are shaped by a complex interplay between intrapsychic and interpersonal.

> Object relations "cannot be understood simply in terms of drive contributants, ego contributants, superego influences, and the impact of the outside world .... It is the complexities of the reactions and inter-reactions within and between all these agencies that ultimately give human relationships their richness and individuality".
>
> (Yorke, 1988, p. 443)

Anna Freud's developmental line for relationships for which successive stages of libidinal development form an inborn, maturational base reflects the aforementioned complexity. The first postulated step is the biological unity of mother-infant, with the mother's narcissism extending to the child, and the child's inclusion of the mother in his narcissistic world. Another step along the line is the ambivalent relationship of the pre-oedipal, anal-sadistic stage, characterized by the ego attitudes of clinging, torturing, dominating, and controlling objects (Freud, 1963).

The basic psychic structures which shape relationships and transference are representations of objects and self. Sandler and Sandler's (1998) notion that unconscious phantasy is represented as wished-for interactions between self and object is evident in the understanding of most CFs. External relationships are derivatives of underlying wishful-phantasy role relationships. The Sandler's regard all wish fulfilment as brought about through some form of actualization. The most common means of making a phantasy actual or real is through action aimed at bringing about a correspondence of what is perceived and what is wished for. The creation of illusions, delusions, hallucinations, daydreams, and symbols are other means of actualization (Sandler & Sandler, 1998).

Assumptions about Developmental Stages

Thinking about development is rooted in Freud's conception of infantile sexuality (Freud, 1905), together with his dynamic concepts of regression, fixation, and *nachträglichkeit*. Development is viewed as a non-linear process in which successive libidinal phases—oral, anal, phallic, latency, and genital—do not supersede one another. *Nachträglichkeit* and its elaboration in the concept of *après coup* by French analysts and in the work of Perelberg (2006) is central to the understanding of mental functioning and development. Perelberg (2006) distinguishes between descriptive and dynamic *après coup*. Dynamic *après coup* refers to "the way in which in Freudian metapsychology later events resignify earlier ones which then emerge with a new meaning … . this is central to the Oedipus complex, structurally inserted between two different notions of time" (p. 1217).

The bi-phasic Oedipus complex is central to development (e.g., Burgner, 1985; Perelberg, 2015b; Robinson & Schachter, 2020). Edgcumbe and Burgner's (1975) differentiation between pre-Oedipal and Oedipal aspects of phallic development and their insertion of a phallic-narcissistic phase is broadly accepted. The crucial nature of the revisiting of the Oedipus complex in puberty (genital phase) is underscored in Moses and Egle Laufer's work (Laufer & Laufer, 1984). CFs regard a present father or father figure as crucial to healthy pre-Oedipal and Oedipal development (e.g., Burgner, 1985).

Anna Freud's concept of developmental lines (1963) informs the thinking of some CFs. For her,

> The basic interactions between id and ego and their various developmental levels, and also age-related sequences of them, which in importance, frequency, and regularity are comparable to the maturational sequence of libidinal stages or the gradual unfolding of the ego functions.
>
> (Freud, 1963, p. 246)

Anna Freud conceived of lines for example leading from irresponsibility to responsibility in body management and from complete dependency in infancy to emotional self-reliance, each with various stations along the way. Setbacks may occur on the way, mostly temporary. Not all progress will be comparable on every line. It is important to note that the temporality of developmental lines, involves fixation and regression, but not *après coup*.

Assumptions about the Body

Generally, CFs distinguish between body and soma (Perris-Myttas, 2020). The soma is the physical, biological organization, manifest in illness and pain and the libidinal body is the representation of soma in the psyche. The soma is the source of the drives which are understood to be at the frontier of psyche and soma. The demand for work on the mind in connection with its relationship with the soma (Freud, 1915) is met in the matrix of the mother and child relationship which facilitates libidinal development and representation.

Formation of representations (initially of a "somatic self") (Sandler & Sandler, 1998) gradually allows for a relative desomatizing and for a move from somatic to verbal expression of experience (Edgcumbe, 1984).

Not all somatic experience is represented. From a structural perspective, unrepresented traces of somatic experience form part of the id. Unrepresented somatic experience can find expression in somatic symptoms or illness (Perris-Myttas, 2020), or in acting out (Pines, 2010). Schachter (1997) importantly points out that unconscious phantasies which become attached secondarily to somatic symptoms should not be confused with phantasies that give rise to somatic symptoms. Hysterical conversion symptoms are understood as symbolic bodily expressions which enlist somatic experience.

Assumptions about Anxieties/Instincts and Defenses

In *The Analysis of Defense: The Ego and the Mechanisms of Defense Revisited,* Joseph Sandler and Anna Freud concluded that any existing capacities and abilities can be used defensively, in addition to the main defense mechanisms which Freud and his inner circle identified (repression, projection, regression, reaction formation, isolation, undoing, introjection, reversal, turning against the self, splitting, and sublimation) and to which Anna Freud added identification with the aggressor, altruism, and elaborated several forms of denial (in fantasy, word, and act) (Sandler & Freud, 1985).

A developmental progression of defense mechanisms is assumed, although more primitive defense mechanisms are never outgrown. Defenses are less structured, less effective, and readily undone in infancy and toddlerhood prior to the establishment of the repression barrier at the end of the Oedipal period (Kennedy et al., 1985).

Contemporary Freudians by and large hold to Freud's distinction between signal anxiety and traumatic anxiety (Freud, 1926). Signal anxiety entails a mechanism whereby small doses of anxiety are generated to alert the ego of threats posed by psychic conflict and to mobilize defenses. With traumatic anxiety, the ego is overwhelmed by an "excitation, whether of external or of internal origin, which cannot be dealt with" (Freud, 1926, p. 81). Freud's conception of anxiety in *Inhibitions, Symptoms and Anxiety* is not regarded as a contradiction or abandonment of his first theory but as a re-evaluation of the limits of the earlier theory (Davies, 2012). According to Davies (2012) Freud himself shows the crucial connection between separation anxiety and castration anxiety, when he describes the latter as the "fear of being separated from a highly valued object" (Freud, 1926, p. 137).

Following Anna Freud (1993), CFs tend to distinguish between defenses motivated and mobilized by signal anxiety (which occurs at a comparatively late stage in development) and defenses against painful affects other than anxiety (that occur at an earlier stage but continue to operate with varying degrees throughout life). Joseph Sandler's work on affect and his notion of establishing and maintaining a "background of safety" also informs the thinking of many CFs (Sandler, 1960).

Assumptions Concerning Etiology

Following Freud, CFs view the psychopathology of everyday life and beyond as the outcome of the conflict between the drives and their vicissitudes and between the id, ego, and superego.

A comprehensive understanding of the compromises forged by conflict and defense requires dynamic, topographical, economic, and genetic perspectives to be brought to bear on what patients bring to the consulting room (Yorke et al., 1989). Due to the multiplicity of factors that shape what is manifest, symptoms are understood to be overdetermined. Following Freud, CFs continue to mine their clinical experience to develop models of specific psychopathologies. Glasser's (1986) notion of the core complex in perversions, Campbell's (1995) work on pre-suicidal states, Perelberg and colleagues' (Perelberg, 1998) investigation of violence and suicide in borderline young men, and de la Sierra's (1995, 2012) writing on addiction are examples.

Freud's postulation of a death drive which does not correspond to any representation but is expressed through the repetition compulsion is important in the thinking of CFs influenced by the work of Rosine Perelberg (2003, 2015a). What is traumatic and engenders helplessness is the excess of what is un-absorbable by representation and inaccessible to symbolization. Compulsive repetition of the infantile traumatic past dominates because of the absence of psychic representation.

Anna Freud's (1989) view of mental health as the harmonious interaction between the psychic agencies which have reached and are maintaining the same level, is central to the thinking of some CFs. Disturbances of development of a qualitative and/or quantitative nature may arise because of deviations from the norm (constitution, structuralization, environmental factors) and/or from the breakdown of synchronization in the unfolding of the drives, the ego functions, the superego, and environmental interventions. When disturbances of the developmental lines are extensive, they can become a pathogenic factor for personality structuring.

Implications for Technique

CFs focus on understanding patients' preconscious and unconscious phantasies through listening to their free associations and dreams and attending to their transference. Parallel to patients' free associations, analysts aim for free-floating attention and to monitor their countertransference (Perelberg, 2009; Robinson & Schachter, 2020; Sandler & Schachter, 2014). Patients are seen as collaborators in the analytic process, which some analysts understand with reference to the notion of the therapeutic alliance (Sandler & Schachter, 2014).

Transference is seen as at the heart of the analytic process; activity and affective investment become organized around it as the analyst offers himself as an object of transference (e.g., Sandler & Schachter, 2014). The present unconscious (preconscious) phantasies of patients are discerned by identifying the dominant affect in the here-and-now. CFs draw on both Freud's formulation of transference as a resistance to the flow of free associations and transference as repetition. Generally, countertransference, defined as the analyst's unconscious responses to the patient's transferences, is distinguished from the analyst's transference to the patient, and from the analyst's affective response to the patient (Sandler & Schachter, 2014). Joseph Sandler's (1976) concept of role responsiveness which describes the actualization of elements of the patient's infantile relationships in the transference, and the associated technical recommendation that analysts also attend with free-floating responsiveness informs the thinking of many CFs about the complexity of mutual influence in the analytic dyad. According to Robinson and Schachter (2020), Baker's (1993) concept of the analyst as a new object is present, explicitly or implicitly, in the thinking of analysts included in their book on the Tradition. According to Baker, the analyst's neutrality constitutes an implicit transference interpretation that facilitates freeing patients from re-enactment of a transference relationship and the discovery of a new object.

Interpretation is central to the therapeutic process and the act of interpreting is seen as embodying the analyst's separateness. Analysts aim to identify the dominant affect in sessions, the underlying conflicts, and the anxiety and the defenses deployed to maintain psychic equilibrium. Interpretations tend to move from the surface to depth, in order to facilitate the patient's engagement in the process, and to avoid overwhelming the patient or pushing him or her into a pseudo-intellectual understanding. Accurate identification and interpretation of anxieties and defenses aim to decrease resistance and further the analytic process. The timing of interpretation is paramount; this entails waiting and listening to the network of the patient's associations as they gradually reveal the current unconscious transference phantasies, conflicts, and affects. Extra-transference interpretations and other interventions are regarded as necessary tools in furthering the process toward interpretation of the particular transference phantasy activated in sessions (Sandler & Schachter, 2014). Dreams are still regarded as one of the royal roads to the unconscious and interpreted in their own right, not only as expressions of transference (Loden, 2003). The role of analysts faced with repetition and absence of representation is not one of interpreting what is already there in the mind of the patient but, rather, one of inaugurating the symbolic domain and the world of representations (Perelberg, 2003). The analyst's use of his or her countertransference experience to inform interpretations that facilitate the work of representation and the construction of meaning *après-coup* is crucial.

2. Contemporary UK Freudians	
Main, general underlying assumptions	• nature is best approached via Wittgenstein's notion of "family resemblances" • CF family rests on Freud's metapsychological perspectives; dynamic, topographical, structural, economic, and developmental • dynamic unconscious can only be apprehended indirectly and partially through its derivatives
Specific theoretical assumptions	
psychic structure	• ego does not exist at birth and is at first a bodily ego, shaped by repeated experiences of physical contact with mother/primary carer • first basic structures are representations of objects and of self • representations are shaped by drives, affects, defense, and phantasy • Oedipal resolution inaugurates repression which takes place *après-coup* and consolidates the structural division of the id, ego, and superego
energy	• drives are seen as the prime motivational forces • dual conception of drives in conflict is shared, but no agreement upon Freud's final drive conception • Freud's thinking about the nature of aggression and destructiveness is partly reflected in the range of views amongst CFs
relationships	• shaped by a complex interplay between the intrapsychic and interpersonal • basic psychic structures shaping relationships and transference are representations of objects and self • unconscious phantasy is represented as wished-for interactions between self and object • wish-fulfillment is brought about through some form of actualization
developmental stages	• thinking about development is rooted in Freud's conception of infantile sexuality together with his dynamic concepts of regression, fixation, and *nachträglichkeit* • *nachträglichkeit* and its elaboration in the concept of *après coup* by French analysts and in the work of Perelberg (2006) is central to understanding mental functioning and development • the bi-phasic Oedipus complex is central to development • Anna Freud's concept of developmental lines informs the thinking of some CFs

(*Continued*)

body	• distinction between body and soma; soma is the physical, biological organization, manifest in illness and pain and the libidinal body is the representation of soma in the psyche • formation of representations (initially of a somatic self) gradually allows for a relative desomatizing and for a move from somatic to verbal expression of experience • not all somatic experience is represented and can find expression in somatic symptoms or illness or in acting out • hysterical conversion symptoms are understood as symbolic bodily expressions which enlist somatic experience
anxieties/instincts and defenses	• any existing capacities and abilities can be used defensively, in addition to the main defense mechanisms which Freud identified and to which Anna Freud added • a developmental progression of defense mechanisms is assumed, although more primitive defense mechanisms are never outgrown • Freud's distinction between signal anxiety and traumatic anxiety • distinguish between defenses motivated and mobilized by signal anxiety (which occurs at a comparatively late stage in development) and defenses against painful affects other than anxiety (that occur at an earlier stage but continue to operate with varying degrees throughout life)
Assumptions concerning etiology	• psychopathology of everyday life and beyond is regarded as the outcome of the conflict between the drives and their vicissitudes and between the id, ego, and superego • due to the multiplicity of factors that shape what is manifest, symptoms are understood to be overdetermined • Freud's postulation of the death drive which does not correspond to any representation but is expressed through the repetition compulsion is important in the thinking of CFs influenced by the work of Rosine Perelberg • Anna Freud's view of mental health as the harmonious interaction between the psychic agencies which have reached and maintain the same level, is central to the thinking of some CFs

(*Continued*)

Implications for technique	• Focus on understanding patients' preconscious and unconscious phantasies through listening to their free associations and dreams and attending to their transference • parallel to patients' free associations, analysts aim for free-floating attention and to monitor their countertransference (including their free-floating responsiveness) • patients are seen as collaborators in the analytic process • interpretation is central to the therapeutic process and tends to move from surface to depth in order to decrease resistance
Subsequent developments of the core concept	N/A

References

Baker, R. (1993). The patient's discovery of the psychoanalyst as a new object. *International Journal of Psycho-Analysis*, *74*, 1223–1233.

Burgner, M. (1985). The Oedipal experience: Effects on development of an absent father. *International Journal of Psychoanalysis*, *66*, 311–320.

Campbell, D. (1995). The role of the father in a pre-suicide state. *International Journal of Psychoanalysis*, *76*, 315–323.

Davies, R. (2012). Anxiety: The importunate companion. Psychoanalytic theory of castration and separation anxieties and implications for clinical technique. *International Journal of Psychoanalysis*, *93*(5), 1101–1114.

de la Sierra, L. R. (1995). Of sentiments and sensations. *British Journal of Psychotherapy*, *12*(2), 229–241.

de la Sierra, L. R. (2012). Countertransference: Our difficulties in the treatment of substance abuse. *Romanian Journal of Psychoanalysis*, *5*(2), 76–92.

Edgcumbe, R. M. (1984). Modes of communication: The differentiation of somatic and verbal expression. *Psychoanalytic Study of the Child*, *39*, 137–154.

Edgcumbe, R., & Burgner, M. (1975). The phallic-narcissistic phase: A differentiation between preoedipal and Oedipal aspects of phallic development. *Psychoanalytic Study of the Child*, *30*, 161–180.

Freud, A. (1963). The concept of developmental lines. *Psychoanalytic Study of the Child*, *18*, 245–265.

Freud, A. (1989). *Normality and pathology in childhood.* Karnac.

Freud, A. (1993). *The ego and the mechanism of defence.* Karnac.

Freud, S. (1905). Three essays on the theory of sexuality. In J. Strachey (Ed. and Trans.), *The standard edition of the complete works of Sigmund Freud* (Vol. 7, pp. 123–246). Hogarth Press.

Freud, S. (1915). Instincts and their vicissitudes. In J. Strachey (Ed. and Trans.), *The standard edition of the complete works of Sigmund Freud* (Vol. 14, pp. 109–140). Hogarth Press.
Freud, S. (1920). Beyond the pleasure principle. In J. Strachey (Ed. and Trans.), *The standard edition of the complete works of Sigmund Freud* (Vol. 18, pp. 1–64). Hogarth Press.
Freud, S. (1923). The ego and the id. In J. Strachey (Ed. and Trans.), *The standard edition of the complete works of Sigmund Freud* (Vol. 19, pp. 1–66). Hogarth Press.
Freud, S. (1926). Inhibitions, symptoms and anxiety. In J. Strachey (Ed. and Trans.), *The standard edition of the complete works of Sigmund Freud* (Vol. 20, pp. 75–176). Hogarth Press.
Glasser, M. (1986). Identification and its vicissitudes as observed in the perversions. *International Journal of Psychoanalysis*, *67*, 9–16.
Kennedy, H., Moran, G., Wiseberg, S., & Yorke, C. (1985). Both sides of the barrier: Some reflections on childhood fantasy. *Psychoanalytic Study of the Child*, *40*, 275–283.
King, P., & Steiner, R. (Eds.). (1991). *The Freud-Klein controversies 1941–1945*. Routledge.
Laufer, M., & Laufer, M. E. (1984). *Adolescence and developmental breakdown: A psychoanalytic view*. Routledge.
Loden, S. (2003). The fate of the dream in contemporary psychoanalysis. *Journal of the American Psychoanalytic Association*, *51*, 43–70.
Perelberg, R. J. (1998). *Psychoanalytic understanding of violence and suicide*. Routledge.
Perelberg, R. J. (2003). Full and empty spaces in the analytic process. *International Journal of Psychoanalysis*, *84*(3), 579–592.
Perelberg, R. J. (2006). The controversial discussions and après-coup. *International Journal of Psychoanalysis*, *87*(5), 1199–1220.
Perelberg, R. J. (2009). On becoming a psychoanalyst. *Psychoanalytic Inquiry*, *29*(3), 247–263.
Perelberg, R. J. (2015a). Excess, trauma and helplessness: Repetitions and transformations. *International Journal of Psychoanalysis*, *96*, 1453–1476.
Perelberg, R. J. (2015b). *Murdered father, dead father: Revisiting the Oedipus complex*. Routledge.
Perelberg, R. J. (2018). *Psychic Bisexuality: A British-French dialogue*. Routledge.
Perris-Myttas, M. (2020). The soma and the body: Navigating through the countertransference. In K. Robinson, & J. Schachter (Eds.), *The contemporary Freudian tradition: Past and present* (pp. 155–175). Routledge.
Pines, D. (2010). *A woman's unconscious use of her body: A psychoanalytical perspective*. Routledge.
Robinson, K. (2015). Remembering, repeating and working through: The impact of the controversial discussions. *British Journal of Psychotherapy*, *31*(1), 69–84.
Robinson, K., & Schachter, J. (Eds.) (2020). *The contemporary Freudian tradition: Past and present*. Routledge.
Sandler, J. (1960). The background of safety. *International Journal of Psychoanalysis*, *41*, 352–356.

Sandler, J. (1976). Countertransference and role-responsiveness. *International Review of Psycho-Analysis, 3*, 43–47.
Sandler, J., & Freud, A. (1985). *The analysis of defense: The ego and the mechanisms of defense revisited.* International Universities Press.
Sandler, J., & Rosenblatt, B. (1962). The concept of the representational world. *Psychoanalytic Study of the Child, 17*, 128–145.
Sandler, J., & Sandler, A. (1994). The past unconscious and the present unconscious. *Psychoanalytic Study of the Child, 49*, 278–292.
Sandler, J., & Sandler, A. (1998). *Internal objects revisited.* Routledge.
Sandler, A., & Schachter, J. (2014). An outline of our contemporary Freudian approach. *British Journal of Psychotherapy, 30*(1), 6–17.
Schachter, J. (1997). The body of thought: Psychoanalytic considerations on the mind-body relationship. *Psychoanalytic Psychotherapy, 11*(3), 211–219.
Yorke, C. (1988). Some thoughts on pre-Oedipal development: A "contemporary Freudian" view. *British Journal of Psychotherapy, 4*(4), 436–446.
Yorke, C., Wiseberg, S., & Freeman, T. (1989). *Development and psychopathology: Studies in psychoanalytic psychiatry.* Yale University Press.

Chapter 3

Klein, Kleinians, and Post-Kleinians: Deeper Layers of the Mind and Projective Identification

Tomasz Fortuna

In this chapter I will focus mainly on the British developments in Kleinian psychoanalysis. Those developments took place in an important context of dialogue and mutual influence between different psychoanalytic traditions since the Controversial Discussions of the British Psychoanalytical Society (1943–1944).

Kleinian analysis is rooted in the ideas of Sigmund Freud and Karl Abraham that paved the way for object-relations theory as a school of thought and a therapeutic technique. Through early processes of splitting, projection, and introjection, the mind is thought to be populated by internal objects with their phantasized intentions and motivations. Those dynamic internalized relationships, between the objects themselves and the self, reveal complex narratives akin to children's play. Influenced by experiences of working with children and her wish to understand severe emotional disturbance, Melanie Klein modified a number of axioms that were firmly located within the classical Freudian psychoanalysis. Further understanding of those deeper layers of the mind, governed by processes of splitting and projection, led to her own model of early development and opened the way to a psychoanalytic approach to psychiatric disorders.

General Assumptions

Although the Kleinian school of psychoanalysis shares common axioms with other branches of psychoanalysis, there are clear ideas that distinguish it from other traditions.

Klein effected a shift from the centrality of libido to the emphasis on anxiety, in the context of life and death drives and associated impulses, as a source of unconscious motivations and psychic defenses. The content and the quality of anxiety acquired a fundamental importance and led to further differentiation of psychotic and non-psychotic anxieties, later associated with psychic positions: *paranoid-schizoid* and *depressive*.

DOI: 10.4324/9781003027768-4

This shift led not only to new perspectives on early development but also a new conceptualization of states of mind, psychopathology, and psychoanalytic etiology, and as a result, changes to psychoanalytic technique.

The ego becomes established in processes of projection and introjection leading to the phantasized presence of internal objects seen as acting according to unconscious relational narratives (phantasies). It is difficult to separate phantasies from internal objects that "come to life" in the context of those narratives imbuing them with intentions, motivations, and human-like characteristics (Bronstein, 2001). This way ego becomes organized in a dynamic way. Indeed, for Klein (Isaacs, 1948; Klein, 1952), unconscious phantasies are the rudimentary mental building blocks of the mind, representing biological drives.

Melanie Klein firmly believed in early forms of object relations from birth, demonstrating the infant's capacity to momentary contact with external reality and primary objects even if in a primitive part-object form. This allowed her to see children's play as an expression of the unconscious narratives and interpret the transference situation to her young patients. Seeing children's play as equivalent to free associations in adults, with inhibitions and resistances respectively, she adopted a similar approach to working with adults. In one of her lectures, Klein writes, "Transference experience repeats former experiences, of both real and phantasy situations, and leads to memories both of real happenings and of emotional attitudes in the patient." (Klein, 2017a/1936, p. 61).

Therefore, internal object relationships are always influenced by processes of splitting, projection, and introjection creating a particular quality and life to the individual's internal landscape. Klein's notion of *memories in feelings* (Klein, 1957) conveys her emphasis on the preverbal experiences and representations that can only be communicated in a form of an emotional experience or re-enactment.

Understanding of the attitude toward reality is an important feature here. Segal (1981) wrote about the difference between an omnipotent phantasy—subjectively considered a fact but delusional in nature—and a thought, which is recognized as a product of one's mind and can be examined against external reality.

Specific Theoretical Assumptions

Nature of Psychic Structure

1 The unconscious phantasy is a basic and immediate psychic representation of the drives and a building block of the mind. Unconscious phantasies are closely linked to internal objects providing them with dynamic relational narratives; here defense mechanisms of the ego are unconscious phantasies too (providing them with their motivations and

aims); as well as processes of thinking, linking of ideas, and acquiring the meaning of the sensuous and emotional experiences. Unconscious phantasies in Kleinian theory can be of different levels of representation (Bell, 2017; Bronstein, 2015; Isaacs, 1948).

2 The dynamic anxiety-defense relationship structures the experience here-and-now in terms of the fleeting states of mind, as well as the more established functioning of the personality. Initially described as developmental stages of the young ego relating to external and internal realities, later in life they organize human experience according to the presence of a particular kind of anxiety and psychic defenses that are mobilized in response. Classically, Klein described the paranoid-schizoid (PS) and depressive (D) positions, where PS is characterized by paranoid anxieties and a sense of danger to self, while D is underpinned by anxieties related to own impulses and the concern for the object.

3 Constitutional factors play an important role. It is not only the environment but also the internal qualities of the mind. The majority of Kleinian analysts agree on the existence of life and death drives as a constitutional factor, and in extension, the presence of libidinal and destructive tendencies (e.g., envy) from the beginning of life. The infantile defensive processes and, in consequence, the development of the ego and a sense of self, will be affected by those constitutional factors. They also operate in the here-and-now contributing to actual experience in the analytic couple.

Sources and Nature of Energy

There is no direct reference to energy in the Kleinian and post-Kleinian models. The life and death drives are sources of impulses interacting with the external world. This interaction leads to the development of defenses modulating the impact of the awareness of reality i.e., psychic pain.

Nature of Relationships

Unconscious phantasies of different levels of concreteness and symbolization provide narratives as a context for relationships between internalized objects and the self and have a significant influence on our perceptions of external and internal realities. Therefore, an interplay of different anxieties, the resulting states of mind and defenses in operation color to a greater or lesser degree the experience of a particular relationship with another person. These phenomena, often underpinned by processes of projective and introjective identification, may facilitate recognition that the other person is independent of our phantasy world, when those processes are truly symbolic in nature. In other words, it is the capacity for an authentic engagement with another person, empathy, and true emotional intimacy that results from more mature and flexible modes of pre-verbal and verbal communication. However, when they are concrete, they seriously interfere with the accurate perception of the other, leading to the narcissistic type of engagement (Rosenfeld, 1983; Sodré, 2004).

Developmental Stages

The interplay between libidinal and destructive impulses and the evoked anxieties lead to initial defenses of splitting and projection. In normal development splitting, projection and introjection are dynamic and balanced and lead to the development and enrichment of the ego. The core of a good (idealized) object provides the basis for feelings of gratitude and generosity. This also helps to manage one's own impulses and tolerate their phantasized murderousness.

The first, paranoid-schizoid, stage of early development is governed by a sense of threat and avoidance of recognition of separateness from the object. This is necessary as the early ambivalence is overwhelming for the infantile ego. Projective and introjective processes are assumed to organize this period of development. The primary object is perceived as a sum of part-objects.

In the second, depressive, phase of development the primary object as well as one's own self begins to be perceived in their complexity (with their good/bad parts) and the ambivalence of feelings toward the objects and the self is better tolerated. Recognition of one's own hateful feelings leads to a sense of guilt, which can result in paranoid anxiety or manic defenses, or be accepted and responded to with a phantasy of reparation. The latter outcome results from the capacity to recognize and accept separateness as well as appreciation of the goodness of the object and the creative link between parents. This can mitigate the narcissistic regressive pull and envious attacks on external and internal objects and linking.

Those two phases of development subsequently interact with each other, and even during the paranoid-schizoid period more complex and coherent momentary perceptions of reality are present.

Symbol formation is closely connected to the development of recognition of separateness from the object and the capacity to tolerate associated anxieties through creating mental representations of the objects and their characteristics. The phantasy of lack of separateness and of possession of the object has to be given up and mourned when the depressive position is reached. Any inhibitions in symbol formation impede thinking and creativity and lead to concrete thinking, *symbolic equation,* where the difference between the symbol and the symbolized is denied (Segal, 1957).

Klein postulated an early emergence of the *Oedipal situation* starting from the momentary recognition of the link between parents from which the infant is excluded. Segal offered a formulation of the early pre-verbal perception of the parental couple: "Mummy—Daddy—Mummy gone." (Segal, 1981,

p. 222). Once tolerated, this leads to the capacity to observe oneself from different perspectives in relationships with others—creating a triangular space (Britton, 1989). Taking the third position (outside the couple) is an important capacity allowing for true emotional experience, helping to avoid over-identification with others, collusion, and enactment.

The early Oedipal situation (an unconscious phantasy and an organizing developmental process) remains central. The capacity to occupy the third position creates a three-dimensional mental space but also organizes the perception of reality.

Anxieties/Instincts/Defenses

The question of anxiety had become a central focus for Klein. Understanding and interpreting anxieties are thought to be important tasks for the analyst. Klein did not speak about drives in the Freudian sense and mainly referred to Freud's later dichotomy of life and death drives. What remains important is the dynamic interplay between the libidinal and destructive impulses that leads to anxieties and defensive responses. For example, satisfaction-frustration, love-hate, and grateful dependence versus envious dependence.

Importantly, anxiety springs from the interaction of two main sources—firstly, the death drive and destructive anti-developmental impulses, and secondly, frustration and unpleasure due to the bodily and external sources, conceived as coming from the primary object. Anxieties about survival are associated with the death drive and paranoid anxieties when this internal destructiveness is deflected and projected outward.

In consequence, in the paranoid-schizoid position we deal with defenses based on splitting, projection and introjection, in a form of omnipotent phantasies (e.g., denial, idealization, projective, and introjective identification). They are directed against the death drive and the anxiety of annihilation.

In the depressive position "they include manic defenses involving triumph over and contempt for the object and obsessional defenses involving control of the object." (Bott Spillius et al., 2011, p. 307). These defenses are related to the perception of the whole object and shield the ego from a sense of loss and guilt in relation to the object. However, the depressive position opens up the way to reparative efforts and the possibility to relinquish the omnipotence.

In the Kleinian model, defenses are also narrative unconscious phantasies and acquire relational context.

There always is a possible regression to more primitive defenses against both paranoid and depressive anxieties. Complex narcissistic defensive organizations maintaining split-off and relocated in phantasy parts (aspects and functions) of the self, internal objects, and the external object, constitute *psychic retreats* (Steiner, 1994) protecting from those anxieties. These complex defenses have a profound effect on the ego, usually resulting in various kinds of impairment of its function.

According to Klein, neurotic defenses such as repression come about when an object can be perceived as a whole-object and "greater integration of the self and object has been achieved and splitting has lessened" (Bott Spillius et al., 2011, p. 307).

Etiology

For Klein, the ego is concerned with its relationship to reality. This capacity is rooted in developmental advances leading to the achievement of the depressive position, i.e., the capacity to tolerate and engage with the complexity of the surrounding reality and own emotional world. The interplay of constitutional factors and the environmental response may mitigate or exacerbate challenges posed by these developmental milestones. Therefore, psychopathology stems from traumatic disruptions to the emotional development leaving fault-lines in the personality. The timing of those traumatic events points to the likely defensive responses to severe distress in the future. Broadly speaking, psychotic pathology is associated with paranoid anxieties (PS) and neurotic with depressive anxieties (D).

Many Kleinian authors (e.g., Britton, 1989; Feldman, 2008; Steiner, 2005) wrote about the difficulties in the management of the Oedipal situation and triangularity, resulting in developmental deficits, especially in the area of thinking, symbolization, and creativity, where the ability to mourn play an important role. The link between parents and the parental couple itself can be denied or seen as threatening or inadequate, at times leading to the experience of a dangerous combined parental object precluding any possibility of seeing the parental couple as caring and supportive.

In these situations, phantasies of splitting and projection offer a narcissistic defensive solution against awareness of separateness from the object, need and longing for the object and envy aimed at its good qualities. A sense of omnipotence and omniscience defensively replaces the reality-testing capacity (Segal, 1981).

If the superego retains its archaic harsh punitive qualities and is unmodified by the good aspects of other internal objects, it puts a serious strain on the functioning of the mind, leading to persecutory guilt and severe emotional disturbance (Klein, 1958).

Technique

In one of her seminars Klein emphasizes changes to psychoanalytic technique, "The two things, the approach to anxiety and the approach to transference, are interlinked; I believe it is only when the approach focused on emotions, particularly on anxiety, that this technique could be developed" (Klein, 2017b/1958, p. 97). And later, "This implies that both the unconscious and the transference situation are considered much more, and from the very beginning" (Klein, 2017b/1958, p. 97).

This attention to unconscious phantasy linked to relevant anxieties and the transference is complemented by clinical attention to the current most dominant anxiety in the particular moment of the session and this needs to be appropriately interpreted (verbally or through attitude and openness). This way the analytic situation can be established and the patient's anxiety reduced.

> If we have an eye to the full urgency of the material presented, we find ourselves obliged to trace not only the representational content but also the anxiety and sense of guilt associated with it right down to that layer of the mind which is being activated.
>
> (Klein, 1997/1932, p. 25)

Klein's attention to the early stages of psychic development and her interest in pre-verbal and pre-symbolic levels of experience drew clinical attention to the wealth of human experience and communication, becoming a part and parcel of our clinical work.

As Bronstein (2015) stated, "We resort to many different pieces of data to infer the nature of the unconscious phantasies that are being enacted in the analytical situation and how they operate." She further reminds us of Klein's notion of memories in feelings as manifestations of "pre-verbal emotions and phantasies ... revived in the transference situation" (Klein, 1957, p. 180) as non-verbal modes of communication. Therefore, attention is being paid not only to the verbal material but also behaviors, attitudes, enactments, and bodily experiences in both the patient and the analyst—interpretation not only of the content but also the function of clinical material. In other words, "... what is not meaningful is not therefore meaningless." (Waddell, 2013, p. 12).

The uncovered complexity of human psychic life requires the analyst to follow the patient's communications and address the appropriate level of experience in the here-and-now transference situation. The focus is on the psychic reality of the patient and the countertransference of the analyst.

The analyst allows the patient to re-experience the transference situation anew in the consulting room, whether the analyst represents (and is actually experienced as) a persecutory or a friendly supportive figure. The patient's experience of emotional attunement and being understood by the analyst serves as a verification of reality and the difference between the transference figure and the analyst. Equally, the limitations have to be recognized too.

Summary and Developments

Kleinian psychoanalysis exemplifies a close relationship between developmental theory, the focus on transference situation, and the clinical technique.

The shift from libido to anxiety led to the notions of psychic positions linking particular anxieties with relevant psychic defenses. Emphasis on the primitive processes of splitting and projection and the unconscious phantasy opened the way to recognition of manifestations of pre-verbal infantile experience represented in the session as memories in feelings.

The developments in the understanding of narcissistic object relations (Rosenfeld, Joseph, O'Shaughnessy, Steiner) led to clinical advances in working with patients suffering from psychoses (Bion, Bell, Bronstein, Hinshelwood, Jackson, O'Shaughnessy), personality disorders (Rey, Steiner), and perversions (Etchegoyen, Joseph, Meltzer). It furthered the study of processes of thinking (Brenman, Segal, Waddell) and life and death instincts (Abel-Hirsch, Bell, Feldman, Joseph, Rosenfeld, Segal).

Advances in the understanding of transference-countertransference relationship, enactment, and empathy demonstrated the role of projective and introjective identification (e.g., Bion, Bott Spillius, Brenman Pick, Joseph, Money-Kyrle, O'Shaughnessy, Sodré) and refined the technique: analyst centered interpretations (Steiner), levels of transference interpretation (Roth), or analysis of grievances (Feldman).

Others developed an understanding of clinical teams and organizations (Bion, Hinshelwood, Jacques, Menzies-Lyth), racist attitudes (Davids), and notions of creativity (Segal), as well as child and adolescent psychoanalysis (Brenman Pick, Bronstein, Joseph, Meltzer, O'Shaughnessy, Segal, Waddell).

The work of W. R. Bion, his notions of containment and linking but also transformations and the particular analytic attitude he advocated are vitally important in the contemporary post-Kleinian practice.

3. Melanie Klein, Kleinians, and Post-Kleinians	
Main, general underlying assumptions	1 Centrality of anxiety: paranoid-schizoid/ depressive positions 2 Unconscious phantasy/internal objects 3 Projective identification
Specific theoretical assumptions	
psychic structure	• Unconscious phantasy/internal objects • Psychic positions • Constitutional factors (e.g., death drive—envy)
energy	• Impulses originating from life and death drives
relationship	• Unconscious phantasy—perceptions of others and reality • Projective/introjective identification

(Continued)

development stages	• Paranoid-schizoid/depressive stages • Early Oedipus • Gratitude, reparation, symbol formation, mourning
body	N/A
anxieties/instincts and defenses	• Death drive vs. frustration • Interplay of internal and external realities • Splitting, projective identification, enactment, manic defenses, repression
Assumptions concerning etiology	• Ego vs. reality • Archaic superego • Developmental fault-lines • Narcissistic defensive organizations—psychic retreats
Implications for technique	• Interpretation of anxiety, unconscious phantasy, transference/countertransference • Attention to preverbal material and enactment
Subsequent developments of the core concept	• Theories of psychosis, personality disorders, perversions • Relevant clinical technique • Organizations, social phenomena, creativity • Child analysis

References

Bell, D. (2017). Unconscious phantasy: Some historical and conceptual dimensions. *International Journal of Psychoanalysis*, *98*, 785–798.

Bott Spillius, E., Milton, J., Garvey, P., Couve, C., & Steiner, D. (2011). *The new dictionary of Kleinian thought*. Routledge.

Britton, R. (1989). The missing link: Parental sexuality in the Oedipus complex. *The Oedipus Complex Today: Clinical Implications*, *54*, 83–101.

Bronstein, C. (2001). What are internal objects? In C. Bronstein (Ed.), *Kleinian theory: A contemporary perspective* (pp. 108–124). Whurr.

Bronstein, C. (2015). Finding unconscious phantasy in the session: Recognising form. *International Journal of Psychoanalysis*, *96*, 925–944.

Feldman, M. (2008). Grievance: The underlying Oedipal configuration. *International Journal of Psychoanalysis*, *89*, 743–758.

Isaacs, S. (1948). The nature and function of phantasy. *International Journal of Psychoanalysis*, *29*, 73–97.

Klein, M. (1952). The origins of transference. *International Journal of Psychoanalysis*, *33*, 433–438.

Klein, M. (1957). *Envy and gratitude: A study of unconscious sources.* Tavistock Publications.
Klein, M. (1958). On the development of mental functioning. *International Journal of Psychoanalysis, 39*, 84–90.
Klein, M. (1997). The technique of early analysis. In *The psycho-analysis of children* (pp. 16–34). Vintage. Reprint of a revised version of the book originally published in 1975 by The Hogarth Press Ltd. London. Revised edition by H. A. Thorner, translation by Alix Strachey. (Original work published 1932).
Klein, M. (2017a). Lecture 4: Clinical illustration of transference and interpretation. In *Lectures on technique by Melanie Klein. Edited with critical review by John Steiner* (pp. 61–70). Routledge. (Original work published 1936).
Klein, M. (2017b). The seminars on technique, 1958. In *Lectures on technique by Melanie Klein. Edited with critical review by John Steiner* (pp. 95–117). Routledge. (Original work published 1958).
Rosenfeld, H. (1983). Primitive object relations and mechanisms. *International Journal of Psychoanalysis, 64*, 261–267.
Segal, H. (1957). Notes on symbol formation. *International Journal of Psychoanalysis, 38*, 391–397.
Segal, H. (1981). Psychoanalysis and freedom of thought. In *The work of Hanna Segal: A Kleinian approach to clinical practice* (pp. 217–227). Jason Aronson.
Sodré, I. (2004). Who's who? Notes on pathological identifications. In E. Hargreaves & A. Varchevker (Eds.), *In Pursuit of Psychic Change. The Betty Joseph Workshop* (pp. 53–65). Routledge.
Steiner, J. (1994). *Psychic retreats: Pathological organizations in psychotic, neurotic and borderline patients.* Routledge.
Steiner, J. (2005). The conflict between mourning and melancholia. *Psychoanalytic Quarterly, 74*, 83–104.
Waddell, M. (2013). Reflections on "meaning" and "meaninglessness" in post-Kleinian thought. In D. Bell & A. Novakovic (Eds.), *Living on the border: Psychotic processes in the individual, the couple, and the group.* Tavistock Clinic Series (pp. 11–27). Karnac Books.

Chapter 4

Fairbairn and the Independent Tradition

John Keene and Graham S. Clarke

The relationships between what has come to be known as the Independent Tradition and the formal political entities known as the "Middle Group" and the Group of Independent Psychoanalysts can be puzzling to those not familiar with the history of the British Psychoanalytical Society. After the conclusion of the Controversial Discussions in 1945, where the theoretical and technical controversy was centrally between the committed followers of Melanie Klein and Anna Freud, the analysts of the middle group became a political force without wanting to be one, since they were the majority and held the political balance in the British Society. As the political structures and training arrangements evolved in the 1950s, the middle group was finally constituted as a group, calling itself the Group of Independent Analysts, one of three constitutional groupings in the society. Thus the Independent Group (for short) became the political and philosophical home of two partially overlapping groups within the Society: those members of the Society who resisted being drawn into the partisan struggles and wished to uphold their freedom to pursue psychoanalysis as a scientific rather than a tribal endeavor by failing to identify as either Freudian or Kleinian, and those who had a key role in the creation and development of the object relations approach in psychoanalysis, which Kohon (1986) helpfully designated the "Independent Tradition." This term has remained useful because some key thinkers of the tradition, such as Winnicott, were determinedly not prepared to join any group.

Keene (2012) suggests that a central concern in Independent thinking is the elaboration of an underdeveloped assumption in Freud's theorizing which seriously overestimated the capacity of average maternal care to fully satisfy an infant's needs, leading to a particular set of defensive maneuvers. This approach was largely pioneered in Europe by the Hungarians, led by Ferenczi, Michael and Alice Balint, and their counterparts in the British Psychoanalytical Society who were eventually concentrated in the Independent Group. These theorists suggest a range of consequences of problems in early relationships, with Winnicott noting failures of ego integration, premature ego development with a preoccupation with "doing"

DOI: 10.4324/9781003027768-5

over "being," quasi-mental defect, schizophrenia, and false-self organizations. Balint adds a primary attachment to objects (people) or to the spaces between them. Winnicott and Balint featured strongly in the clinical discussions while Fairbairn, geographically separated in Scotland, provided a compelling reconfiguration of some of Freud's underlying assumptions.

Fairbairn: Introduction

Fairbairn followed Ferenczi in seeing omnipotence and internalization as desperate defenses against helplessness, dependence, and the emergence of overwhelming primitive anxieties, in the context of objectively bad experiences with external objects. Of particular significance are the consequences if the mother fails to convince the infant through spontaneous and genuine expression that she cares for him or her as a person. Fairbairn's paper on schizoid phenomena (1940/1952a), a major contribution to the understanding of borderline phenomena, suggested that this leads to part-object relationships to the breast and its functions, rather than to the mother as a person. (Klein recognized Fairbairn's work in calling her earliest phase "paranoid-schizoid" rather than just the paranoid phase.) Crucially, the mother's rejection or distaste for the child's passionate "libidinal" true self desires, its infantile "love" for the mother and her body, lead to a sense of futility and shame in the infant. A combination of possessiveness and emotional indifference is also potentially unmanageable, except by depersonalization and de-emotionalization of the relationship. Regular defenses against this situation are an over-valuation of internal processes and ideas. Similarly, amassing possessions, physical, bodily, and mental, defends against the experience of emptiness within. Intellectualization, with or without erotization and perverse elements, substitutes for the desired relationships with the parents. Primitive elements of these are split off and relationships inside are full of secret control and grandiosity. The playing of roles and a preference for "showing" rather than giving create an essentially narcissistic way to manage the anxieties concerning emptiness, loss, and the surrender of control.

General Underlying Assumptions

Fairbairn's critique of Freud's libido theory, developed in a series of papers (Fairbairn, 1940/1952a, 1941/1952b, 1943/1952c, 1944/1952d) collected in 1952 under the title *Psychoanalytic Studies of the Personality,* echoed Balint's (1935/1952) in pointing out that the maturity of object relationships is in no way guaranteed by the reproductively appropriate use of the genital organs, just as an infant who was well fed could fail to thrive for psychological reasons. Fairbairn saw the early psychoanalysts' emphasis on the erotogenic zones as resulting from a misplaced stress on instinctual discharge and a corresponding lack of a theoretical place for the need for relationships which led Fairbairn to assert that "libido," as described by Freud, should be regarded as "object-seeking" rather than purely "pleasure-seeking." The revised view sees the function of libidinal pleasure and the erotogenic zones as providing signposts to the object.

Fairbairn also found Klein's version of Freud's life and death instincts, in which the infant is the battleground for a primal clash between loving and hating urges, psychologically unconvincing and less than useful in understanding the complexities for the infant of maintaining relationships with objects which have combinations of exciting and frustrating aspects. Fairbairn's work with abused children and the victims of war showed him how individuals will persist in relationships with objectively bad figures to whom they are attached, identify with them, and support them in preference to being alone, suggesting a primary instinct for attachment and maintaining relationships which, in many situations, would take preference over matters of pleasure and pain. Fairbairn's account of the infant's necessary attachment to bad objects in the interest of survival provides a straightforward explanation for the repetition compulsion, which avoids Freud's contortions on the subject. Fairbairn's is a thoroughgoing model of the internalization of aspects of real relationship experiences, whereas many Kleinians have espoused a model of internal object relations in which the objects are generated from the drives and projected [cf. Hamilton, 1982].

Wider biological and psychological accounts of motivation showed that human instinctual behavior divides into two broad categories. The first covers the regulation of internal tensions caused by physiological needs: hunger and thirst, evacuation of bodily waste products, and, eventually, sexual release. These appetitive instincts, in which there is a build-up of need and tension, which is released by a consummatory pleasurable act, are the paradigm Freud had adopted for his account of all instincts. Freud was well aware of situational (i.e., external) threats to the individual, as he noted that different psychological defenses were required to deal with internal dangers because fight or flight, which are the prime options for external dangers, were not available. Fairbairn criticized Freud's last schema of the life and death instincts, with its emphasis on the strength of internal tensions, because it gave a poor account of those drives which are situational rather than appetitive. For Fairbairn, it seemed more appropriate to regard aggression as primarily a situational drive, in that it is a response to danger, frustration, or threat to self or to people to whom one is attached. In Fairbairn's model, the appetitive drives and the situational ones, including aggression, are all developments of inherited dispositions, which refutes the old accusation that Fairbairn did not believe in instincts.

Fairbairn felt that Freud's conception of the ego as a structure without its own energy, which develops on the surface of the psyche for the purpose of regulating id-impulses in relation to the demands and constraints of external reality, did not adequately describe the situation. He felt that it made more sense conceptually to see the central ego, or self, as the agency which experiences needs, has desires, and has to manage both internal and external reality in trying to satisfy these, negotiating the conflicts that are aroused in the process. His reworking of Freud's structural theory removed Freud's unhelpful distinction between energy and structure and created a model based fully on object relationships and the ways in which they become internalized unconscious schemas, or models of reality in the mind.

Fairbairn's model sees the external reality of caregivers as a major source of the objects that become internalized in the infant's mind. The young infant, in its absolute dependence, has to find a way of adapting to its objects to get its needs met, or it would face death. Internalization is a way of dealing with unmanageable aspects of reality by bringing them inside the self, where they can be modified by wish-fulfilling phantasy, which is, by its nature, omnipotent. In this, it is always the relationship that is internalized and the most unbearable aspects repressed. Once repressed, the central ego, or self, can unconsciously identify itself with either the self or object side of the relationship. There are structural consequences that follow, as loving parts of the self, which are in relation to loving objects, have to be kept apart (dissociated) from the hating parts of the self, which are connected to the depriving, frustrating, or cruel aspects of external objects. Fairbairn refers here to the accepted and the rejected objects, following Freud's observations that there is a wish to hold on to and incorporate the good object while those generating bad experiences are to be rejected and evacuated. The relationships to the bad, rejecting, and rejected objects have to be held out of consciousness by repression, consuming emotional resources, and impoverishing the ego/self. The conscious and preconscious ego contains the parts of the self and its relationships to both good and bad objects that can be tolerated in consciousness.

Fairbairn suggests that the hatred of these purified, frustrating, and rejecting aspects of the object is the emotional source of repression. It is turned against both the experience of the self in relation to the bad object and also against the loving, libidinal parts of the self, with its urges to seek out libidinally satisfying relationships with good objects. This forms the basis of fundamental splits in the personality, which, for Fairbairn, are the basal layer of the personality. The primitive superego, therefore, contains both a cruel and rejecting element and an antilibidinal element, which acts as a "fifth column" within the personality, sabotaging benign functioning. Even in relatively healthy and integrated individuals, this factor is liable to come to prominence when stress and anxiety in the individual threatens more balanced and sophisticated functioning since it attacks healthy and loving impulses. This fifth column functions just as Rosenfeld later described his internal mafia, mocking any attempts to believe in and seek out good objects, arguing that the rewards of triumph and manipulation are safer and superior to a doomed belief in love and goodness.

This revised picture of the mental apparatus should not be seen as rigid, but comprised of many layers of self and object representations from different experiences with objects at different developmental stages. Bowlby's (1969) description of the child's need to develop multiple models of the world which are derived initially from repeated sequences of interactions with caregivers around particular patterns of need, anxiety, and gratification closely parallels Fairbairn's conception although he argues that "attachment" is a better term for what Fairbairn is describing than "dependence." Fairbairn's view of the internalized schemas of the relationship to reality implied that all objects in dreams represent different versions of the self and its objects. Dreams, at an important level, always represent elements of the current state of internal reality.

Fairbairn (1941/1952b) saw the classically described neuroses as various ways of structuring the psyche's attempts at managing the threat of the eruption of these schizoid phenomena from the basal layer of the personality. Schematically, he sees these as depending on the predominant preferences in the ego/self as to where the split-off good and bad objects are felt to be located. Thus, for the phobic individual, or, perhaps more accurately, "an individual in a phobic configuration," both good and bad objects are felt to be outside the self and the depleted self urgently seeks for the good object but always fears getting the bad object instead. In paranoia, the good object is clearly felt to be inside, and is, therefore, an object of envy and hostility from an external world entirely peopled with bad objects. The obsessional has good and bad retained inside, but, in wishing to keep the good and evacuate the bad, is constantly persecuted by the thought of losing the good by mistake and by doing untold damage in the evacuation of the bad. The hysteric projects the good because it is associated with unmanageable sexuality, but has to constantly seek external objects to deal with the bad that remains inside.

Fairbairn's work emphasizes important differences between depressive affects arising from different situations. The first is a depressive sense of futility in the infant from the early oral stage which follows if he feels his libidinal urges and desires are not well received by the mother, while depression is, as classically described, a consequence of guilt at his angry responses in the later oral (biting) stage.

A second clinically important distinction is between the sense of guilt itself and the "moral defense" where an individual takes on the sense of blame and guilt for some adverse interpersonal situation in order to keep the belief and hope alive that their objects are fundamentally benign and loving, and can become good to them if they are better. Fairbairn noticed this particularly in his work with abused children who tended to blame themselves for their abuse rather than accept the reality that they may often have been hated or unfairly punished by their parents.

Specific Theoretical Assumptions

Over 20 years or so, Fairbairn gave a number of synopses of the characteristics and processes of his object relations theory, the final version of which was published in 1963 in IJPA.

1 An ego is present from birth.
2 Libido is a function of the ego.
3 There is no death instinct, and aggression is a reaction to frustration or deprivation.
4 Since libido is a function of the ego and aggression is a reaction to frustration or deprivation, there is no such thing as an "id."
5 The ego, and therefore libido, is fundamentally object-seeking.
6 The earliest and original form of anxiety, as experienced by the child, is separation-anxiety.
7 Internalization of the object is a defensive measure originally adopted by the child to deal with his original object (the mother and her breast) in so far as it is unsatisfying.
8 Internalization of the object is not just a product of a phantasy of incorporating the object orally but is a distinct psychological process.
9 Two aspects of the internalized object, viz. its exciting and its frustrating aspects, are split off from the main core of the object and repressed by the ego.
10 Thus there come to be constituted two repressed internal objects, viz. the exciting (or libidinal) object and the rejecting (or antilibidinal) object.
11 The main core of the internalized object, which is not repressed, is described as the ideal object or ego-ideal.
12 Owing to the fact that the exciting (libidinal) and rejecting (antilibidinal) objects are both cathected by the original ego, these objects carry into repression with the parts of the ego by which they are cathected, leaving the central core of the ego (central ego) unrepressed, but acting as the agent of repression.
13 The resulting internal situation is one in which the original ego is split into three egos—a central (conscious) ego attached to the ideal object (ego-ideal), a repressed libidinal ego attached to the exciting (or libidinal) object, and a repressed antilibidinal ego attached to the rejecting (or antilibidinal) object.
14 This internal situation represents a basic schizoid position which is more fundamental than the depressive position described by Melanie Klein.
15 The antilibidinal ego, in virtue of its attachment to the rejecting (antilibidinal) object, adopts an uncompromisingly hostile attitude to the libidinal ego, and thus has the effect of powerfully reinforcing the repression of the libidinal ego by the central ego.

16 What Freud described as the "superego" is really a complex structure comprising (a) the ideal object or ego-ideal, (b) the antilibidinal ego, and (c) the rejecting (or antilibidinal) object.
17 These considerations form the basis of a theory of the personality conceived in terms of object-relations, in contrast to one conceived in terms of instincts and their vicissitudes.

(Fairbairn, 1963)

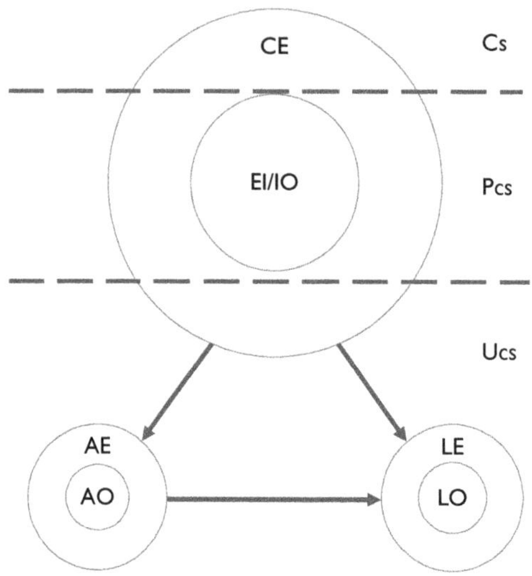

Figure 4.1 Based on Figure 1 from Fairbairn's 1944/1952d paper. The labels for the different dynamic endopsychic structures were later modified. In his 1954 paper on Hysterical States Fairbairn introduces the Antilibidinal Ego and Object and in his 1963 Synopsis of his theory he uses the following: In the Unconscious (Ucs) part of the mind: The Internal Saboteur became the Antilibidinal Ego (AE). The Rejecting Object became the Antilibidinal Object (AO). The Libidinal Ego (LE) remains the same throughout. The Needed Object becomes the Exciting Object in 1952 and then in later accounts the Libidinal Object (LO). In the Preconscious (Pcs) part of the mind: He places the Ideal Object (I.O.)/Ego Ideal (E.I.) in the Preconscious (Pcs) part of the Central Ego (CE). [Author's addition to original diagram based upon the 1944/1952d text.] In the Conscious (Cs) part of the mind: The Central Ego (CE) remains the same throughout. The Central Ego or Self also contains Preconscious and Unconscious aspects which are part of the unrepressed, everyday, unconscious, and preconscious, aspects of our internal world. The vectors (arrows) represent aggression used for repression as per item 13 of Fairbairn's synopsis (1963).

Fairbairn's Legacy

Fairbairn's influence theoretically and clinically is widespread but not always acknowledged. His geographical isolation from the rest of the British Psychoanalytical Society meant that in the UK, he mainly engaged personally with psychotherapists and analysts with connections to Scotland, Suttie (1935/1960), Macmurray (1957, 1961), and Sutherland (1989), in particular, who along with, Guntrip (1961, 1968), from the North of England, shared and developed his ideas. In that respect one could consider him an "isolated" independent. Despite this, his contribution to psychoanalytic metapsychology and to clinical issues in early disturbance and trauma has been hugely significant inside and outside the evolving independent tradition. (For accounts of the latter see Kohon, 1986, 2018; Rayner, 1990, pp. 9–10; Williams et al., 2012.)

Assessing Fairbairn's contribution to psychoanalysis, Sutherland said,

> I believe [...] it is entirely accurate to say that he was the first to propose in a systematic manner the Copernican change of founding the psychoanalytic theory of the human personality on the experiences within social relationships instead of the discharge of instinctual tensions originating solely within the individual (1989, p. 163).

One of the most useful commentaries on the development of Fairbairn's model of endopsychic structure is to be found in John Padel's paper, "The Contribution of W. R. D. Fairbairn (1889–1965) to Psychoanalytic Theory and Practice," produced for the *European Psycho-Analytic Foundation Bulletin* and published as Chapter 21 in Clarke and Scharff (2014).

Grotstein and Rinsley's *Fairbairn and the Origins of Object Relations* (1994) provides perspectives from across the world as do Greenberg and Mitchell in their *Object Relations in Psychoanalytic Theory* (1983). Greenberg and Mitchell consider that Fairbairn "provides the purest and clearest expression of the shift from the drive/structure model to the relational/structure model" (p. 151) while James Grotstein (1991, 1994) described Fairbairn's theory of endopsychic structure as "the unsurpassed metapsychology of child abuse and of multiple personality" (1991, p. 140) and "the most apposite paradigm yet proffered for child-abuse, child molestation, post-traumatic stress disorder and multiple personality disorder" (1994, p. 123).

In the same period Joseph Sandler and colleagues writing in *The Patient and the Analyst* described Fairbairn's theory as the best available account of resistance and super-ego development as described by Freud.

> Later developments particularly stimulated by Fairbairn's work on the relation between object relations and resistance, have led object relations theorists to think less in terms of Freud's structural theory and to conceive of intra-psychic life essentially in terms of internal object

> relationships. Superego resistance is seen by object relations theorists in terms of the relation to and interaction with an internalized critical, or even persecutory, figure. The connection between internal object relationships is beautifully described by Fairbairn (1958), who points out that "in a sense, psychoanalytical treatment resolves itself into a struggle on the part of the patient to press-gang his relationship with the inner world through the agency of transference, and a determination on the part of the analysts to effect a breach in this closed system and to provide conditions under which in the setting of a therapeutic relationship, the patient may be induced to accept the open system of outer reality."
>
> (Sandler et al., 1973/1993, pp. 112–113)

Strikingly, Ronald Britton, a British Kleinian, provides a fitting concluding quotation in the 2nd edition of his book *Sex, Death and the Superego.*

> When I began reviewing my ideas on the need to reconstruct the underlying metapsychological assumptions of psychoanalysis, I thought of myself taking a new path, but I soon found out I was stepping into the footsteps of an earlier pioneer, Ronald Fairbairn … Fairbairn tried to join in the famous Controversial Discussions between Klein's followers and those of Anna Freud (1941–1945) with a very brief statement of his theory in writing. It was concise, clear and enormously relevant to the discussion. It was ignored completely. Perhaps since the discussions were a sort of trial of Melanie Klein as a psychoanalytic heretic, it was not a good moment for her to join in his dismantling of Freud's libido theory." (2021, pp. 2–3).

4. Fairbairn and the Independent Tradition	
Main, general underlying assumptions	1 An initial active self, dependent upon the real world 2 Dynamic internal world, reality oriented 3 Dynamic internal world learns from relationship experiences 4 All explanations in terms of dynamic internal objects and ego structures
Specific theoretical assumptions	
psychic structure	Internal ego-structures and internal objects as residues of earlier object relationships
energy	Energy cannot be separated from structure
relationship	Crucial concept: everything mediated by relationships

(Continued)

development stages	From infantile dependency through transitional stage to mature dependency with differentiated objects/others
body	Thoroughly embodied
anxieties/instinct and defenses	All mediated via the internal world of dynamic structures
Assumptions concerning etiology	Deficit theory of structure generated by shortfall in environmental affordances
Implications for technique	Gain access to closed system of internalized bad objects and transform them, reduce splitting, and dissociation to a minimum
Subsequent developments of the core concept	Widely used foundation of object relations theory

References

Balint, M. (1952). Critical notes on the theory of the pregenital organizations of the libido. In *Primary love and psycho-analytic technique* (pp. 37–58). Tavistock. (Original work published 1935).

Bowlby, J. (1969). *Attachment: Attachment and loss* (Vol. 1). Hogarth.

Britton, R. (2021). *Sex, death and the superego*. (2nd ed.). Routledge.

Clarke, G. S., & Scharff, D. E. (2014). *Fairbairn and the object relations tradition*. Karnac.

Fairbairn, W. R. D. (Ed.). (1952a). Schizoid factors in the personality. In *Psychoanalytic studies of the personality* (pp. 3–27). Tavistock, Routledge & Kegan Paul. (Original work published 1940).

Fairbairn, W. R. D. (Ed.). (1952b). A revised psychopathology of the psychoses and psychoneuroses. In *Psychoanalytic studies of the personality* (pp. 28–58). Tavistock, Routledge & Kegan Paul. (Original work published 1941).

Fairbairn, W. R. D. (Ed.). (1952c). The repression and the return of bad objects (with special reference to the "war neuroses"). In *Psychoanalytic studies of the personality* (pp. 59–81). Tavistock, Routledge & Kegan Paul. (Original work published 1943).

Fairbairn, W. R. D. (Ed.). (1952d). Endopsychic structure considered in terms of object relationships. In *Psychoanalytic studies of the personality* (pp. 82–136). Tavistock, Routledge & Kegan Paul. (Original work published 1944).

Fairbairn, W. R. D. (1952e). *Psychoanalytic studies of the personality*. Tavistock, Routledge & Kegan Paul.

Fairbairn, W.R.D. (1954). Observations on the nature of Hysterical States. *British Journal of Medical Psychology*, *27*(3), 106–125.

Fairbairn, W.R.D. (1958). On the nature and aims of psychoanalytical treatment. *International Journal of Psycho-Analysis, 39*(5), 374–385.

Fairbairn, W. R. D. (1963). Synopsis of an object-relations theory of the personality. *International Journal of Psychoanalysis, 44*, 224–225.

Greenberg, J., & Mitchell, S. (1983). *Object relations in psychoanalytic theory.* Harvard University Press.

Grotstein, J. S. (1991). [Review]. Hughes, J. M., Reshaping the psychoanalytic domain: The work of Melanie Klein, W. R. D. Fairbairn, and D. W. Winnicott. *Psychoanalytic Quarterly, 60*, 136–140.

Grotstein, J. S. (1994). Notes on Fairbairn's metapsychology. In J. Grotstein & D. Rinsley (Eds.) *Fairbairn and the origins of object relations* (pp. 112–150). Free Association Books.

Grotstein, J., & Rinsley, D. (Eds.). (1994). *Fairbairn and the origins of object relations.* Free Association Books.

Guntrip, H. (1961). *Personality structure and human interaction.* Hogarth.

Guntrip, H. (1968). *Schizoid phenomena, object-relations and the self.* Hogarth.

Hamilton, V. (1982). *Narcissus and Oedipus: The children of psychoanalysis.* Chs. 2, 3, and 4. Routledge & Kegan Paul.

Keene, J. (2012). Reflections on the evolution of independent psychoanalytic thought. In P. Williams, J. Keene, & S. Dermen (Eds.), *Independent psychoanalysis today* (pp. 3–61). Karnac. 10.4324/9780429475832

Kohon, G. (Ed). (1986). *The British school of psychoanalysis: The Independent Tradition.* Free Association Book.

Kohon, G. (Ed). (2018). *British psychoanalysis: New perspectives in the Independent Tradition.* Routledge.

Macmurray, J. (1957). *The self as agent: The form of the personal* (Vol. I). Faber and Faber.

Macmurray, J. (1961). *Persons in relation: The form of the personal* (Vol. II). Faber and Faber.

Rayner, E. (1990). *The independent mind in British psychoanalysis.* Free Association Books.

Sandler, Dare, & Holder. (1993). *The patient and the analyst.* Revised and enlarged edition. Karnac Books. (Original work published 1973).

Sutherland, J. (1989). *Fairbairn's journey into the interior.* Free Association Books.

Suttie, I. D. (1960) *The origins of love and hate.* Pelican Books. (Original work published 1935).

Williams, P., Keene, J., & Dermen, S. (Eds.). (2012). *Independent psychoanalysis today.* Karnac.

Chapter 5

Winnicott and the Winnicottians[1]

Frances Thomson-Salo

Donald Winnicott (1896–1971), a British pediatrician and psychoanalyst, wrote extensively over several decades but, while influencing significant transformations in psychoanalysis, he did not gather a school around him.

Main Assumptions

Mother[2]-infant Relationship and Object Use

The mother-infant relationship begins with devoted maternal preoccupation and holding care (Winnicott, 1971/2005, pp. 130–138) creating a loving, empathic environment. This supports the normal maturational processes of curiosity, autonomy, creativity, empathy, and dreaming so that an infant can develop in a "personal beginning."

An infant's conception of the mother as a whole person is primarily established through good experiences during excitement. As the "environment mother" holds her infant in quiet states, and in excited states is treated as a "ruthlessly" devoured object (the "object mother"), the infant gradually realizes that mother and infant are the same in both states. The mother gives her infant the illusion that the world can be created out of need and imagination, later taking her infant through a process of disillusionment, which makes the demands of reality bearable until creativity can develop. The drives to love and be aggressive begin to join at about five months.

An infant establishes a self of "unit status," physically within the body's skin and psychologically integrated, feeling that there are personal riches inside the self, and the mother has become a "whole object." Anxiety about ambivalence becomes tolerable, and maternal holding of the situation enables an infant's experience of guilt to be transformed into a concern which is shown in gestures that are intended to make reparation for wishes and actions (Winnicott, 1965, pp. 73–82). Consolidation of separateness is facilitated, as well as moves toward the reality principle, a capacity to play alone (Winnicott, 1971/2005, pp. 44–61), and to fantasy. Experiences of object use, and concern, underpin all subsequent relationships. The most

DOI: 10.4324/9781003027768-6

difficult path in emotional development, from object relating to object use in unconscious fantasy, requires the continual destruction of the object relation (to a breast which is not yet a separate phenomenon), followed by the survival of the object which now has more robust externality (Winnicott, 1971/2005, pp. 101–111). The process is: "I love and simultaneously destroy you in fantasy and you have value for me because you survived my destruction." Object use (the object surviving hatred) means the object can be a life tool in the world of shared external reality.

True Self as Isolate Communicating from Choice and the Sense of Aliveness

The sense of self, particularly the true self (Winnicott's leading developmental concept), is crucial to mental and emotional well-being (Winnicott, 1965, pp. 140–152). The aim of development is that the innermost, centrally alone self is only reached by living and cultural experience and is not to be violated.

Early body experiences with the mother and the environment contribute to an emerging sense of self through attuned mirroring and spontaneous feelings being welcomed, which gives the confidence to express feelings, protects the illusion of omnipotence, and prepares for the shock of losing this illusion. Inevitable parental unreliability supports the emergence of the self. The true self is a subject that possesses personal authenticity and creativity yet is always partly hidden. The sense of being alive, feeling real in mind and body, experiencing intuitive feelings, and being in touch with others and one's own body—that is, a personal way of being—is essential to this sense of being alive. Creative internalizations and excitement about being alive make life worth living.

Transitional Objects and Phenomena

From about four months onward, the mother-infant unity transitions to a mother-and-infant state, a potential space with transitional objects and transitional phenomena (Winnicott, 1971/2005, pp. 1–30). This state of mind (infant and mother are both one, and two) embodies a paradox not to be challenged. The transitional object represents an infant's transition from a state of merger toward separateness, forming a link to the absent mother by becoming attached to an object (like a teddy bear), neither part of the self nor the world, yet both, simultaneously presented to the infant but also created by the infant, and is both dream and real. The object survives being cherished and punished and the infant comes to understand that maternal absence, provided it is brief, need not be catastrophic.

Transitional phenomena spread over into the arts, culture, and imaginative living, and gradually become de-invested. Playing is a transformational component of creative living (living fully). Only in playing does a person feel most alive, a creative and spontaneous self, able to enjoy the world's pleasures, which is essential to maintaining an authentic, sustaining self. Creativity is linked with *doing* (that is, the male element, which is associated with activity), but is dependent on *being* (the female element).

Creativity and Playing

Everything an infant does and feels is a creative act, which means aliveness: the world has no meaning unless it is created and discovered (Winnicott, 1971/2005, pp. 76–100). Play with a transitional object is an important bridge between self and other and is foundational to genuineness in all relationships. Playing is neither inside nor in the external world, which makes it hazardous and exciting. An infant is never asked whether a teddy is real or an imaginative creation so that experiencing its transitional status between imagination and the real world can continue. Infants gradually bring their spontaneous self into play with others.

Specific Theoretical Assumptions

Psychic Structure

An ego organizes defenses early, and from about 2 months onward, an infant can hold a moment of concern. A superego develops in the first year, which protects the objects whom an infant loves from primitive love which aims only to satisfy instinctual impulses; the resulting guilt is transmuted into concern, and reparative wishes develop whereby an infant feels that they can make a contribution back to the world. Concepts of the unconscious are less prominent in this conceptualization.

The Nature of Relationship

An infant's relationship with a good-enough mother is the template for all future relationships.

The most difficult path in emotional development, from object relating to object use in unconscious fantasy, involves the continual destruction of the object relation followed by the survival of a more robust real object.

From about one year onward, a child reaches 3-person triangular relationships. Relationships with paternal figures become important in resolving Oedipal conflicts when an infant's violent fantasies may turn to hate. This hate can now appear freely, as the hated person, who is already well-known and loved, is able to defend himself. Experiencing the Oedipus complex contributes to an infant developing reflective capacity and increasingly nuanced relationships.

Whatever the natal sex, an infant's pure female element relates at birth to the breast by *being* the breast (becoming a subjective object), and their pure male element by active relating or passive being related to (Winnicott, 1971/2005, pp. 76–100). The self emerges based on relating in terms of being, from this early primary identity. The process of separation establishes the basis for gender. In normal bisexuality, a child is usually identified with each parent but can be mainly identified with one parent who may be differently gendered; cross-identifications between toddlerhood and adolescence are normal (Winnicott, 1971/2005, pp. 139–161).

Developmental Stages

The aim of development is the true and false self, with personal authenticity and creativity, reached by living and cultural experience. The main theoretical concepts are the true and false self, object use, transitional phenomena, playing, and creativity.

Good-enough parents enable infants to realize their inherited potential. Early developmental stages are prebirth, unintegration, unit status, stage of concern, and Oedipal conflicts. In feeding, the mother and infant share an experience in which the infant feels alive. From about four months onward, transitional objects appear; from about five months onward, love and aggression begin to be united. As the object assumes more reality, anxiety stemming from ambivalence can be tolerated because a mother holds the situation over time, which enables an infant's boldness in drive expression and feeling that they can contribute to the world, and in this way offset any guilt. Around the time of weaning an infant achieves unit status, with everything felt to be contained in the self, including personal riches, and guilt is transformed into a sense of concern.

Oral activity starts ruthlessly, followed by the emergence of the anal and the phallic drives. From 1½ years onward, genital excitement becomes predominantly important.

Aggression is part of the life force of a newborn whereas the destructive drive which emerges later creates the quality of externality.

From about 5 months onward, aggressive and libidinal impulses are fused. An infant develops three lines of communication, firstly, forever silent internal subjective communication of the infant, permanently non-communicating and unfound (Winnicott, 1965, pp. 179–192). Second is pleasurable communication with language, with a third intermediate transitional form, from playing to cultural experience. Only communication with subjective phenomena gives the feeling of real.

While early sexuality and fantasy contribute to a sense of self, erotic desire and creative expression, however, involve the sense of a core vulnerability, that is, exposure of the true self.

Assumptions about the Body

Maternal holding assists an infant's secure psychosomatic integration: a 1-year-old infant feels they are living in their own body, in psyche-soma coexistence. Bodily changes bring psychic changes, for example in puberty girls begin to fantasize about conceiving, and boys about penetrating. The body as a central marker of identity continues to be at the center of adult clinical work.

Anxieties/Instincts and Defenses

Sources and Nature of Instincts

Instincts and the unconscious are subsumed in the true self in a creative body, with a primary drive for development. Oral activity starts ruthlessly; in excited breastfeeding, a boy may experience erections, a girl may experience vaginal activity. Oral experiences quickly carry an infant's capacity for relating to objects, culminating in a love relationship between two whole persons, infant and mother. Anal and phallic drives demand satisfaction; gradually, erections and clitoral excitement assume their specific importance; from about 1½ years, genital excitement becomes predominantly important. Periods of instinctual excitement are largely unconscious (such as a boy's wish to penetrate the loved one, aggressive fantasies toward the father which arouse castration fear, and a girl's rivalry with her mother which arouses fear of retaliation for wanting to steal her babies).

Aggression is part of a newborn's life force, whereas the destructive drive creates the quality of externality. From about five months, aggressive and libidinal impulses begin to be fused.

Developmental Line of Defenses

A developmental line of defenses is initiated by primitive agonies, such as falling forever (self-holding) or loss of a capacity to relate to objects (autistic states), and psychotic illness defends against these agonies. Disintegration into a chaotic state is a sophisticated defense against anxiety about a failure of holding and is within an infant's omnipotence (defending against the fear of attack, and preventing organized paranoid patterns).

Subsequent defenses are of a splitting nature: when a mother inadequately protects her infant's sense of illusion, the true self is based on omnipotent relating to the subjective world, and the false self, a most successful defense organization protecting it, relates with compliance. Instead of an infant's personality based on subjectively arising feelings and thoughts, the false self unconsciously introjects the behavior of others, to seem like those who dominate their world. The more extreme false self defends against overwhelmingly unsafe, intrusive caregiving. Seriously troubled patients can appear to be real, while inwardly suffering a sense of emptiness.

An infant anxiously sensing severe maternal depression and unable to enjoy an illusion of omnipotence might try hard to be a "good infant." The common denial of depression in children underlies exaggerated liveliness and anxious restlessness. In the manic defense, depressive anxiety about guilt for instinctual experiences is denied; the central fact that is denied is death in the inner world. Defenses against depressive trends operate in manic-depressive psychoses, defense by splitting and loss of reality sense in schizophrenia.

Repression initiates mature defenses.

Assumptions Concerning Etiology

Early devastating experiences of the holding environment's failure, when an infant's ego is incapable of understanding and integrating abandonment, trigger primitive anxieties. Defense "freezes" the failure situation which is the breakdown that an adult fears to (re-)experience; some infants short-circuit primitive agonies by generating psychotic defenses.

The core catastrophe is the annihilation of the self by intrusion. If a mother cannot be good-enough, the consequences for the child may be chronic anxiety, obsessive behaviors, addiction, and feeling outside their life. If a mother is absent too long, memory of the internal representation fades. With traumatic failure a false self can develop to protect the true self; a split lacking creative originality may result in a sense of futility, an unlived life at the core of chronic disturbance, with the person searching for a life that feels real, even if it leads to death. The risk in trauma is to become aware of being helplessly small: an infant who becomes too aware of real-world dangers will not learn optimally.

Infants may internalize their mother's depression hoping to relieve her. Infant depression manifests in loss of liveliness, psychosomatic issues, and a risk of developmental delay.

Neurosis arises between 2 and 5 years when a child's powerful instinctual experiences, like castration anxiety arising from Oedipal death wishes, may lead to clinical states. Masturbation commonly disappears, defending against intolerable anxiety.

The antisocial tendency reveals a breakdown in good-enough parenting when the parent, a child's first "possession," is lost. The child compensates by stealing, looking for a protective father, and destroying the environment. Delinquent behavior or running away may be the true self's cry for help; otherwise, the child becomes inhibited in love, depressed, depersonalized, and eventually only feels real when violent.

Older children can present with an organized manic-depressive illness resembling adult illness and persecution.

Psychosomatic disorders, with an underlying psychotic anxiety, have many determinants. Close links between body, identity, and self are revealed in bodily symptoms and body modification.

Implications for Technique

Psychoanalysis is viewed primarily as ontological (being involved in playing, toward becoming more fully oneself) rather than epistemological (seeking the symbolic meaning of play, and gaining knowledge). With the mother-infant relationship as a template, the analyst and patient live an experience together, psychoanalysis protecting the privacy of the self in making personal sense. The psychoanalytic exchange enables a patient to experience more fully their own sense of aliveness, to self-analyze, to engage, to play (e.g., a sense of humor). An analyst aims to be authentic, to interpret transference and the unconscious, and to respect a patient's wish not to communicate.

Psychoanalysis provides a potential space where children or adults can be surprised by their own self-awareness. Insight is an experience of creative discovery, which is more important than interpretations which can interrupt a transference.

Some patients, mainly those who are psychotic, need to regress to early childhood dependence to repair a trauma; then what is particularly important is a reliable setting adjusted for those for whom transitional space may not exist. Interpretation (sometimes silent) needs to be carefully "managed;" the analyst may interpret the feared breakdown that has already been experienced. An analyst needs to be aware of their hate or fear over a long time. When regression allows development to restart, this liberates the true self to reach a patient's life goals.

In brief psychotherapy, a therapist may provide a bridge, without viewing insight as the only acceptable result. Children have a primary wish to be understood and to understand themselves; the experience of playing, often healing, is more important than interpreting the play. Psychodynamics can be discerned in impulsive line drawings, "Squiggles," (Winnicott, 1971/2005, pp. 139–161), even in children seen infrequently, as in "the Piggle," (Winnicott, 1978). Parents are often involved in therapy. From the first session, play is diagnostic, an inability to play points to pathology. Children with antisocial difficulties cannot always use psychoanalysis and the most use should be made of initial consultations.

Level of Attention to Transference

"Playing" extends Freudian notions of transference as play repeats the mother-child dynamics. Enjoyment of play leads to the child understanding its meaning and feeling understood without interpretation being imposed.

With adult neurotics, transference neurosis, the Oedipus complex, and superego development are analyzed.

Interpretation aims to reconstruct early unacknowledged developmental needs in a collaborative model, enabling a patient to change themselves. Analysts should only treat those with early disturbances whom they can carry through Oedipal conflicts in the transference *and* severe regression to dependence. With "dissociation" of male and female elements, a patient may need to find primary unity with the analyst in the transference. When psychoanalysis reaches the depths of their personality, destructively interpreting what is "not me" too close to the core self delays deep change; if an analyst can wait, a patient can arrive at an understanding with joy and creativity.

Countertransference

Analysts need to manage their own depression to contain that projected by a depressed patient; also to be able to love without fear of its destructive effects or it would be difficult to be able to analyze a patient's fear of the possible draining effects of their love. Crucially, countertransference illuminates feeling vulnerable to the deathliness or deadness of a patient's inner world and objects, and to hating the patient (Winnicott, 1965, pp. 158–165). Enactments in the countertransference are important self-communication to the analyst.

Developmental Process Thinking

Psychotherapy facilitates the unfolding of play to initiate therapeutic change and a patient's developmental process (rather than interpretation) determines the analysis. Psychoanalysts are initially as vulnerable as a mother who is identified with her infant who is temporarily dependent on her for an emergent true self; a child has a strong ego because the analyst gives ego support. Regression to dependence is the return to psychic functioning with the self undifferentiated from the object and it is not to be interpreted as defense.

Field

A focus on creative apperception could contribute to a field theory of the analyst's role and understanding of how the dyad interacts to reach analytic goals. Maternal provision creates a psychological-interpersonal field which an infant could enter, a potential space between infant and parent being a sense of a safe interpersonal field in which to be playful, while simultaneously connected to other people.

Subsequent Development of Some Core Concepts

Neuroscientists concur that motherhood results in a reorganization of their brain and psyche and that newborns have an active mirror neuron system and seek to engage others. Intentional neonatal activity is a key contributor to the sense of self and others, a core sense of self from birth, which is intentional, empathic, and moral. Development of children's sense of ownership and agency at the embodied level necessitates the interpersonal encounter.

Research into the exquisite sensitivity of infants to the nuances of maternal communication confirms the intergenerational transmission of disturbance, like the long-term impact on mental health of postnatal depression or anxiety: adolescents have a fourfold increase in the risk of depression. Maternal guilt and anxiety can militate against accepting the universality of maternal ambivalence. Maternal hostility is predictive of a child's less active control and more negative construction of experience.

In infant-parent psychotherapy, infants are equal partners in the interaction. My position agrees with the focus in infant research and neuroscience on an infant as a sociable person from birth.

5. Winnicott and the Winnicottians	
Main, general underlying assumptions	1 Mother-infant relationship, object use 2 True self as isolate, aliveness 3 Transitional objects and phenomena 4 Playing, creativity
Specific theoretical assumptions	
psychic structure	• The unconscious is a less prominent concept. • An ego organizes early defenses and can hold a moment of concern. A superego developing in the first year protects love objects from ruthless love.
energy	N/A
relationship	• An infant's relationship with a good-enough mother is the template for all future relations. The most difficult path in emotional development, from object relating to object use in unconscious fantasy, involves the continual destruction of the object relation followed by survival of a more robust real object. • From 1 year, 3-person triangular relationships are reached. • Cross identifications in toddlerhood and adolescence are normal.
development stages	• The aim of development is the true self, with personal authenticity and creativity, reached by living and cultural experience. • In feeding, mother and infant share an experience of being alive. From 4 months, transitional objects appear; about 5 months love and aggression become fused. Around weaning, an infant achieves unit status, the self-containing everything including personal richness, and guilt transformed into concern.

(Continued)

	• An infant develops 3 lines of communication: subjective communication communicating from choice, pleasurable communication using language, and an intermediate form, from playing toward cultural experience. In playing a child/adult feels most alive and creative.
body	• By 1 year, an infant develops secure psychosomatic integration; bodily changes bring psychic changes. The body, a central marker of identity continues at the center of adult clinical work.
anxieties/instincts and defenses	• Sexual and aggressive instincts are present from birth. • Developmentally defenses are initiated by primitive agonies, which psychotic illness may defend against. Subsequent defenses are of a splitting nature: a false self defends against maternal intrusive internal reality. In the manic defense, depressive anxiety about guilt for instinctual experiences is denied. • Mature defenses appear after repression.
Assumptions concerning etiology	• Early devastating experiences of the environment's failure, when an infant's ego cannot integrate abandonment, primitive agonies are triggered which can be defended against by "freezing" the failure situation (the breakdown that an adult fears [re]experiencing). Some infants short-circuit this with psychotic defenses. • The core catastrophe is the annihilation of the self by intrusion. A pathological false self may lead to death. • Neurosis arises from 2 years with anxiety about instinctual experiences: disappearance of masturbation defends against anxiety. • The antisocial tendency reveals a breakdown in good-enough parenting. • Older children can present with manic-depressive illness and persecution. • Psychosomatic disorders, overlaying psychotic anxiety, are multi-determined. Body symptoms or modification reveal close links between body, identity, and self.
Implications for technique	• In psychotherapy, the model is the mother-infant relationship with analyst and patient sharing an alive experience, an ontological rather than epistemological perspective.

(*Continued*)

	• Children often experience playing as more important than interpretation. • Psychoanalysis protects the self's privacy to make personal sense. The frame is a potential space where child or adult can be surprised by self-awareness, creatively discovering insight. An analyst interprets transference and the unconscious, respecting a patient's wish not to communicate. • Some patients need to regress to repair a trauma; an analyst sometimes interprets the feared breakdown.
Subsequent developments of the core concept	• Neuroscientists concur motherhood results in a reorganization of brain and psyche. A mirror neuron system suggests a core sense of self from birth. Development of children's sense of ownership and agency at the embodied level necessitates the interpersonal encounter. • Research into infants' sensitivity to maternal communication confirms intergenerational transmission of disturbance. • In infant-parent psychotherapy, infants are equal partners.

Notes

1 I am grateful to those whose work I have drawn on, who, because of space restrictions, are not acknowledged; any shortcomings are mine.
2 "Mother" may stand for parents or parental substitutes.

References

Winnicott, D. W. (1965). *The maturational processes and the Facilitating Environment*. Hogarth Press and The Institute of Psycho-Analysis.

Winnicott, D. W. (1978). *The piggle: An account of the psychoanalytic treatment of a little girl.* The Hogarth Press and The Institute of Psycho-Analysis.

Winnicott, D. W. (2005). *Playing and reality*. Routledge Classics. (Originally published in 1971).

Chapter 6

Bion, Bionians, and Post-Bionians: The Relational and the Unrepresented

Tomasz Fortuna

Initially a member of the Klein group, Wilfred R. Bion made an original contribution to psychoanalytic theory and technique. His experience in working with emotional trauma and psychosis led to the extension of the notion of projective identification and the development of concepts such as the container-contained (1959) and the later ideas on the use of countertransference. These contributions found their firm place in the post-Kleinian framework and gave root to newer developments. This chapter offers a reflection on Bion's contribution from the British Object Relations perspective.

Besides clear references to Freud (the pleasure and reality principles and the origins of thought) and Klein (the drive for knowledge, psychic positions, and the role of projective identification), Bion reached out to mathematics, philosophy, poetry, and social sciences. In his pre-psychoanalytic work with groups, Bion (2014a/1961) noticed the two-tier mental functioning reflecting a conflict between the drive to comprehend external and internal realities and the wish to avoid the resulting conflicting emotional experiences. Adopting his binocular vision, the clinician attempts to observe both levels of mental functioning. This constant mental struggle to evade or modify psychic pain had become the central focus of his work.

Bion's vast contribution to psychoanalysis includes his theory of group processes, the role of containment in the development of thought and psychic growth, and his understanding of psychotic functioning. It continues to be alive and inspires current psychoanalytic trends.

General Assumptions

Bion declared that it is the thought (emotional experience) that requires a thinker (mind). For him, sensuous proto-mental experiences need modification in order to acquire a meaning and as a model of this process he took the mother-infant couple. This container-contained model opened the way to further exploration of early development, non-verbal modes of communication, and the theory of clinical encounter e.g., selected fact and the role of intuition.

DOI: 10.4324/9781003027768-7

Projective identification, a defensive phantasy initially described by Melanie Klein, which has become the basis for Bion's container-contained model, acquired a communicative interpersonal dimension, in spite of its unconscious motivations. Now the infant, or patient, projects an unsettling emotional experience (the contained ♂) and the mother, or analyst, takes it in her mind (the container ♀), unconsciously identifies with the projected aspect of the mind, and responds accordingly in the process of actualization of the initial phantasy or offering a relevant meaning. This shift, and later recognition of the essentially ineffable nature of emotional truth (or O), led Bion to a modification of psychoanalytic technique and his focus on the emotional experience in the session. The role of our senses as a research tool, and our attachment to the grounding cognitive phenomena, such as memory, expectations, and comprehension, were now seen as obstacles to the intuitive contact with the ultimate reality of the patient (Bion's O). Although important in our psychic apparatus and mental life, all representations of this reality that are available to us were considered to be transformations by Bion. The further they move in abstraction the further away they are from the original source. This constitutes quite a conundrum for the clinician who has to move between an unsettling, unrepresented as yet, experience and a relational context of internal objects and phantasies that can be interpreted (Bion's K).

"In studying the thinking of emotional experiences or transformation in K, Bion developed a theory including concepts such as α-function, β-elements, constant conjunction, PS-D, selected fact and container contained." (Vermote, 2019a, p. 140). However, following the above developments, his concept of change had also shifted. At this point for Bion, "fundamental psychic changes (transformations in O) happen at a not yet represented, or undifferentiated psychic level" (Vermote, 2019a, p. 140).

After he discovered a new area of psychoanalytic investigation, Bion started looking for appropriate research tools. In this context Bion insisted on creating optimal conditions and discipline for the analyst to promote emotional development and to comprehend the ultimate psychic truth (O), which can only be intuitively intimated in the session, since it is timeless and infinite. In the next step, the ultimate reality can only be approximated by the use of thinking and representations embedded in our interpersonal and finite mode of perception. This of course is an integral part of our mental functioning and clinical technique that enables symbolization and verbal interpretation of psychic experience.

Specific Theoretical Assumptions

Nature of Psychic Structure

1 In Bion's important model, the container-contained ♀♂, constitutional factors play a role in shaping the relationship between the mother and

her baby. The capacity for containment versus tolerance of frustration constitutes a dynamic axis of interaction. In his earlier work, envy, seen as a constitutional factor related to death drive, is the source of attacks on the creative link to the object (Bion, 1957, 1959).

2 Bion's clinical experience led him to the conclusion that the true nature of emotional experience is a-sensuous and characterized by infinity and timelessness. Psychic change T(O) occurs in this unrepresented psychic domain he named O. The ineffable ultimate psychic reality can only be intimated emotionally through intuition and represented in a series of transformations at different levels of abstraction and verbalization T(K). The constant elements, invariants in the series of transformations, offer an indication of the nature of psychic truth and enable the creation of meanings in a form of interpersonal unconscious narratives.

3 The mental functioning can be divided into domain K (thinking) and domain O (experiencing). Since the emotional experience from O is as yet unrepresented (or undifferentiated), it requires further elaboration and representation, acquiring a sense of time and location, and a relational context. This way an experience of an indescribable void can be felt as loneliness and longing for the object and as such interpreted.

4 In dreaming, the sensuous external and bodily experiences (β-elements) and the internal a-sensuous emotions can be transformed into α-elements in order to acquire a meaning and be further represented and symbolized. For Bion dreaming is not limited to a night dream, as it continuously occurs on the unconscious level (dream-work-α). In his model of functions, α-elements are the building blocks of the semi-permeable contact barrier dividing the mind into the conscious and the unconscious. It is a dynamic and not an anatomical structure, and results from thinking processes. Later on in Bion's work, this divide shifts in between the O and the K domains of experience. One can see here connections to Kant's theory of noumenon (unknown) and phenomenon (experienced).

5 Unconscious phantasy, and its interpretation, remain important for Bion in his early work. However, the narrative guiding projective identification and the container-contained dynamic relationship is seen in his later work as representations (K) resulting from the emotional experience from O in the process of transformations. It describes the intuitive connection between the subject and the object, linking, learning, and growth when uncertainty can be tolerated and new metaphors are needed. This creative connection may succeed or not. On the K level of thinking and representation, unconscious phantasy is a continuous activity, which has the function of organizing the rich experience of relationships between internal objects.

Sources and Nature of Energy

Although there is no direct reference to energy in his work, owing to the Kleinian influence, Bion recognized the life and death drives as sources of psychic impulses interacting with the external world. He later conceptualized them as the emotional relational links of L (love), H (hate), and K (getting-to-know).

Nature of Relationships

Transference, experienced in the context of projective and introjective processes, and the role of unconscious phantasy continue, in Bion's view, to shape one's state of mind and perceptions of others and the surrounding reality (see this section in the Klein chapter in this book). The relational nature of those phenomena had been, however, an essential aspect of his theory.

In his later work, Bion gradually puts more emphasis on the intuitive aspects of communication and the experience of dreaming taking place between two people, including psychoanalysis (e.g., Cassorla, 2018). The discovery of the ultimate psychic reality that can only be intimated and mutually experienced from the domain of O moves us a step earlier before the sense-based mental elaboration of relationships occurs.

Developmental Stages

In his model of container-contained ♀♂, Bion spoke about the early experience of the breast as an active container full of milk, loving and hateful feelings, actively working through experiences—offering and withholding.

"The part-object relationship is not with the anatomical structures only but with function, not with anatomy but with physiology, not with the breast but with feeding, poisoning, loving, hating." (Bion, 1959).

This complex relationship between the mother and her infant leads to the development of the internal representations of object relationships and the capacity to modify anxieties (α-function) and learn from experience. For Bion, there is the interplay and oscillation of the paranoid and depressive positions (PS ↔ D) which gives an opportunity for this ongoing process of meaning-creating and learning. This takes place in an open receptive state of mind, *reverie,* in a presence of a containing mind able to work through, modify, and symbolize emotional experiences. In the clinical context, *patience (PS)* offers a chance for evolution that may bring a sense of coherence, *security (D)*, from which the analyst can speak to his patient (Bion, 1970). Britton (1998) extended it further stating that one never returns to exactly the same position (PS/D) if learning takes place.

Developmentally, prior to the oscillations between PS and D, experience is governed by a sense of threat and avoidance of recognition of separateness from the object, underlined by the anxieties and defenses of the paranoid-schizoid position. The appearance of the depressive position leads to a sense of guilt characterized by the recognition of one's own destructive impulses; it can result in reverting to paranoid anxiety or manic defenses, or alternatively accepted and responded to with a phantasy of reparation.

The hypothetical α-function operating in the container-contained ♀♂ model leads to the development of the contact barrier and differentiation of the mind into conscious and unconscious, enabling processes such as repression. This is an important contribution connecting early development governed by processes of splitting and projection with later mental functions described by Freud.

The meaning-creating ability of the mind is described by Bion as the capacity for linking (Bion, 2014b/1962). That is a capacity for connecting experiences, thoughts, and their representations. A passionate relationship with the object can therefore be characterized by a trio of links: L (love), H (hate), and K (knowing and being known). This is a combination of Freud's principles of mental functioning and Klein's epistemophilic instinct. Loving and hateful feelings operate in synergy and facilitate emotional engagement with and learning about the object. The anti-developmental forces are described as negative links -L, -H, and -K, and are characterized by disengagement, lack of learning, and attack on perceptions of reality.

Linking has also become the basis for his theory of thinking where the linking and evolution of pre-conceptions with their realizations or frustrations lead to conceptions and conflicts.

Bion (1957) made a distinction between the psychotic and the non-psychotic parts of a personality. Although the earliest stages of development were referred to as psychotic, by Klein, it meant that there was an insufficient development of the reality principle. When Bion however used the term psychotic, he meant a pathological aspect of the personality that operated self-destructive fragmentation of the ego functions that comprised the reality principle after it had been developed.

Anxieties/Instincts/Defenses

A Anxiety remains a central focus for Bion and it is closely related to the experience of reality. Bion saw the problem with external reality arising from various sources: (i) the separation from an object; (ii) the humiliation of recognition of dependence evoking envious attack on constructive linking; and (iii) the threat from an object holding projected dangerous parts of the self which could retaliate against the projector.

Bion, in the Klein tradition, accepted inherent experiences of anxiety and means of defense, including splitting, projection, and introjection. Thus, anxiety is dealt with by fragmentation and evacuation of parts of the self, or developmentally by modification through help from a suitable and effective container.

One of the important anxieties he described stems from a phantasy of the ego-destructive superego. He attributed this especially harsh precursor of Freud's structure as arising very early and from the introjection of an external object into which the subject had projected his own violent and destructive parts of self and a failure of containment and modification of relevant anxieties.

B Later, Bion formulated a dynamic structure in the mind and in group processes in which a new idea threatened a disruption of the mind by requiring various pre-conceptions to be rejected as redundant and to reconstruct the possibility of a new system of meanings. He saw this as an example of the alternation of PS $\leftrightarrow$ D, and that this disruption can feel like a catastrophic change in one's mental functioning—literally as one's mind "going to pieces." Later, he described it in a context of a creative or inhibiting tension between a group *establishment* and an innovative individual *mystic* (Bion, 1970).

Bion advocated receptiveness, *reverie*, toward these potentially disruptive changes any mind has to face. He understood the resistance to this highly unsettling effect of new experiences and perceptions and regarded this ability to withstand this threat as the achievement of creative minds. Following poet John Keats, he adopted the term *negative capability* for this ability. These are the conditions for emotional development and psychic growth, and in the clinical context, they relate equally to the patient and the analyst.

Etiology

Bion saw emotional suffering, as arising from numerous causes:

i The lack of an effective container, in development or in the analysis, results in the predominance of psychotic defenses (e.g., evacuation of emotional experiences, enactment, and the role of retaliatory ego-destructive superego). Looking at it from another angle, it is a failure of communicative function in the analytic couple where the capacity for dreaming and working through is insufficient, and verbal and non-verbal communications are rejected. The container-contained relationship is parasitic and precludes psychic growth.

ii Envious attacks on the container-contained linking with fragmentation, evacuation, and projective identification. Here Bion includes constitutional factors related to the tolerance of frustration, temperament, and death drive.

iii The avoidance of reality by attacking and dismantling the functions of the reality principle, generating omniscient arrogant attitudes, loss of reality testing, and rejection of truth. Here the reversal of α-function leads to the production of pseudo β-elements lacking a real sense data, emotional depth, and resonance (β-screen), leading to the concretization of experience and thinking.

iv As a consequence of the above, the dominance of unconscious phantasy as a replacement for reality becomes merely delusions and hallucinations.

Technique

For Bion, O is the ultimate, ineffable, unknowable reality, the "inexpressible truth of one's experience" (Ogden, 2008, p. 17)—akin to Lacan's concept of the Real and to Kant's thing-in-itself. The idea of *becoming O* emphasizes the fact that it cannot be known rationally within domain of K but appreciated through direct experience. In a session, becoming O of the patient offers a chance to grasp the emotional truth of what is going on unconsciously in the analytic couple, entering a state of passivity (reverie) in order to receive an unconscious and direct impact—as Freud's unconscious-to-unconscious communication. O/being is opposed to K/knowing, where the latter indicates more abstract and intellectual understanding. In clinical work, the analyst continuously goes through the sequence of O → K → O → K, a process of continuous oscillation between immersion and interactivity (see Civitarese, 2008, 2013).

Increasingly through his career, Bion attempted to refine the technical approach he used. Having been the Kleinian, to define most clearly the communicative form of projective identification and its role in the interpersonal life of a subject, he aimed at freeing the exchanges between patient and analyst. The aim was to enable based on intuition interchange in the domain of O. This involved recommending practicing reverie by abolishing possible obstructions to receptivity, which he defined most explicitly as *memory and desire* (Bion, 2014c/1965). He increasingly saw the capacity to link two thoughts and two minds as the core of growth, and this meant the intuitive and communicative impact of one on another rather than the more abstract representations of knowledge. Out of this receptive state of mind would evolve a new thought which, after Poincare, he called the *selected fact*—the result of the free play of mind that allowed an unrestrained roving. He also conceived of a binocular vision as a movement between one perspective (vertex) and another, or a reversible perspective as one finds in optical illusions where a vase can suddenly change to the outline of two faces or a diminished lighting illuminate a detail invisible in a bright light.

This means that the analyst must allow himself to be emotionally moved in a way directed by the patient's communications, and to respond and interpret with an authentic conviction based on his belief of what he has creatively received. This is a dialectic relationship from which originates *language of achievement*—a communication capable of reflecting the previously unrepresented experience that took place in the relational context.

Further Developments

Bion's thought continues to have a significant influence on analytic schools. Vermote (2019b) offers a succinct overview of these developments. I will refer to just a few of these lines of development.

In the British context, there is an implicit presence of Bion's ideas such as the containment and the theory of thinking (Bell, Brenman Pick, Bronstein, Feldman, O'Shaughnessy, Sodré). This includes work on the selected fact, triangulation, and uncertainty (Britton, Steiner). Meltzer and more recently Abel-Hirsch and Mawson wrote about Bion's later contribution, as did some American authors (Caper, Eekhoff, Levine). Grotstein extended and elaborated a number of Bion's concepts. Transformations, dreaming, and the work from O received a lot of attention (Cassorla, Civitarese, Ferro, Fix Korbivcher, Horowitz, Pistiner de Cortinas, Reiner, Sandler) as well as Ogden's important contribution to the analytic third. Ferro and Civitarese established the analytic field perspective. Symington and Lombardi extended Bion's conceptualization of psychosis and Durban described the autisto-psychotic states. Vermote created a model of the mind with its implications for technique, dividing psychic functioning and communication into three zones: finite rational thought, mixed finite-infinite, and fully infinite zone of pure experience.

6. Bion, Bionians, and Post-Bionians	
Main, general underlying assumptions	1 Concept of container-contained ♀♂ and α-function 2 Theory of groups—avoidance of psychic pain (reality) 3 Theory of thinking of emotional experience and transformations 4 Psychic truth (O) and the role of intuition
Specific theoretical assumptions	
psychic structure	• Domains of O (experiencing, unrepresented, infinite) and K (thinking, representations seen in a relational context, finite) • Process of transformations (from O and K) and models of functions (α)
energy	• Emotional links of L (love), H (hate), and K (getting-to-know) in relation to the object
relationships	• Unconscious phantasies and the perception of others and the reality • Relational model of containment • The trio of links L (love), H (hate), and K (knowing and being known)

(Continued)

developmental stages	• Development seen in the context of the container-contained (α-function) • Capacity for thinking and linking and tolerating reality • Psychic growth through the emotional experience
body	N/A
anxieties/instincts and defenses	• Anxieties related to the experience of internal and external reality (e.g., separateness from the object, dependency and vulnerability, the threat from a persecutory object (superego)) • Fear of catastrophic change vs. negative capability. • Defenses such as splitting, evacuation, and fragmentation.
Assumptions concerning etiology	• Lack of an effective container, envious attacks, the retaliatory ego-destructive superego, active avoidance of reality, dominance of the unconscious phantasy • Reversal of α-function resulting in concretization and β-screen • Linking and dreaming replaced by splitting, evacuation, and action
Implications for technique	• Containment in the container-contained ♀♂ model • Eschewing of memory and desire; selected fact • The role of intuition and emotional experience from O • Oscillation between domains of O and K
Subsequent developments of the core concept	• Developments in the theory of thinking and containment • Development of various aspects of transformations • Focus on the experiential domain of O • Theories of psychosis and autism • Analytic third and Psychoanalytic Field

References

Bion, W. R. (1957). Differentiation of the psychotic from the non-psychotic personalities. *International Journal of Psychoanalysis*, *38*, 266–275.

Bion, W. R. (1959). Attacks on linking. *International Journal of Psychoanalysis*, *40*, 308–315.

Bion, W. R. (1970). The mystic and the group. In *Attention and interpretation. A scientific approach to insight in psycho-analysis and groups* (pp. 62–71). Tavistock Publications.

Bion, W. R. (2014a). Experiences in groups and other papers. In C. Mawson (Ed.), *The complete works of W. R. Bion Vol. IV* (pp. 95–245). Karnac. (Original work published 1961).

Bion, W. R. (2014b). Learning from experience. In C. Mawson (Ed.), *The complete works of W. R. Bion Vol. IV* (pp. 247–265). Karnac. (Original work published 1962).

Bion, W. R. (2014c). Memory and Desire. In C. Mawson (Ed.), *The complete works of W. R. Bion Vol. VI* (pp. 7–26). Karnac. (Original work published 1965).

Britton, R. (1998). *Belief and imagination: Explorations in psychoanalysis*. Routledge.

Cassorla, R. M. S. (2018). *The psychoanalyst, the theatre of dreams and the clinic of enactment*. Routledge.

Civitarese, G. (2008). Immersion versus interactivity and analytic field. *International Journal of Psychoanalysis*, *89*, 279–298.

Civitarese, G. (2013). Bion's "evidence" and his theoretical style. *Psychoanalytic Quarterly*, *82*, 615–633.

Ogden, T. (2008). Bion's four principles of mental functioning. *Fort Da*, *14*, 11–35.

Vermote, R. (2019a). Attention and interpretation. In D. Birksted-Breen (Series Ed.), *Reading Bion*, The New Library of Psychoanalysis Teaching Series (pp. 140–168). Routledge.

Vermote, R. (2019b). The further development of Bion's ideas. In D. Birksted-Breen (Series Ed.), *Reading Bion,* The New Library of Psychoanalysis Teaching Series (pp. 228–233). Routledge.

Chapter 7

John Bowlby, Attachment Theory, and Attachment-Based Psychoanalytic Psychotherapy

Orit Badouk Epstein

> "Many of the most intense of all human emotions arise during the formation, the maintenance, the disruption, and the renewal of affectional bonds ...."
> – John Bowlby, 1979

Main, General Underlying Assumptions of Attachment Theory

Attachment theory was founded on John Bowlby's observation that we are all hardwired to attach, and that attachment plays a primary role in humans and other primates in a way that facilitates survival and identity formation. Since its inception in the 1940s, attachment theory has been striving to understand human emotions and behaviors through evolutionary mechanisms that affect child development and relationships throughout life. The theory is founded on the following assumptions:

1 Attachment is a protective survival mechanism against abandonment, separation, and loss that is part of our biology.
2 We all need an attachment figure to feel safe and secure. This early synchronized interaction between the care-seeking child and their caregiver, is a primal mechanism that is also essential for affect regulation.
3 Through the attachment relationship, we develop a representation of ourselves and others which Bowlby called internal working models (IWM). These are mental representations of the self in relation to the other and are a core determinant of interpersonal relationships and behavior.
4 Attachment is needed throughout the life cycle: from the cradle to the grave, we all need a secure base as well as recognizing the role grief plays in the lifecycle.

As a young family psychiatrist and psychoanalyst, Bowlby carried out an observational study on the effects on young children who had been evacuated during World War II and put into the care of strangers. In Bowlby (1944), he published his paper "Forty-Four Juvenile Thieves" in which he

DOI: 10.4324/9781003027768-8

witnesses that antisocial behavior in juveniles was rooted in early attachment disruptions. This led him to challenge the Freudian drive theory and metapsychology, and Klein's view that an infant becomes emotionally linked to his mother because she feeds him/her. He thought that psychoanalysis had underestimated the role of environmental trauma in generating neurosis. In perceiving human experiences as representations of real-life events, Bowlby aimed to find scientific evidence to underpin his early observations. Following the Darwinian idea of the "'environment of evolutionary adaptedness' in which protection from predation through attachment conferred selective advantages for vulnerable human infants" (Holmes & Slade, 2018, p. 7), Bowlby borrowed his ideas from ethology and showed a keen interest in the work of the ethologist Harry Harlow's (1958) experiments with Rhesus monkeys and Konrad Lorenz's experiments with geese (1961), both of which emphasize the strong bonds between offspring and parents in a range of animal species. Using this as a model, he argued that the way a biological organism behaves is through a feedback loop/mechanism between the body, the brain, and the environment.

The opposing themes of attachment, separation, and loss are a central tenet of Bowlby's attachment theory and provide a framework to understand underlying issues in children and adults following environmental and relational adversities. It recognizes the primary protective role of an attachment figure and the importance of a stable and trusting relationship for the child's emotional and physiological development that will enable the child to develop a sense of security and a sense of a coherent self. In the absence of such relationships and in times of uncertainty and fear, the separation from the caregiver can elicit intense distress that is transformed into grief and mourning whenever the loss becomes permanent. To support his observations, Bowlby hired the social worker, James Robertson (1953) to film children in hospitals, noticing their distress when they were separated from their parents. The care-seeking dependent dyad with the caregiver, which is dependent on the caregiver's response, could be seen to lead to three phases of a child's reaction to separation:

1 Protest – related to separation anxiety, according to Bowlby (1973) it is the anger of hope whenever the child is seeking comfort, trying to get the caregiver's presence and attention back.
2 Despair – related to chronic unresolved grief, when separation and abandonment have been dismissed and frowned upon, the child's anger will be transformed into what Bowlby considered as the anger of despair (1973).
3 Detachment – denial of attachment needs and reorganization of the self around the caregiver's absence, often results in a strong self-reliance.

Later, empirical research by Mary Ainsworth (1962) supported Bowlby's theory and it has broadened an understanding of important areas of human development beyond the classic psychoanalytic domain. In short, "Attachment theory and research speak to fundamental questions about human emotion, relationships, and development." (Duschinsky, 2020, p. vii).

Specific Theoretical Assumptions

Assumption about the Nature of Psychic Structure

Both attachment and psychoanalytic theories seek to understand human behavior and psychological wounds. Freud's formulation of meta-psychology was to define the theoretical assumptions on which psycho-analysis was founded. His account of human sexuality and descriptions of the pleasure and reality principle, however, is more imagined in relation to the vulnerable and needy infant. By locating attachment theory in the context of psychoanalysis, Bowlby had no issues in accepting the psycho-dynamic structure of the mind. He postulated a new concept of instinctual behavior within which the attachment relationship is a primary survival mechanism that was distinct from feeding and the expression of sexuality. Attachment for Bowlby was intrinsic to human nature and is not some childhood phase that needs to be outgrown with maturity. Bowlby saw human behavior as not merely existential angst and the inner pain which underpins it, but rather as a result of an outer threat around separation, rejection, and abandonment, all of which will decrease the biological chances of survival and will contribute to the formation of the self. Attachment theory nonetheless is also interested in how the environment influences the inner world of the child. Bowlby then attempted to bring together some of the psychoanalytic ideas which object relations theories have been concerned with. Influenced by Kenneth Craik's book *The Nature of Explanations* (1943), Bowlby added that the proximity the child seeks from an attachment figure will also construct an internal working model of the self and of the self with the other.

> The function of these models is to simulate happenings in the real world, thereby enabling individuals to plan their behaviors with all the advantage of insight and foresight. The more adequate and accurate the simulation, of course, the better adapted is the behavior based on it likely to be.
>
> (Bowlby, 1988a, p. 4)

Internal working models may seem similar to the psychoanalytic term "internalization." However, IWMs are neither entirely outside nor entirely inside the person, rather it is what occurs in the space in between them, as Daniel Stern put it, it is an "experience-of-being with" (1998).

Assumption about Sources and Nature of Energy

According to Freud, instinctive behavior is rooted in the sexual instinct which, when reaching a certain level will require discharge. Bowlby disagreed with this as he considered that it was not based in scientific evidence. Nonetheless, we can say that Bowlby's model of an instinctive behavior is activated by both external and internal conditions of the child's capacity for care-seeking.

Assumption about the Nature of the Relationship

Attachment runs through the entire life cycle and relationships can be understood in attachment terms. As a care seeker, the child always relies on the caregiver's proximity and affective responsiveness. Attachment Theory offers an interactive pattern rather than assuming an intrinsic property of the infant. It provides a relational context to a plethora of emotions that is often a reaction to relational disruptions around separation, loss, and abuse. The attachment system gets activated and dysregulated whenever the child feels stress or fear and when receiving poor or no affective responsiveness from their parent or another significant attachment figure.

Bowlby's ideas led to a new school of empirical research in developmental psychology. The developmental psychologist and researcher, Mary Ainsworth became Bowlby's lifelong collaborator in the studies of separation and disruptions in the parent-child relationship. Ainsworth (1969) devised the Strange Situation Procedure for examining attachment, exploratory, and affiliative behaviors in infants and children which is closely linked to the attachment. What she found

> did not support the Freudian notion of a passive, recipient, narcissistic infant in the oral phase. Rather, she was impressed by the babies' active search for contact with the mother when they were alarmed or hurt, when she moved away, or left even briefly.
>
> (Ainsworth & Bowlby, 1991, p. 6)

What emerged from the procedure were patterns of care-seeking interactions between parent and infant. Ainsworth's attachment classifications powerfully demonstrated the impact of separation which was responsible for the discrepancies created between actual psychic reality and defensive behavior in insecure children. These patterns are:

- A – avoidant attachment pattern.
- B – secure attachment pattern.
- C – ambivalent attachment pattern.
- D – disorganized-disoriented attachment pattern—added later by Main and Solomon (1986, 1990).

The "secure base," (Ainsworth, 1982) related to the secure attachment pattern, is the person and place we return to whenever we feel threatened, stressed, or ill. Essentially, it is the confidence the child will develop in the relationship with a sensitive and available caregiver who enables them to relax, explore, seek pleasure, and play. From a mentalizing point of view, the symbolic function is crucially dependent on the synchronized and harmonious relationship between parent and infant. Secure attachment thus is the capacity to recognize interpersonal frustration yet be able to regulate affects and monitor thoughts and feelings in a collaborative manner.

Furthermore, the explosion of mother-infant research laboratory observations that occurred from the 1970s, in particular the work of The Boston Group: Stern, Beebe, Lachmannn, Tronick, add Lyons-Ruth and others, emphasized the importance of the caregiver's responsive attunement and interactions with the infant and provided additional data on the interpersonal rather than the intrapsychic world of the infant.

Assumption about Development Stages

Bowlby's developmental model is a nurturing hypothesis, placing the quality of parental caregiving and other environmental influences at the center of the development of the personality. Bowlby disagreed with Freud's notion of libidinal phases. He also opposed Klein's views which made assumptions that aggression was innate and used terms derived from psychopathology to describe normal processes (Marrone, 1998, p. 41).

Longitudinal studies have shown that children classified as secure at a year old, still show signs of security later in life. However, despite the prediction of stable attachment patterns, one's attachment status can change over the course of a lifetime depending on life's trajectories. Inspired by the biologist C. H. Waddington (1957), Bowlby used the concept of "developmental pathways" of personality throughout life, through an array of discreet and non-discreet pathways. The choice of pathways is determined by the qualitative interaction between the individual and his surroundings. For example, a child who grows up in conditions of emotional security and stability is likely to follow an optimal pathway, whereas a less secure child, whose environment cannot provide such conditions, is likely to follow a sub-optimal pathway.

Subsequently, Mary Main and Ruth Goldwyn (1980) devised the Adult Attachment Interview which is an autobiographical semi-structured interview that surprised the unconscious into self-revelation. It has shown that there is a consistent correlation between the outcome of the Strange Situation Procedure linking infant security and parental attachment status. Furthermore, the Minnesota longitudinal study (1976), followed 267 families over 50 years and provided striking findings about the persistence of the attachment patterns and the impact of intergenerational trauma and childhood adverse effects (Sroufe, 2005).

Assumption about the Body

For Bowlby, an attachment bond with a safe and loving caregiver is the key to psychological and physiological well-being. The maintenance of physical proximity by a young animal to an adult is evident in most mammalian species and this is similarly the case in humans. Offering the child physiological security, and the child's need for physical proximity to the parent at the same time makes the body equally relational. The experience of persistent separation, loss, and other attachment disruptions is embodied and can affect the regulatory and exploratory attachment systems such as with sleep, feeding, sexual desire, and many other physiological symptoms. Attachment theory provides a sharp lens through which we can further understand the client's persistent somatic ailments and complaints. Pathological mourning in children and adults has been found to be connected to a variety of autoimmune deficiencies. There is a growing body of literature that has studied the psychological immune system which points to the attachment system being deeply rooted in neurobiology (Holmes, 2001; Luyten & De Meulemeester, 2017). Many affects and their disorders can be attributed to psychological worry and illness which can be viewed in terms of attachment history. Taking into consideration an attachment perspective on the medical treatment of a patient with somatic issues can greatly increase the effectiveness of that treatment.

Assumption Concerning Etiology

Bowlby saw the roots of psychopathology as something which originates in a loss that is then followed by mourning and unresolved grief. "The theory, fundamental to social psychiatry, suggests that relationships and their difficulties might influence psychiatric disorders in three distinct but interrelated ways" (Holmes, 1993, p. 179):

1 The absence, severance, or disruption of attachment bonds.
2 The internalization of early disturbing attachment patterns.
3 Later life adversities can tip over the already vulnerable person and bring about a breakdown.

The evidence in general shows that insecure attachment is a critical developmental precursor of psychopathology. In the presence of childhood adversity and sub-optimal developmental pathways, psychopathology is seen as having a direct link to the poor attachment conditions the child often experienced, during his formative years. In his paper "On Knowing What You Are Not Supposed to Know and Feeling What You Are Not Supposed to Feel," Bowlby (1988b) wrote about how traumatic and abusive experiences, could lead to segregating systems of knowing and not-knowing in what would now be considered to be dissociation. This happens in situations where the child was subjected to intense pressure to "forget" what happened in the past, either by the use of threats, denial, and/or the infliction of sexual, physical, and emotional pain.

Implications for Technique

Attachment theory and attachment-based therapy offers a theoretical basis for the therapeutic relationship always encompassing external and internal realities.

In his book *A Secure Base*, (1988b, p. 138) Bowlby outlined five therapeutic tasks for an attachment-based psychoanalytic therapist in which the client can explore, elicit, modify, and integrate their IWM. These are as follows:

1 Provide the client with a secure base from which they can explore, both past and present relationship and life experiences.
2 Assist and encourage the client to form healthy relationships.
3 With the help of transference and countertransference, the therapist is encouraged to examine her relationship with the client.
4 Encourage the client to accept that their perception of themselves and expectations is based on their perceptions of their parents and what they were told by them.
5 Enable the client to develop their reflective functioning and see how much of their past relationships have tainted their view of present relationships.

The secure base offered in therapy enables the move from insecurity to earned security. This can be used as a measure of outcome of successful therapy. In the words of Jeremy Holmes:

> Attachment theory is not just another brand name in psychotherapy. Successful psychotherapy depends on the capacity to hold to a secure base and to be open to the exploration of new ideas. That is one of the essential and possibly deceptively simple, messages of attachment theory (1996, p. xvi).

Problems of Attachment Theory and Your Own View

In one of her letters to Bowlby, Ainsworth (1968) wrote,

> Attachment has become a bandwagon. There are so many people now interested in research in this area, and so many approaches, both theoretical and methodological. I am afraid that people will leap in a

half-baked way, that findings will be equivocal or conflicting and that perhaps interest will move away from "attachment," dismissing it as one more area that did not "pan out."

As an attachment-based psychoanalytic psychotherapist, what I see as a "half-baked approach" to attachment-based therapy is the tendency of some schools of psychotherapy to manualize and create a short-term program which may alleviate some symptoms for a short period yet ignore the fundamental tenet of what Bowlby intended, which is that in order to have a good and sustainable mental health, we all need an attachment figure and a long-term trusting relationship.

A common critique of attachment theory is with the usage of the attachment classification as a simplistic fourfold typology. Human behavior is indeed more complex and simply putting people into boxes based on these categories would be a misrepresentation of the theory. The insecure attachment patterns are a relational defensive strategy rather than personality traits. Thus, "Attachment patterns are self-perpetuating developmental tracks that maintain some predictability in an uncertain interpersonal world." (Holmes, 1996, p. 11). In my own practice, I find the classification to be a useful heuristic that can be used as a shortcut to the transference/countertransference dynamics presented mostly during the initial stages of the therapy.

A History of the Development of the Core Concepts of the Objective School

The collaboration between Bowlby and Ainsworth was followed by an explosion in attachment research. Other important figures in the field are Inge Bretherton, Everett Waters, the Steeles, Shaver, and Cassidy Crittenden, Sroufe. Mary Main, a student of Ainsworth, who with Goldwyn, (1980) devised the Adult Attachment Interview and with Judith Solomon (1986, 1990), identified a fourth attachment pattern which they called the disorganized-disoriented attachment status. Their findings along with Judith Solomom Erick Hesse, Carol George, Karlen Lyons-Ruth, and Pat Crittenden, were radical as they identified the impact of fear and the maltreatment of children, placing these firmly on the map of childhood development. The longitudinal approach of the Minnesota studies conducted by Alan Sroufe et al. in the early 1970s, was another major milestone showing the persistence of attachment patterns through observations over 40 years. Other vital research has been the work of Fonagy et al in the 1990s on the link between secure attachment and mentalization and the work of the neuroscientist and psychoanalyst Alan Schore on the link between attachment and affect regulation in the early 2000s.

7. Bowlby and Attachment Theory	
Main, general underlying assumptions	1 Emphasis on the biological function: attachment as a survival mechanism and what happens when separation, fear, and loss take over. 2 Attachment is a survival mechanism essential for affect regulation and good reflective functioning. 3 Through the attachment relationship we develop internal working models which are core determinants of interpersonal relationships and behaviors. 4 Attachment is needed throughout the life cycle.
Specific theoretical assumptions	
psychic structure	Influenced by evolution, behavioral, and psychoanalysis theories, attachment theory seeks to understand human behavior, as it occurs via the interactions between the parent (caregiver) and the child (care seeker) and how the environment shapes the inner world of the child.
energy	N/A
relationships	The child relies on the caregiver's affective responsiveness. Attachment theory offers an interactive view of relationships rather than assuming that this is intrinsic within the infant and is validated through empirical research. The emerging relationship patterns are secure, avoidant, ambivalent/preoccupied, and disorganized.
developmental stages	Bowlby's developmental model places the nurturing quality of caregiving and other environmental factors at the center of the development of the personality.
body	A safe and loving attachment bond between the child and the caregiver is the key to psychological and physiological well-being.
anxieties/instinct and defenses	Bowlby perceived that defense mechanisms are not internally generated, rather they are a response to an environment which failed to protect, attune, and repair the child's negative experiences. The ill-effects of deprivation can produce long lasting anxieties, effect personality development and the capacity to sustain healthy relationships.
Assumptions concerning etiology	Bowlby saw the roots of psychopathology as something which originates in loss that is then followed by mourning and unresolved grief.

(*Continued*)

Implications for technique	The secure base offered during therapy is meant to help the client reduce their symptoms, reorganize their IWM, and improve their relationships.
Subsequent developments of the core concept	Bowlby's attachment theory provided the building blocks for the subsequent development of theory in the following areas: infant observation, neuroscience research showing the plasticity of the brain, mirror neurons, affect regulation, and mentalization.

References

Ainsworth, M. D. S. (Ed.). (1962). The effects of maternal deprivation: A review of findings and controversy in the context of research strategy. In *Deprivation of maternal care: A reassessment of its effects* (Public Health Papers, No.15, pp. 87–195). World Health Organization.

Ainsworth, M. (1968). Letter to John Bowlby, 27 April 1968. *Wellcome Collection Archive*, PP/BOW/K.4/12.

Ainsworth, M. D. S. (1969). Object relations, dependency and attachment: A theoretical review of the infant-mother relationship. *Child Development*, *40*, 969–1025.

Ainsworth, M. D. S. (1982). Attachment: Retrospect and prospect. In C. M. Parkes & J. Stevenson-Hinde (Eds.), *The place of attachment in human behviour* (pp. 3–30). Basic Books.

Ainsworth, M., & Bowlby, J. (1991). An ethological approach to personality development. *American Psychologist*, *46*(4), 333–341.

Bowlby, J. (1944). Forty-four juvenile thieves: Their characters and home-life. *International Journal of Psycho-Analysis*, *25*, 19–53.

Bowlby, J. (1973). *Attachment and loss: Separation.* (Vol. 2). Basic Books.

Bowlby, J. (1979). *The making and breaking of affectional bonds.* Tavistock Publications.

Bowlby, J. (1988a). Developmental psychiatry comes of age. *American Journal of Psychiatry*, *145*(1), 1–10.

Bowlby, J. (1988b). *A secure base: Clinical applications of attachment theory.* Routledge.

Craik, K. (1943). *The nature of explanation.* Cambridge University Press.

Duschinsky, R. (2020). *Cornerstone of attachment research.* Oxford University Press.

Harlow, H. F. (1958). The nature of love. *American Psychology*, *13*, 673–685.

Harlow, H. F. (1961). The development of affectional patterns in infant monkey. In B. M. Foss (Ed.), *Determinants of infant behaviour*, Vol. 1. Wiley.

Holmes, J. (1993). *John Bowlby and attachment theory.* Routledge.

Holmes, J. (1996). *Attachment, intimacy, autonomy. Using attachment theory in adult psychotherapy.* Jason Aronson.

Holmes, J. (2001). *The search for the secure base.* Routledge.

Holmes, J., & Slade, A. (2018). *Attachment in therapeutic practice.* Sage.

Luyten, P., & De Meulemeester, C. (2017). Understanding and treatment of patients with persistent somatic complaints through the lens of contemporary attachment theory. *Attachment: New Directions in Psychotherapy and Relational Psychoanalysis Journal, 11*(3), 205–222.

Main, M., & Goldwyn, R. (1980). *Adult attachment scoring and classification system.* [Unpublished Manuscript]. University of California at Berkeley.

Main, M., & Solomon, J. (1986). Discovery of new insecure-disorganized-disoriented attachment pattern. In T. B. Brazelton & M. Yogman (Eds.), *Affective development in infancy* (pp. 95–124). Ablex.

Main, M., & Solomon, J. (1990). Procedures for identifying infants as disorganized/disoriented during the Ainsworth Strange Situations. In M. Greenberg, D. Cicchetti, & E. M. Cummings (Eds.), *Attachment in the preschool years: Theory, research, and intervention* (pp. 121–160). University of Chicago Press.

Marrone, M. (1998). *Attachment and interaction.* Jessica Kingsley Publishers.

Robertson, J. (1953). *A two-year-old goes to hospital.* [Film]. Concord.

Stern, D. (1998). *The interpersonal world of the infant.* Basic Books.

Sroufe, A. L., Egeland, B., Carlson, E. A., Collins, A. W., (2005). *The development of the person. The Minnesota study of risk and adaptation from birth to adulthood.* The Guilford Press.

Waddington, C. H. (1957). *The strategies of gens.* Allen and Unwin.

Chapter 8

Lacan and the Lacanians: The Lacanian Unconscious

Patrick Landman

We take this formula "Lacanian unconscious" in the sense of the Lacanian conception of the unconscious.

The Unconscious is Structured as a Language

Lacan's reading is difficult, even for native French speakers, and his theses often seem to move, which can give the reader a feeling of incoherence; the constant advances of his teaching have often embarrassed his readers, but also his students; there are constantly additions and complements, and at the moment when there seems to be an explicitation of a concept, there may be a reversal of Lacan's thought. But in the uninterrupted flow of his thought, there are some formulas that have emerged such as: "*The unconscious is structured like a language*" (Lacan, 1981, p. 251, 2011).

This formula seems to constitute Lacan's main hypothesis concerning the Freudian unconscious.

Many have questioned Lacan's fidelity to Freudian theory, in particular when Lacan affirmed that the unconscious is structured like a language. Is he in the Freudian lineage? Some claim that the Lacanian conception of the unconscious extends the Freudian conception as it is formulated in the *traumdeutung* (Freud, 1953a, b) and the later articles, whereas others think that Lacan invented a new unconscious or reinvented the unconscious (Soler, 2015).

We must leave this question open and try instead to grasp what Lacan wanted to express with this compact, striking, and almost incomplete formula. Lacan formulated it several times during the decades of his teaching until he reformulated his conception of the unconscious in his last years.

We can, for example, begin by asking ourselves the following question: what are the main consequences that we must draw from this notion, from this hypothesis that the unconscious is structured like a language?

First of all, the fact that the Lacanian unconscious is not principally, and perhaps not at all, the place of primary instincts or of the most archaic drives, nor is it the most obscure part of us, but that it presents itself as a

DOI: 10.4324/9781003027768-9

structure and that it contains, as its principal elements, signifiers in the manner of language. Lacan refused the vocabulary of passions, some will reproach him for moving away from affects in his conception of the unconscious even if he devoted a year of seminars to the anguish which is the affect par excellence. We can also say that the Lacanian unconscious is not the habitat of the subject nor the heart of the being. Language is rather, in a way, the habitat of the being.

The unconscious marks its print on the subject, the language which constitutes it impregnates the subject who is born in a bath of language which precedes it. The subject is as spoken as it is speaking.

With this unconscious language, the situation that the subject lives in is not based on the subject. Lacan had a conception opposed to phenomenology, the subject is in the situation of language because of the unconscious. The unconscious is structured but it is only verified and proven in the practice of the treatment; it does not have an ontological status; rather, it has an ethical status because it is, in a way, established by the act of the analyst.

If the unconscious is structured like a language, it is expressed in some language, and access to this unconscious is a matter of translation. All languages are not equal for translating the unconscious, according to Lacan, and he evoked the particular difficulty with English. Lacan worried about English becoming a universal language. Why would English be less propitious than other languages to translate the language of the unconscious? Lacan did not say so explicitly but the hypothesis that is proposed is because of the double structure of the origin of this language, both Saxon and Romance, whereas other languages have a single dominant origin.

Lacan proposed a triad to account for psychic life; this triad, as its name indicates, includes three components: the symbolic, the imaginary, and the real.

We must examine how this triad is expressed in the unconscious.

First of all, the real.

The Lacanian Unconscious has a Real Dimension, an Imaginary Dimension, and a Symbolic Dimension

The translation of the language of the unconscious, like any translation, leaves a remainder, and it is this remainder that is the part of the real in the unconscious. The Lacanian unconscious, which includes signifying chains or chains of signifiers, does not belong only to the symbolic; the symbolic does not cover the whole unconscious. There is a remainder that is inaccessible through language; this is what Lacan called the real. This real corresponds in part to the Freudian notion of the dream's umbilicus. Lacan developed this notion of the real of the unconscious or at least gave indications in the last part of his teaching. The question has often been raised as to whether this unconscious real is sexual in nature. It seems that we can answer positively from two other propositions of Lacan's repeated on several occasions;

"There is no sexual relation" and "language babbles about the sexual." The sexual comes as a remainder and as a limit to the power of language and thus to the power of the symbolic.

The Lacanian unconscious has an imaginary face in relation to the unconscious fantasy, a kind of narrative that supports both the subject's desire and his symptoms. The imaginary unconscious, the foundation of the unconscious fantasy, crystallizes in the phase of development that Lacan identified as crucial in the constitution of the self, namely the mirror stage. The illusion of mastery at the moment of the mirror produces an effect of misrecognition in which the unconscious fantasy is lodged. In the psychotic structures where one notes a porosity of the ego, a weakness of the ego, it is possible that the unconscious fantasy is not really constituted, it leaves the place in the moments of crisis to a delusional construction. Freud showed the relations of certain delusions with unconscious fantasy, megalomaniac fantasy, homosexual fantasy, etc.

The imaginary face of the unconscious, the unconscious fantasy, is an important therapeutic resource. This resource had already been exploited by the hypnotic technique, which Freud considered too authoritarian, and he substituted free association. Psychoanalytic psychodrama makes extensive use of the imaginary through interpretative play.

The Lacanian unconscious is also, if not essentially, of a symbolic nature. The signifying chains that constitute it are offered for interpretation during the treatment. This focus on the symbolic dimension of the unconscious led Lacan to change the framework of psychoanalytic cures. A signifier is by its very nature different from other signifiers. From this specificity of the signifier, particular techniques of intervention in the course of the treatments, such as scansion or the interruption of a session, even a short one, in order to punctuate a signifier that had appeared in the patient's associations, were developed. These technical changes earned Lacan the disapproval of many colleagues, although they were consistent with his conception of the unconscious. Interpretation saw its role diminished in Lacanian cures because it was a technique that relied a priori more on signification, on the unconscious signifieds, than on the signifiers as such.

The unconscious structured as a language brings with it certain consequences in the conception of the direction of psychoanalytic cures. In the same way, language has a place of Other in relation to the subject, hence Lacan's affirmation that in parallel to the interaction between the patient's ego and the analyst's ego there is another interaction of a symbolic nature between the subject who has the place of the analysand and the psychoanalyst who occupies for a certain time the place of the Other. This is the nature of the transference because the psychoanalyst is supposed to know. This is Lacan's famous definition of the transference: the subject is supposed to know.

The Second Lacanian Unconscious: The Real Unconscious, the Unconscious *Jouissance*

Lacan seems to have perceived the insufficiency of this supposition that the unconscious is structured like a language. A re-assessment was necessary. Lacan had a structuralist moment, he relied on Saussure's and Jakobson's linguistics as well as on Levi-Strauss' structural anthropology. But the device of psychoanalysis rests on the subject of the word and the word is similar to an act, the analysand who is a subject is very different in this respect from the mythant. Language can designate a particular language and a word expressed in this language to constitute a discourse but what we collect in a cure is the word and not the discourse. Certainly, the great psychic structures are psychosis, neurosis, and perversion, which Freud borrowed from psychiatry, reveal to us perhaps different modalities of inhabiting language, but what is expressed in the cures is the word of the subject in search of a subjective truth that is always singular and not to be confused with the truth itself. In the psychoanalytical treatment the subject makes constructions as Freud showed and these constructions can allow him to emancipate himself. The signifiers of the unconscious are integrated into a narrative and they emerge in the course of speech, but Lacan, after Freud, questioned the stumbling blocks of the technique based on punctuation, scansion, and interpretation. Freud had spoken of a "beyond the pleasure principle" and of the death drive leading to repetition. Lacan introduced the concept of *jouissance*, an untranslatable word, and this new notion will lead to a new Lacanian approach to the unconscious. This concept designates a psychic modality opposed to pleasure because it provides a particular satisfaction that does not really allow a discharge of the excitation.

Indeed, the symptom that in neurosis results from a compromise between the different psychic instances, some of which are unconscious, does not disappear most of the time under the effect of the action on the signifiers. Lacan thought that the action of the signifiers on the language unconscious does not reach another dimension of the unconscious that we could designate as the real unconscious or the *jouissance* unconscious.

Lacan's hypothesis: before being impregnated by signifiers, the subject in his early childhood is bathed in an atmosphere of melody and speech that give rhythm to his biological life and construct his psychic life, especially his subjectivity and his interaction with the Other. This melody, these sounds, Lacan called them an untranslatable neologism: *lalangue.*

Lacan produced this neologism because of the proximity of the word *lalangue* with the Latin word *lallare* which means to sing. *Lalangue* evokes a melodious language sung before the syntax. But this *lalangue* is not the mother tongue as we usually conceive it, it is in relation with the care brought to the body of the baby, it is a language punctuated with events of the body of pleasure as well as traumas. The *lalangue* is not completely assigned to a particular language, it transcends the multiplicity of languages, and it is translinguistic rather than universal. Meaning is absent from *lalangue*. *Lalangue* is not structured, it does not form a corpus, it shapes the unconscious of the subject even before he or she engages in language. *Lalangue* is constituted of scattered differences devoid of meaning, it precedes the entry into the signifier, it is the support of a *jouissance*. Of course there are words heard but they do not fix any meaning, only events of the body to which they are associated.

The Real Unconscious and the End of the Analysis

It is classic in many schools of thought in psychoanalysis to consider that the end of the analysis consists in the lifting of the major part of what has been the object of the repression because it is the model of hysteria that dictates this theory. Hysteria is the basis of Freud's discovery and it is from cases of hysteria that Freud built his very elaborate theory of repression. Although Freud spoke of winning over the repressed, he nonetheless advocated taking up a new slice of analysis regularly, because the repressed never gets rid of itself and tends to be reconstituted. The lifting of the repression tends to be confused with the lifting of amnesia; it is the traumatic model, the painful memories are forgotten, the impulses but also the affects that are unacceptable for the subject are repressed, mainly everything that relates to incest and parricide. Only memories remain, called screen memories, they condense the essence of the repressed, they are enigmatic, even opaque, condensed, and often of a very banal narrative.

The work of the psychoanalytical treatment will go in the direction of an unfolding of the meaning contained in these memories, they are carriers of unconscious signifiers and *jouissance* unknown by the subject.

I am thinking of a patient who recounted the following screen memory.

> I must have been three years old, I was at my maternal grandmother's. I was walking on the beach with her, I was barefoot and the water was covering my feet. I don't understand why I remember this, it seems like an immense banality.

But when I ask him to try to specify the elements of this memory, a fact comes back to him: I was walking at the place where the sea and the earth were separated and when they were reunited on my feet, I felt a great satisfaction. He understands then that he was worked by the signifier separation, that the screen memory testifies to his preoccupation of the time, that about the parental separation, of his desire that it does not take place and that he is in the center of this reconciliation. The screen memories allow access to the unconscious signifiers.

Without minimizing the importance of these screen memories or slips of the tongue, Lacan, from his conception of the real unconscious, said that the psychoanalytical treatment aims at an off-sense, at snippets of *jouissance* locked up in symptoms or social and cultural apparatuses appearing in dreams without it being possible to attribute a meaning to them. These snippets are the testimony of the incarnation of *lalangue* in the symbolic space, in signifiers that even emptied of their meaning remain enigmatic, because these snippets possess a dimension of *hors sens*.

If we follow Lacan in this way, if we give credence to this hypothesis of a nonsense unconscious, we have to admit that winning over repression, however noble this objective may be, cannot constitute the only objective of the psychoanalytic treatment, because the nonsense part of the unconscious is not accessible to interpretation. So how to aim at an acceptable end of the analysis?

The answer, or more exactly, Lacan's answers are not univocal, after having spoken of an end of analysis as identification with the symptom in the sense that the symptom is what is most intimate to me, we must naturally understand what remains of the symptom after the psychoanalytic treatment and not the symptom that will have led the subject to undertake an analysis, the symptom that made him suffer, that constituted the heart of his complaint. The analytic treatment has passed by but the remainder is what belongs to my being and emancipated from the alienation that operated in the symptom, freed from the particular formal envelopes that surrounded this symptom, I can identify myself with what remains in the symptom, I can legitimately assume this part of my being that is my singularity and thus I am able to inscribe my desire with less impediment, fewer hindrances, fewer inhibitions.

The other way for the end of a psychoanalytical treatment is to find the way of one's desire.

The psychiatrist works with the reference of the normal man, which we know is a fiction, that no one will meet him, but it is this normal man that the psychiatrist's patient must get closer to in order to conform to the heavy demands imposed by society. The normal man is the one who accepts to pay his tribute of renunciation to the *jouissance* by submitting himself to the social part of his superego. The patient of the psychoanalyst seeks to clarify his desire, a desire with an indeterminate meaning, a large part of which was unconscious to him, and to inscribe it in actions and spaces of intimate and social life. The psychoanalytic treatment has the power to support this search for the path of desire if it operates with an ethic that banishes authoritarianism, directivism, and the manipulation of transference love. The analyst's desire is not reduced to a therapist's desire, it does not put healing or recovery as the central axis of the psychoanalytic cure; we know that Freud thought that some recoveries were resistant to the cure, that these recoveries were aimed at sparing the difficult work that a psychoanalytic cure requires. Lacan spoke of healing as coming "in addition to."

Lacan formulated a third way for the end of the psychoanalytical treatment, which seems to be related to his conception of the unconscious as real unconscious. The end comes about through the exhaustion of the process, which was already the intuition of Sandor Ferenczi. The analytic process aims at emptying the *jouissance* that is contained in the symptom but also at putting an end to it by exhaustion of the *jouissance* that is contained in the transference, The transference and therefore the treatment ends by exhaustion on the condition that certain accidents of this transference are avoided that can lead to its premature end because the repetition at work has not been observed by the patient, the destitution of the subject supposed to know is not parricide, and the end of an analysis must not be confused with a passage to the oedipal act. It goes without saying that for the cures of psychotics the questions are posed differently because of the major risk that the use of interpretations poses for a subject who is often interpretative, especially as these interpretations can lead the psychotic toward a delusional transference: the Other that the psychoanalyst embodies takes *jouissance* from me or toward an erotomanic transference: the Other that the psychoanalyst embodies loves me.

To empty the *jouissance* to exhaust the process is not enough; it is necessary to add another operation: the subject at the end of a psychoanalytical treatment should be able to observe a modification of his relation to the *jouissance*. Lacan saw in this a kind of psychic marker of the end of analysis or at least an indicator of decisive change. The phenomenological expression of this modification of the relation to *jouissance* is very variable but it can be heard when a patient has succeeded in moving on.

Mental health is not the absence of symptoms but it is rather to inscribe one's desire emptied of the cumbersome *jouissance* of the symptom, which is the best guarantee of health, it is not homeostasis, it is not all restful, but it offers a satisfaction guaranteeing that one is on the right track. Moreover Lacan spoke of the satisfaction of the end of the analysis.

So does a Lacanian unconscious exist in the sense of a specific Lacanian theory of the unconscious? I would tend to answer "yes" by reformulating Lacan's main theoretical suppositions while affirming that the Lacanian unconscious is not very far from the Freudian unconscious as the neuronal unconscious can be.

- The unconscious is structured like a language.
- The unconscious is composed of three dimensions: the real, the imaginary, and the symbolic.
- The unconscious is real: forged by the *lalangue* and the *jouissance* of the body.
- The analytical technique must not only be made of interpretations, scansions, and punctuations on the signifiers but must operate on the *jouissance*.

- The analysis reaches its end through the elucidation of desire, the evidence of *jouissance*, the modification of the subject's relation to *jouissance*, and finally, the appearance of satisfaction at the end of the analysis.

8. Lacan and the Lacanians	
Main, general underlying assumptions	1 The unconscious is structured like a language. 2 The unconscious is composed of real, imaginary, and symbolic. 3 Real unconscious and *lalangue*
Specific theoretical assumptions	
psychic structure	N/A
energy	N/A
relationships	N/A
developmental stages	Mirror stage and imaginary
body	N/A
anxieties/instincts and defenses	N/A
Assumptions concerning etiology	N/A
Implications for technique	Interpretation, punctuation, scansion, hollow out the *jouissance*
Subsequent developments of the core concept	N/A

References

Freud, S. (1953a). The interpretation of dreams. In J. Strachey (Ed. and Trans.), *The standard edition of the complete works of Sigmund Freud* (Vol. 4–5, pp. ix–627). Hogarth Press.

Freud, S. (1953b). Constructions in analysis. In J. Strachey (Ed. and Trans.), *The standard edition of the complete works of Sigmund Freud* (Vol. 23, pp. 255–270). Hogarth Press.

Lacan J. (1981). *Les psychoses: Séminaire livre III* [The psychoses: Seminar book III]. Seuil.

Lacan, J. (2011). *Ou pire: Séminaire XIX* [Or worse: Seminar book XIX]. Seuil.

Soler, C. (2015). *Lacan: l'inconscient réinventé* [Lacan: The unconscious re-invented]. PUF.

Chapter 9

New York Freudian Group, US Freudians, and Contemporary Freudians

Leon Hoffman

History

The New York Psychoanalytic Society and the American Psychoanalytic Association were both founded in 1911, with blessings from Freud, who had come to America in 1909. A. A. Brill, the leader of the New York, was the first practicing analyst in the United States and the first to translate Freud into English. In addition to promoting psychoanalytic ideas among professionals, Brill was active in disseminating psychoanalytic ideas to the public. He was a principal consultant to Edward Bernays, who was Freud's nephew and founder of the field of public relations.

For the next 20 years, potential psychoanalysts went to Europe for formal training (Berlin, Vienna, and Budapest). As the demand grew, the New York Institute was founded in 1931, the first in the United States. The tripartite training model (training analysis, supervision, didactics), which continues to the present, was developed by Max Eitingon, co-founder of the Berlin Institute.

From the 1930s until after World War II, a large number of émigrés from Nazi Europe became leaders at the Institute: Berta Bornstein, Robert Bak, Kurt Eissler, Edith Jacobson, Marianne Kris, Margaret Mahler, and Herman Nunberg. Heinz Hartmann, Ernst Kris, and Rudolf Loewenstein were the founders of ego psychology. For the next several decades, the teaching of Freud and ego psychology was the predominant paradigm. During the last quarter of the 20th century, the work of Jacob Arlow, stressing the concept of unconscious fantasy, and that of Charles Brenner, refining the construct of conflict and compromise formation, became the leading theoretical perspective. Sander Abend, Martin Willick, Michael Porder, and Arnold Richards continued to refine these ideas, which morphed into modern conflict theory (MCT), first cited by Brenner in 1994. Theodore Jacobs promoted the integration of interactive elements into the predominant intrapsychic model of treatment. Child and adolescent analysts refined the value of defense analysis, particularly of unpleasant affects, developed by Bornstein. Analysis of defenses became a staple of technique.

DOI: 10.4324/9781003027768-10

Main, General Underlying Assumptions

1 Ubiquity of unconscious fantasy: impact on development, character, interpersonal interactions, and symptoms.
2 Understanding patient's presentation from the perspective of conflict and compromise formation.
3 Understanding transference and countertransference in the analytic situation and real-life interactions.
4 Addressing and analyzing defenses.

Specific Theoretical Assumptions

Arlow stressed the importance of understanding the nature of a patient's unconscious fantasy in his/her mental representations and its impact on a person's object choice, a central function of analytic work (Arlow, 1969a, 1969b, 1980, 1987). This conception is similar to the construct of emotion schema (Bucci et al., 2016).

Arlow and Brenner (1964) highlighted the centrality of Freud's (1923, 1926) structural theory. Brenner expanded these ideas into conflict and compromise formation theory, summarizing in *The Mind in Conflict* (1982) and *Psychoanalysis or Mind and Meaning* (2006). Brenner (2006) argued that analytic and extra-analytic evidence support the hypothesis that conflict and compromise formations are ubiquitous in both normality and pathology.

Brenner (1982) eschewed the concept of "drives," noting that one only observed "drive derivatives." When one observes patients' wishes, they are always inextricably linked with relationships. In contrast to interpersonal and relational psychoanalysts (Bromberg, 2009; Levenson, 1981), Brenner, like Arlow, stressed the impact of the mental representations of people in a patient's life, not only the "real" interactions with others.

Arlow and Brenner stressed the importance of analyzing the transference, in contrast to interpersonal and relational analysts who maintain that the agent of change involves understanding the real interaction between patient and analyst. Brenner (1982) stressed that transference is a universal experience of all mental life and is not unique to psychoanalysis. "What is unique about transference in psychoanalysis ... is the fact that the transference is analyzed ..." (1987, p. 103). Both transference and countertransference are viewed as compromise formations (Brenner, 1985).

Nature of Psychic Structure and Assumptions About Developmental Stages

The first three assumptions encompass the understanding of the nature of psychic structure—the balance of forces in the mind—and that early development impacts later life.

Abend (2005) expanded on the utility of unconscious fantasy and conflict and compromise formation, arguing that the concept of defense is part and parcel of psychic conflict: an unconscious force in the mind, opposing the expression of a forbidden wish (1981). Bornstein (1945, 1949, 1951; Hoffman, 2007, 2014) and Paul Gray (Goldberger, 1996; Gray, 1996) had the greatest influence on the development of defense analysis. Bornstein stressed the value of interpreting defenses against painful feelings in children, an elaboration of Anna Freud's (1936/2018) work.

Implications for Technique as a Result of the Assumptions about Anxieties/Instincts and Defenses

As a result of all the assumptions, particularly the importance of the power of defenses, the analysis of defenses is central to technical approaches.

Assumptions about the Nature of Relationships

Clinicians continue to try to understand the mutative factors in psychotherapy and psychoanalysis: addressing intrapsychic conflicts or the real interaction between analyst/therapist and patient. Freud (1912) coined the term the "unobjectionable" part of the transference, which is admissible to consciousness, persists, and "is the vehicle of success in psychoanalysis exactly as it is in other methods of treatment" (p. 195), the therapeutic/working alliance. Debates ensued about the value of this construct in psychoanalytic work. Abend (1996a, 1996b) argued, like Brenner (1979), that in analysis the idea of the therapeutic alliance should be subsumed under the analysis of transference. Leo Stone (1967, 1981, 1996) likened the therapeutic alliance to the "mature transference;" and, Stein (1981) argued that those aspects of the initial therapeutic relationship which seem rational and unconflicted become part of the transference neurosis as the analysis proceeds.

David Wolitzky (1996) aptly summarized the essence of the disagreements: some were concerned that the nurturance of the therapeutic alliance would lead to excessive gratification; others expressed concern about excessive deprivation from too rigid a stance (p. 233). These discussions have been mirrored in the general psychotherapy literature. Zilcha-Mano (2017) differentiated a "trait-like" component to the therapeutic alliance (a patient's capacity to form an alliance with people, including the therapist) from a "state-like" component that evolves during treatment.

Jacobs (1993, 1996, 2002a, 2002b, 2002c; Koritar et al., 2010) noted that analysts needed to incorporate understanding the nature of the real interaction between analyst and patient, noting that the analyst's countertransference "constitutes an invaluable pathway for the investigation of the process" (Jacobs, 1999, p. 591). The analyst's awareness of countertransference improves the capacity for appropriate interpretation about the nature of the patient's intrapsychic conflicts (Jacobs, 2002c). The data that the analyst extracts from the interaction and her subjective responses promote more effective interpretations of the patient.

Subsequent Development of the Concepts

Richards and Richards (1995) highlighted differences and similarities among various theories. Self-psychologists avoided dealing with patients' aggression and ego psychologists moved away from the construct of penis envy in feminine psychology. The Kleinian theory became closer to ego psychology with its focus on aggression and early envy—more respected than the concept of penis envy. Self-psychologists focused on the real relationship with the early mother, whereas relationists and interpersonalists focused on the real relationship in the analytic dyad (pp. 451–453). They argue that MCT and Kleinian theory share a common ground of unconscious conflicts, in contrast to self-psychologists, relational, and intersubjective analysts. This is in contrast to Wallerstein's (1990) assertion that there is "common ground" among all analysts. In sum, there is a real difference between understanding the meaning given to "real" events versus maintaining that "the interpersonal therapist must grapple with the *real* matrix of events and personalities in which every therapy is embedded" (Levenson, 1981, p. 492). Can these perspectives be reconciled? When is one approach or another most appropriate?

Contemporary Intellectual Climate

Throughout its history, the New York Psychoanalytic Society & Institute (NYPSI) has been known as among the most "classic" psychoanalytic institutes. Beginning in the 1990s there has been an evolution in teaching and extramural activities. The in-depth study of the origins of psychoanalysis in the works of Freud has continued. Studying Freud's development serves as a model for present-day critical thinking of contemporary clinical challenges, including how much of contemporary theoretical debates are often framed as either following or challenging Freud's assertions and clinical findings. This degree of intensity is likely not part of many curricula throughout the United States.

The part of the curriculum geared specifically to the study of Freud's texts, in a more or less chronological order, constitutes about 10% of the course work over 4 years. Additionally, many courses include readings from Freud. However, the bulk of the teaching is eclectic. Clinical situations (both in supervisions and in clinical seminars) are approached in an open-ended way, trying to understand the meaning of a patient's production. Although many of the faculty ascribe to the importance of MCT, many clinical and theoretical discussions include various contemporary psychoanalytic perspectives:

(modern) Kleinian, self-psychology, relational, object-relational, close process monitoring, and modern ideas of development. Many faculty consider themselves to be eclectic in their approach. There are courses in critical thinking, research methodology, neuropsychoanalysis, ethics, cultural diversity, and a variety of courses on psychotherapies.

In a poll of the faculty in 2020, twenty-four out of forty-three endorsed MCT (with ten including a variety of other models); nine endorsed eclectic; four endorsed ego psychology, object relationships, Kernbergian theory. Two endorsed interpersonal/relational; two endorsed Kleinian (plus one from the MCT group); and two noted the importance of understanding the complex unconscious mechanisms that needed to be considered. Some stressed the importance of Laplanche and Bionian Field Theory. If one considers the numbers who endorsed another perspective while endorsing MCT, fully 2/3 of the faculty at NYPSI who responded to the questionnaire, supposedly the bastion of old-fashioned classic psychoanalysis, utilize a variety of theories in addition to or other than MCT.

This finding is similar to that of Mendelsohn et al. (1992). They "unexpectedly" found "classicists" (members of Boston and NY Institutes) were significantly more heterogeneous in their views than the interpersonal analysts (members of William Alanson White Institute). The classical analysts generally disagreed among themselves and showed a wide range of views; the interpersonalists tended to present greater agreement on theory and technique (p. 373).

This finding of eclecticism is comparable to Rudden and Bronstein (2015). Of seventeen cases presented by North American psychoanalysts at a Comparative Clinical Methods Working Party of the IPA, eight focused only on transference, four managed the therapeutic relationship in some form, and five utilized mixed models. They noted that

> within each of these categories were represented several different schools of thought – contemporary Freudian, Kleinian, self psychological, relational, or a mixture of these paradigms. It was of interest that within each of these overarching schools of thought, individual analysts tended to think and work in unique ways that did not always closely reflect their overarching paradigm (p. 699).

The Future: An Attitude of Research

Abend (2002), who was first "convinced of the advantages of thinking about cases, technique, and theory from the vantage point of his own training and experience" (p. 46), became more persuaded that his preferred mode was the most effective. Yet, his ideas came to be enriched by "an expanding, more pluralistic intellectual stage" (p. 48). This enrichment does not conform to

Cooper (2008), who likened pluralism in contemporary psychoanalysis to a "multiplicity of authoritarian orthodoxies." Bernardi (2005) noted that pluralism allows each analyst to recognize that there is no ideal model, not a "true" psychoanalysis, but could choose a way of working most beneficial to each patient. He also warned of "a dark side of pluralism that appears when it is chosen without adequate critical analysis of the advantages and disadvantages of its different theoretical and technical approaches" (p. 659).

Scientific debates among analysts are difficult because questioning theoretical and technical assumptions and perspectives generates strong feelings of uncertainty and reactivates "remnants of the transference dating back to analytic training and institutional life," with narcissistic conflicts mobilized (Bernardi, 2002, p. 855). When analysts compare theories, they look for similarities rather than critically examine differences (Bernardi, 2005). For true integration to occur, "each party's premises and hypotheses" need to be questioned (Bernardi, 2002, p. 858). Systematic research on process and outcome are needed.

A review of the curriculum of NYPSI illustrates the multiplicity of psychoanalytic perspectives. I highlight the critical thinking sequence which is designed to encourage inquiry; it includes a course on neuroscience and psychoanalysis and one on systematic empirical work. In the 1990s, a Neuropsychoanalysis Center and a journal were established (Nersessian & Solms, 1999). The Pacella Research Center includes a Clinician/Researcher Collaborative Process Seminar which aims to bridge the gap between science and practice in psychotherapy and psychoanalysis, utilized in the teaching of candidates.

The Pacella Research Center has developed a database of twenty-three analyses and psychotherapies, including eight analytic cases and nine completed psychotherapy cases. This data set is enabling us to evaluate outcome and process measures, mainly linguistic measures, which can become a useful tool for teaching and research. A special issue of the *Journal for Psycholinguistic Research,* "Connecting Feelings, Thoughts and Words: The Referential Process in Theory, Research and Clinical Studies" (2021) is edited by Bucci, Maskit, Murphy, and Hoffman. Finally, several manuals have been produced by members of NYPSI: Barbara Milrod (Busch et al., 2012; Milrod, 1997), Leon Hoffman (Hoffman et al., 2016), Sabina Preter, Theodore Shapiro, and Barbara Milrod (2018), and Tehela Nimroody and colleagues (2019a, 2019b). These studies in psychodynamic psychotherapy are valuable applications of basic psychoanalytic theory.

Coda

Rudden and Bronstein (2015) mirror the most important message for psychoanalysis:

> For science of any kind, there must be evidence and a commitment to the observation of subjective and objective facts. We must allow ourselves to openly discuss differences, to compare our methods and our actual work, and truly allow ourselves to doubt, search for evidence, and think (p. 699).

A challenge for the field is to try to develop a "theoretically neutral" way to systematically compare how analysts make decisions, both theoretically and in practice (Hoffman, 2008, p. 1025).

9. New York Freudian Group, US Freudians, and Contemporary Freudians	
Main, general underlying assumptions	1 The ubiquity of unconscious fantasy 2 Conflict and compromise formation 3 Transference and countertransference 4 Addressing and analyzing defenses
Specific theoretical assumptions	
psychic structure	Mind in conflict
energy	Neuroscience
relationship	Relationship vs transference
development stages	Ongoing development
body	Always present
anxieties/instincts and defenses	Defenses against painful affects
Assumptions concerning etiology	Conflict
Implications for technique	Addressing Conflict
Subsequent developments of the core concept	Incorporation of various theoretical strands as well as attitude of importance of research and the study of neuroscience

References

Abend, S. (1981). Psychic conflict and the concept of defense. *Psychoanalytic Quarterly*, *50*, 67–76.

Abend, S. (1996a). The problem of therapeutic alliance. *Journal of Clinical Psychoanalysis*, *5*(2), 213–226.

Abend, S. (1996b). Response. *Journal of Clinical Psychoanalysis, 5*(2), 237–240.
Abend, S. (2002). In retrospect. *Psychoanalytic Inquiry, 22*(1), 43–54.
Abend, S. (2005). Analyzing intrapsychic conflict. *Psychoanalytic Quarterly, 74*(1), 5–25.
Arlow, J. (1969a). Fantasy, memory, and reality testing. *Psychoanalytic Quarterly, 38*, 28–51.
Arlow, J. (1969b). Unconscious fantasy and disturbances of conscious experience. *Psychoanalytic Quarterly, 38*, 1–27.
Arlow, J. (1980). Object concept and object choice. *Psychoanalytic Quarterly, 49*, 109–133.
Arlow, J. (1987). The dynamics of interpretation. *Psychoanalytic Quarterly, 56*, 68–87.
Arlow, J., & Brenner, C. (1964). *Psychoanalytic concepts and the structural theory*. International Universities Press.
Bernardi, R. (2002). The need for true controversies in psychoanalysis. *International Journal of Psychoanalysis, 83*(4), 851–873.
Bernardi, R. (2005). What after pluralism? Ulysses still on the road. *Psychoanalytic Inquiry, 25*(5), 654–666.
Bornstein, B. (1945). Clinical notes on child analysis. *Psychoanalytic Study of the Child, 1*, 151–166.
Bornstein, B. (1949). The analysis of a phobic child: Some problems of theory and technique in child analysis. *Psychoanalytic Study of the Child, 3*, 181–226.
Bornstein, B. (1951). On latency. *Psychoanalytic Study of the Child, 6*, 279–285.
Brenner, C. (1979). Working alliance, therapeutic alliance, and transference. *Journal of the American Psychoanalytic Association, 27S*(Supplement), 137–157.
Brenner, C. (1982). *The mind in conflict*. International Universities Press.
Brenner, C. (1985). Countertransference as compromise formation. *Psychoanalytic Quarterly, 54*, 155–163.
Brenner, C. (1987). Working through: 1914–1984. *Psychoanalytic Quarterly, 56*, 88–108.
Brenner, C. (1994). Response to D. Boesky's discussion of "The mind as conflict and compromise formation". *Journal of Clinical Psychoanalysis, 3*, 523–527.
Brenner, C. (2006). *Psychoanalysis or mind and meaning*. Psychoanalytic Quarterly Monograph.
Bromberg, P. (2009). Truth, human relatedness, and the analytic process: An interpersonal/relational perspective. *International Journal of Psychoanalysis, 90*(2), 347–361. DOI: 10.1111/j.1745-8315.2009.00137.x
Bucci, W., Maskit, B., & Murphy, S. (2016). Connecting emotions and words: The referential process. *Phenomenology and the Cognitive Sciences, 15*(3), 359–383.
Bucci, W., Maskit, B., Murphy, S., & Hoffman, L. (Eds.). (2021). Connecting feelings, thoughts and words: The referential process in theory, research and clinical studies. [Special issue]. *Journal of Psycholinguistic Research, 50*.
Busch, F., Milrod, B., Singer, M., & Aronson, A. (2012). *Manual of panic focused psychodynamic psychotherapy–extended range* (Vol. 36). Routledge.
Cooper, A. (2008). American psychoanalysis today: A plurality of orthodoxies. *Journal of the American Academy of Psychoanalysis and Dynamic Psychiatry, 36*(2), 235–253.
Freud, A. (2018). *The ego and the mechanisms of defence*. Routledge. (Original work published 1936).

Freud, S. (1912). The dynamics of transference. In J. Strachey (Ed. and Trans.), *The standard edition of the complete works of Sigmund Freud* (Vol. 12, pp. 97–108). Hogarth Press.
Freud, S. (1923). The ego and the id. In J. Strachey (Ed. and Trans.), *The standard edition of the complete works of Sigmund Freud* (Vol. 19, pp. 1–66). Hogarth Press.
Freud, S. (1926). Inhibitions, symptoms and anxiety. In J. Strachey (Ed. and Trans.), *The standard edition of the complete works of Sigmund Freud* (Vol. 20, pp. 75–176). Hogarth Press.
Goldberger, M. (Ed.). (1996). *Danger and defense: The technique of close process attention*. Jason Aronson.
Gray, P. (1996). Undoing the lag in the technique of conflict and defense analysis. *Psychoanalytic Study of the Child, 51*, 87–101.
Hoffman, L. (2007). Do children get better when we interpret their defenses against painful feelings?. *Psychoanalytic Study of the Child, 62*, 291–313.
Hoffman, L. (2008). Book review: *Psychoanalysis or mind and meaning*. By Charles Brenner. New York: Psychoanalytic Quarterly, 2006, 140 pp., $25.00. *Journal of the American Psychoanalytic Association, 56*(3), 1016–1027. DOI: 10.1177/0003065108323654
Hoffman, L. (2014). Berta Bornstein's "Frankie". *Psychoanalytic Study of the Child, 68*, 152–176.
Hoffman, L., Rice, T., & Prout, T. (2016). *Manual of regulation-focused psychotherapy for children (RFP-C) with externalizing behaviors: A psychodynamic approach*. Routledge.
Jacobs, T. (1993). The inner experiences of the analyst: Their contribution to the analytic process. *International Journal of Psychoanalysis, 74*, 7–14.
Jacobs, T. (1996). Analysis, mutual analysis, and self-analysis. *Canadian Journal of Psychoanalysis, 4*(2), 255–277.
Jacobs, T. (1999). Countertransference past and present. *International Journal of Psychoanalysis, 80*(3), 575–594. DOI: 10.1516/0020757991598783
Jacobs, T. (2002a). Impasse and progress in analysis: Some reflections on working through in the analyst and its role in the analytic process. *Journal of Clinical Psychoanalysis, 11*(2), 295–319.
Jacobs, T. (2002b). Once more with feeling: On working through in the analyst and its role in the analytic process. *Psychoanalytic Inquiry, 22*(4), 599–616. DOI: 10.1080/07351692209349005
Jacobs, T. (2002c). Secondary revision: On rethinking the analytic process and analytic technique. *Psychoanalytic Inquiry, 22*(1), 3–28. DOI: 10.1080/ 07351692209348970
Koritar, E., Jacobs, T., Bolognini, S., Ungar, V., Rolland, J., & Turgeon, A. (2010). The core of the analytic process. *Canadian Journal of Psychoanalysis, 18*(1), 141–146.
Levenson, E. (1981). Facts or fantasies: The nature of psychoanalytic data. *Contemporary Psychoanalysis, 17*, 486–500.
Mendelsohn, R., Bucci, W., & Chouhy, R. (1992). Transference and countertransference: A survey of attitudes. *Contemporary Psychoanalysis, 28*, 364–385.
Milrod, B. (1997). *Manual of panic-focused psychodynamic psychotherapy*. American Psychiatric Publishing.
Nersessian, E., & Solms, M. (1999). Editors' introduction. *Neuro-Psychoanalysis, 1*(1), 3–4.

Nimroody, T., Hoffman, L., Christian, C., Rice, T., & Murphy, S. (2019a). Development of a defense mechanisms manual for children's doll play (DMCP). *Journal of Infant, Child, and Adolescent Psychotherapy*, *18*(1), 58–70.
Nimroody, T., Hoffman, L., Christian, C., Rice, T., & The Pacella Research Center of the New York Psychoanalytic Society and Institute. (2019b). Defense mechanisms manual for children's doll play (DMCP) coding manual. https://www.tandfonline.com/doi/suppl/10.1080/15289168.2018.1565005/suppl_file/hicp_a_1565005_sm2717.pdf
Preter, S., Shapiro, T., & Milrod, B. (2018). *Child and adolescent anxiety psychodynamic psychotherapy: A treatment manual*. Oxford University Press.
Richards, A. D., & Richards, A. K. (1995). Notes on psychoanalytic theory and its consequences for technique. *Journal of Clinical Psychoanalysis*, *4*(4), 429–456.
Rudden, M., & Bronstein, A. (2015). Transference, relationship and the analyst as object: Findings from the North American Comparative Clinical Methods Working Party. *International Journal of Psychoanalysis*, *96*(3), 681–703.
Stein, M. (1981). The unobjectionable part of the transference. *Journal of the American Psychoanalytic Association*, *29*, 869–892.
Stone, L. (1967). The psychoanalytic situation and transference: Postscript to an earlier communication. *Journal of the American Psychoanalytic Association*, *15*, 3–57.
Stone, L. (1981). Notes on the noninterpretive elements in the psychoanalytic situation and process. *Journal of the American Psychoanalytic Association*, *29*, 89–118.
Stone, L. (1996). Discussion of Abend. *Journal of Clinical Psychoanalysis*, *5*(2), 235–236.
Wallerstein, R. (1990). Psychoanalysis: The common ground. *International Journal of Psychoanalysis*, *71*, 3–20.
Wolitzky, D. (1996). Discussion of Abend. *Journal of Clinical Psychoanalysis*, *5*(2), 227–234.
Zilcha-Mano, S. (2017). Is the alliance really therapeutic? Revisiting this question in light of recent methodological advances. *American Psychologist*, *72*(4), 311–325.

Chapter 10

American Ego Psychology

Les Fleischer

American ego psychology is not the dominant force in psychoanalysis that it was from the 1930s through the 1970s, but its focus on all domains of ego functioning and its flexibility of technique are useful guides for contemporary psychoanalysis. Modern ego psychology has the potential to unite diverse schools of psychoanalysis, incorporating knowledge from developmental psychology, cognitive neuroscience, and psychiatry (Eagle, 2020; Marcus, 2017; Rangell, 1988).

Although American ego psychology, like much of contemporary psychoanalysis, has splintered into different branches, it is possible to explicate its core assumptions and methods. Grounded in Sigmund Freud's tripartite structural model and Anna Freud's work on defenses, the founders of American ego psychology were emigrés from Europe who escaped the holocaust (Richards & Lynch, 1998). Their heirs included defense analysts, modern conflict theorists, developmentalists, ego psychology-object relationists, and modern ego psychologists (Marcus, 1999).[1]

Basic Assumptions/Core Tenets

The ego is a complex, coherent self-regulatory system that mediates conflict between the inner world and external reality. It is "the organ of adaptation" and its processes and functions are essential for survival (Hartmann, 1939, p. 48).

"Adaptation to reality and emotional experience is one of the (primary) mediating tasks of the ego" (Marcus, 1999, p. 844). The ego organizes, mediates, synthesizes, and integrates each individual's psychic reality (Marcus, 2017). Intra- and inter-systemic conflicts are ubiquitous and inevitable. Compromise and synthesis are key ego functions.

People are born with innate ego functions that mature according to a developmental timetable that is affected by nature (temperament/inborn capacities) and nurture (environment/experience/ identifications) (Hartmann, 1939).

The ego is an active, dynamic structure that operates consciously and unconsciously, with much of its activity unconscious. Ego functions like

DOI: 10.4324/9781003027768-11

perception, motility, memory, and attention have primary autonomy but can secondarily become involved in conflict (Hartmann, 1939).

Psychic Structure

The id, ego, and superego include the dynamic contents of affects, drives, unconscious fantasies, and object relations (Marcus, 1999). The conflict between the structures reflects different motivations, compromises, affects, object relations, drives, and defenses. Ego defenses protect against noxious internal and external stimuli and stresses (Freud, 1936/1966). The ego aims at synthesis between competing structures, affects, and motivations (Marcus, 2018).

Energy

There are "hypothetical, quantifiable forces, analogous to physical energy that drive all mental activities, [which] account for the intensity of motivational states, affects, and other mental experiences" (Auchincloss & Samberg, 2012, p. 77). Energy is subject to accumulation, discharge, change of function, and laws of conservation (Freud, 1923). The ego neutralizes energy from the libidinal and aggressive drives for all its functions. For example, neutralized libido transforms love into friendliness and hate into healthy competitiveness. While energic concepts are often considered irrelevant in contemporary analysis, the concept of intensities and the idea that people are "driven" to repeat problematic actions, relations, or trauma implicitly suggest that some type of "energy" or force is operating (Marcus, 2018).

Relationships

The development of object relations is affected by the ego and vice versa. Building psychic structures involves internalizing interpersonal/affective interactions. Satisfactory object relations in the average expectable environment promote optimal ego development while dysfunctional object relations negatively affect ego growth. However, outcomes are complex and associated with endowment and temperament, along with interaction with the environment (Hartmann, 1939). Object-relational theories have increasingly integrated object relations into ego psychological paradigms, although some contemporary theorists argue that these two theoretical paradigms are incompatible (Greenberg & Mitchell, 1983).

Development

Development is considered an internally driven process in interaction with reality experience, relationships, and the environment. Unsatisfactory object relations, environmental stresses, illness, trauma, or intrapsychic conflict can result in developmental arrest or regression. American ego psychologists extended Freud's model of psychosexual development to cover the entire lifespan, with increased emphasis on pre-oedipal development, adolescence, adulthood, and psychosocial factors—including reality, interpersonal dynamics, and culture (Erikson, 1964).

Body

The ego develops from the earliest bodily sensations and self and object representations are initially derived from bodily experiences (Hoffer, 1950). Bodily functions gradually come under the ego's control, and healthy or pathological ego functioning is attached to bodily states. Societal demands and prohibitions are often in conflict with bodily drives and development. Emotional, sexual, and body development are tied together and affected by the ego's capacity for synthesis (Marcus, 2020).

Anxieties, Instincts, and Defenses

Anxiety, conflict, defense, and compromise formations are ubiquitous processes in human mental life. The conflict model uses the impulse/defense configuration. There is a developmental sequence of danger situations/calamities that is tied to object relations (loss of the object, loss of love, castration, superego anxiety). Defenses can simultaneously serve multiple functions, including protection from drives and affects, while promoting adaptation. While there is a hierarchy of defenses associated with different levels of pathology, any mental event can function as a defense (Brenner, 2006).

Etiology

The ego has certain innate capacities/apparatuses that mature according to its own developmental timetable in an average expectable environment (Hartmann, 1939). While ego development is lifelong, early childhood is critical in the development of cognitive, affective, and object-relational capacity. Innate biological deficiencies, genetics, illness, trauma, intrapsychic conflict, or their combination can damage ego capacities. Ego psychologists debate the role of the environment and intrapsychic conflict as opposed to biological factors in the etiology of mental illness—particularly regarding psychosis (Arlow & Brenner, 1964; Marcus, 2017). Contemporary American ego psychologists have mostly adopted a stress/diathesis model, recognizing the complex interaction between endowment, genetic, psychogenetic, and psychosocial factors involved in pathogenesis.

Technique

Accurate assessment of all ego-functioning domains provides the foundation for treatment planning and technique. The technique is flexible, determined by diagnosis, and based on the unique characteristics of the patient's ego (Bellak, 1975; Marcus, 2017). The analysis of defense and resistance plays a central role, including close process analysis, plus analysis of inner conflicts, affects, transference/countertransference, unconscious fantasies, and drive derivatives. Mobilization of the patient's observing ego, focused on helping patients understand how the mind works, is central. Attention to illness states and their impact on autonomous ego functions enhances work with very ill patients. All treatments involve analyzing unconscious, pre-conscious, and conscious ego activities. Ego psychological therapies include expressive and supportive approaches or their combination.

American ego psychology played a key role in widening analytic therapy's scope. The use of parameters, and the flexible use of insight, support, and interpretation of conflict, facilitated effective treatment with a wide population of patients. While the combined use of psychopharmacological treatments and psychotherapy expanded psychoanalytic work, ego psychologists emphasize the development of insight to strengthen ego functioning.

Selected American Ego Psychologists and Their Contributions

Heinz Hartmann

Widely considered the founder of American ego psychology, Heinz Hartmann created an elegant, complex model of the mind, founded on natural science, while incorporating knowledge from the social sciences, psychology, philosophy, and medicine (Rangell, 1965). He preserved and expanded Sigmund Freud's economic, structural, dynamic, developmental, and adaptational points of view in his model of mental functioning which includes depth psychology, psychopathology, and a general psychology. He addressed the interdependence between theory and technique, and offered some technical recommendations based on classical ego psychological principles—attention to the internal and external world, ego functions, character, inter-systemic and intra-systemic conflict, defense, health, and adaptation. Like Freud, he advocated for adherence to general principles but emphasized the importance of flexible techniques based on each patient's unique psychological structure and ego functioning (Hartmann, 1952).

Hartmann focused on "the conflict-free avenues [spheres] of reality adapted development"—the ego apparatuses (neurocognitive capacities) that are primary autonomous functions, including perception, thinking, motility, and memory (1939, p. 12). These innate functions are derived outside of conflict and develop according to a unique developmental timetable in an average expectable environment. Impairment or dysfunction in the ego apparatuses (caused by biological or environmental damage) impacts the ego's capacity to master the drives and conflict and affects its defense structure (Freud, 1936/1966). The primary autonomous ego functions can secondarily be drawn into conflict, losing their freedom from the drives and reality. Functioning that arises from conflict can become secondarily autonomous from a change of a function. Hartmann (1939) warned that it is wrong to assume that a current behavior can be reduced to its childhood precursors since its aims, purpose, and meaning undergo a change of function over time.

His increased focus on conflicts within the ego between different ego attributes or ego functions enhanced psychoanalysis. The "synergistic and antagonistic relations" between structures had important implications for conceptions of health or pathology (Hartmann, 1952, p. 34). While the resolution of intrapsychic conflict is impossible, the ego's ability to mediate satisfactory compromise formations and its capacity for synthesis and adaptation are associated with health.

Hartmann et al. (1949) enhanced our understanding of aggression, alongside libido, as a driving force affecting all psychic structures and development. They highlighted the ego's ability to neutralize aggression for adaptive aims. If the ego cannot manage aggression, pathological outcomes may occur.

Hartmann combined the traditional analytic focus on unconscious conflict and the reconstruction of psychogenetic experience with greater attention to ego processes. The increased focus on the ego's autonomy, functions, and processes enriched diagnosis and treatment.

Anna Freud: Defense Analysis

Anna Freud's focus on defense, resistance, and ego processes became a staple of American ego psychology. While Sigmund Freud (1923) increasingly focused on ego processes, the analytic community lagged behind, particularly around technique (Busch, 2013; Gray, 2005; Hartmann, 1952). Her attention to the ego shifted the analyst's method of observation and technique. She emphasized that analysis was based on work with the ego and the entire psychic apparatus. Her identification of major defense mechanisms increased the focus on mental processes, including defenses against drives and affects (Freud, 1936/1966). She introduced a tentative classification of defenses that were useful for understanding the adaptive and maladaptive nature of defenses and their developmental trajectory. Anna Freud's (1963) conceptualization of developmental lines also outlines the development of ego functions—a major contribution to modern ego psychology.

Paul Gray's (2005) microanalysis of the defensive processes expanded upon Anna Freud's defense analysis. Busch's (2013) emphasis on engaging the analysand's observing ego is rooted in Anna Freud's ego analysis.

Wurmser's (2007) concentration on superego analysis preserved her focus on all components of the psychic apparatus.

Charles Brenner and Jacob Arlow: Modern Conflict Theory

Charles Brenner and Jacob Arlow were the architects of modern conflict theory, the dominant paradigm in North American psychoanalysis from the 1970s through the '80s. This approach focused on compromise formation, conflict, and unconscious fantasy. While based on Sigmund Freud's structural theory, the model jettisoned energic concepts and concentrated on meaning. Drives are manifested in drive derivatives expressed in wishes that are in conflict with affects, fears, defenses, and moral aspirations, under the umbrella of an unconscious fantasy (Brenner, 2006). Building on Waelder's (1936) work on the multi-determined nature of symptoms, Brenner focused on mental conflict's ubiquity in normality and pathology. Retaining Freud's focus on the oedipal conflict's centrality, his attention to the childhood calamities (loss of love, the object, castration anxiety, and superego anxiety), and to anxiety and depressive affect, located instinctual anxieties in a relational context (Richards & Lynch, 1998).

For Brenner, analysis cannot eliminate psychic conflict, but successful analysis results in shifts in compromise formations that allow for greater pleasure and satisfaction, and decreased guilt and anxiety. Though informed by structural theory, Brenner (2006) argued that the presence of id, ego, and superego cannot be empirically supported, so he eschewed the tripartite structure. He developed a theory offering a unique formulation for each individual's conflicts between their wishes and fears. Other modern conflict theorists claim that structural concepts are clinically useful (Boesky, 1988).

Arlow (1969) advanced our understanding of unconscious fantasy as a central motivational force, emphasizing that unconscious fantasies (conscious or unconscious daydreams) profoundly influence human mental life. Fantasies are stories formed in childhood and based on real experience, constitutional factors/temperament, and the naive perceptions of childhood. All perceptions are filtered in part through this lens (Erreich, 2015). Pathogenic unconscious fantasies can have a deleterious impact on a person's life. Identification, analysis, and modification of unconscious fantasies are a key component of the modern conflict approach.

Edith Jacobson, Otto Kernberg, and Roy Schafer

The American ego psychologists/object relations theorists include a diverse range of theorists who attempted to integrate ego psychology with object relations theories. Among the most prominent are Edith Jacobson, Otto Kernberg, and Roy Schafer. Building on the work of Sigmund Freud and

Hartmann, Jacobson (1964) developed a complex meta-psychological developmental framework that focused on how the drives, affects, and innate biological factors interact with reality to create self and object representations and superego elements (Marcus, 1999). She retained structural theory, including energic concepts, while emphasizing the importance of ego synthesis.

Jacobson advanced our understanding of affects and moods, emphasizing that pathological mood states are associated with a constitutional predisposition and early trauma, which affect structural development (Auchincloss & Samberg, 2012). She viewed moods as discharge products of the drives that reduce tension and have motivational force. They mature according to a developmental timetable and, in normal states, contribute to self-regulation. In pathological states, they distort reality and impair self-object relations.

Jacobson (1964) emphasized the importance of superego development on mood and self-esteem regulation; discrepancies between the ego ideal and ego are associated with self-directed aggression, mood fluctuations, and depressive states.

Kernberg (2016) used Jacobson's model as the foundation for his ego psychological object relations theory. While he retained the importance of sexual and aggressive drives, object relations are the building blocks for the drives and intra-psychic structure. His diagnostic framework differentiates between psychotic, borderline, and neurotic levels of character organization. His transference-focused therapy is an effective treatment for borderline conditions.

Schafer (1968) enhanced understanding of complex ego processes, motives, and function. He deepened our knowledge of internalization, introjection, and identification. He located object relations within the entire intrapsychic structure and examined how reality and fantasy affect internalized objects. Motive became a major force rather than just biological drive—affect, object relations, wish, fantasy, compromise formation, and mastery were dynamic forces organized by the ego.

Erik Erikson: The Developmentalists

Building on the work of Anna Freud and Joseph Sandler, developmentalists utilized infant observation and other extra-analytic data to expand our theory of pre-oedipal development and clinical processes. Erikson's (1964) epigenetic theory of human development expanded Freud's theory of psychosexual development with an increased focus on familial, cultural, relational, and social factors interacting with innate biological capabilities across the entire lifespan. Erikson's work on dreams enhanced knowledge of the manifest content of dreams as an explication of ego functioning.

Eric Marcus: Modern Ego Psychology

Eric Marcus is the foremost expert on modern ego psychology—a comprehensive scientific theory of the mind interested in all aspects of mental function and their application to illness. Building on the work of Sigmund Freud, Hartmann, and Bellak, modern ego psychology integrates psychoanalytic theory, descriptive psychiatric diagnosis, ego dysfunction, neurosciences, developmental psychology, and pharmacology to create an integrated framework for treating mental illness (Marcus, 2017). It focuses on ego functioning and its role in symbolic representations, including emotional processes, contents, and themes—especially the ego's capacity to "synthesize or integrate experiences from varying levels of consciousness and different levels of organization" (Auchincloss & Samberg, 2012, p. 72).

According to modern ego psychology, in severe mental illness, emotional experience (primary process/affect) impinges on reality experience because it damages autonomous secondary processes (logic, words, perception, learning) (Marcus, 2017). A thorough evaluation of the mind's structures and processes—namely, a review of ego dysfunction—illuminates pathological processes. Accurate diagnoses of ego dysfunction enable clinicians to develop effective treatment plans, combining medication and psychotherapy to repair damaged ego function and facilitate adaptation. Marcus (2017) explains how different medications effect mental structures and how medications combined with psychotherapy can repair or alleviate ego dysfunctions characteristic of mental disorders.

Identifying day residue thoughts or events that triggered symptom formation, engaging the observing ego, and enhancing reality testing are key components of the therapeutic process (Marcus, 2017). Interpretation expanded to interpreting preconscious experience involving how the ego organizes experience affected by illness, which helps patients master internal and external reality. The interpretation of defenses against autonomous ego functions and personality dynamics that impinge on the therapeutic alliance are crucial. Helping patients understand their illness, its impact on ego function, and its emotional impact, significance, and meaning helps them to manage their reality experience, may pre-empt illness states, and strengthens ego functioning.

One of Marcus's (2017) major contributions involves his refinement of Sigmund Freud's *thing presentation*—involuntary neuro-mental phenomena that combine affect with perception, resulting in a symbol/experience that condenses wishes, fears, conflicts, and aspects of reality. Thing presentations include an underlying story containing emotionally meaningful themes. They are also a *felt* quality of experience—usually intense. Thing presentations are mostly unconscious but may enter preconsciousness or consciousness in dreams, fantasies, art, architecture, human sexual experience, or metaphors. In psychoses, or very ill patients, the patient experiences the thing presentation (e.g., a hallucination) concretely as *real*. In character disorders, thing presentations are expressed in rigid attitudes or behaviors. In severely disturbed patients, thing presentations dominate the mental experience, often triggered by a day residue event—they are rigid, repetitive, and stereotypical. Using medication and therapy, the analyst attempts to translate the thing presentation into words, enhancing reality testing and ego development.

Analytic therapy decodes emotions/symbolism, symptoms, and psychotic language (Marcus, 2017). Modern ego psychology offers a general psychology that examines the ego's representational, affect symbolizing, and integrative functions in pathology and health (Aragno, 2008).

Present State and Future Developments

Although American ego psychology has some core tenets, its many branches are not unified. It lacks a well-articulated theory of personality or the self (Marcus, 1999). The motivational power of affects, object relations, or ego motives has also not been adequately addressed (Eagle, 2020). However, despite these limitations, modern American ego psychology may be best positioned to unify all of the psychoanalytic schools, while incorporating knowledge from extra-analytic sources.

Its focus on affect, affect-symbolizing processes, and the impact of early experiences on adult functioning correlates with advances in neuroscientific and developmental research on affect, brain function, and the association between environment, temperament/inheritance, and the social environment (Eisenberg, 1995; Marcus, 2017; Solms, 2019). Modern ego psychological attention to unconscious mental experience, structures, and dynamic emotional themes and processes enriches the descriptive psychiatric focus on observable, conscious behaviors and symptoms (Marcus, 2017). The focus on mental disorders' impact on ego functioning is useful for treating specific illnesses. However, modern ego psychology is at the nascent stage of integrating ego psychology with the neurosciences, developmental psychology, and psychiatry.

Although scholars debate whether it is possible or even desirable to have a comprehensive meta-theory of psychoanalysis, in my opinion, American modern ego psychology has the greatest potential to unite diverse streams of psychoanalysis. Because ego psychology is a meta-theory, clinical theory, and general psychology, and because it addresses all aspects of mental functioning and experience and its perspective correlates with the neurosciences, developmental research, and psychiatry, it should follow that modern ego psychology has the best chance of one day providing the framework for a unified psychoanalytic theory.

10. American Ego Psychology	
Main, general underlying assumptions	1 The ego is a self-regulatory system that mediates conflict between the inner world and environment. 2 The ego is "the organ of adaptation." 3 People are born with innate ego functions that mature according to a developmental timetable. 4 The ego operates consciously and unconsciously.
Specific theoretical assumptions	
psychic structure	The core intrapsychic structure consists of id, ego, and superego.
energy	There are hypothetical, quantifiable forces, analogous to physical energy that drive all mental activities.
relationship	Development of object relations is affected by the ego and vice versa.
development stages	Development is an internally driven, interactive process.
body	The ego is rooted in the body.
anxieties/instinct and defenses	Conflict involves the impulse/defense configuration.
Assumptions concerning etiology	Ego capacities can be damaged by genetics, illness, trauma, intrapsychic conflict, or their combination.
Implications for technique	Technique is flexible, determined by diagnosis.
Subsequent developments of the core concept	American ego psychology concepts are correlated with the findings of neurosciences, developmental research, and psychiatry.

Acknowledgments

I am grateful to Dr. Eric Marcus and Dr. Madhu Vallabhaneni for their valuable suggestions.

Note

1 There is overlap between the categories and the theorists, and this categorization does not delineate the growth of the paradigm. For comprehensive overviews of the historical development of American ego psychology, see Marcus, 1999; Richards & Lynch, 1998; Wallerstein, 2002.

References

Aragno, A. (2008). *Forms of knowledge: A psychoanalytic study of human communication*. International Psychoanalytic Books.

Arlow, J. A. (1969). Unconscious fantasy and disturbances of conscious experience. *Psychoanalytic Quarterly*, *38*(1), 1–27.

Arlow, J. A., & Brenner, C. (1964). *Psychoanalytic concepts and structural theory*. International Universities Press.

Auchincloss, E., & Samberg, E. (Eds.). (2012). *Psychoanalytic terms and concepts*. Yale University Press.

Bellak, L. (1975). Ego function assessment and analysability. *International Review of Psychoanalysis*, *2*, 413–427.

Boesky, D. (1988). The concept of psychic structure. *Journal of the American Psychoanalytic Association*, *36*(S), 113–135.

Brenner, C. (2006). *Psychoanalysis or mind and meaning*. Psychoanalytic Quarterly.

Busch, F. (2013). *Creating a psychoanalytic mind: A psychoanalytic method and theory*. Routledge.

Eagle, M. (2020). Toward an integrated psychoanalytic theory: Foundation in a revitalized ego psychology. *Clinical Social Work Journal*, *48*, 257–266.

Eisenberg, L. (1995). The social construction of the human brain. *American Journal of Psychiatry*, *152*(11), 1563–1575.

Erikson, E. (1964). *Childhood and society*. Norton and Society.

Erreich, A. (2015). Unconscious fantasy as a special class of mental representation. *Journal of the American Psychoanalytic Association*, *63*(2), 247–270.

Freud, A. (1963). The concept of developmental lines. *Psychoanalytic Study of the Child*, *18*(1), 245–265.

Freud, A. (1966). *The ego and the mechanisms of defense* (Rev. ed.). In *The writings of Anna Freud* (Vol. 2, pp. 3–179). International Universities Press. (Original work published 1936).

Freud, S. (1923). The ego and the id. In J. Strachey (Ed. and Trans.), *The standard edition of the complete works of Sigmund Freud* (Vol. 19, pp. 3–66). Hogarth Press.

Gray, P. (2005). *The ego and analysis of defense* (2nd ed.). Jason Aronson.

Greenberg, J. R., & Mitchell, S. A. (1983). *Object relations in psychoanalytic theory*. Harvard University Press.

Hartmann, H. (1939). *Ego psychology and the problem of adaptation*. International Universities Press.

Hartmann, H. (1952). Technical implications of ego psychology. *Psychoanalytic Quarterly*, *20*(1), 31–43.

Hartmann, H., Kris, E., & Loewenstein, R. (1949). Notes on the theory of aggression. *Psychoanalytic Study of the Child*, *3*(1), 9–36.

Hoffer, W. (1950). Development of the body ego. *Psychoanalytic Study of the Child*, *5*(1), 18–23.

Jacobson, E. (1964). *The self and the object world*. International Universities Press.

Kernberg, O. F. (2016). New developments in transference focused psychotherapy. *International Journal of Psychoanalysis*, *97*(2), 385–407.

Marcus, E. R. (1999). Modern ego psychology. *Journal of the American Psychoanalytic Association*, *47*(3), 843–871.

Marcus, E. R. (2017). *Psychosis and near psychosis: Ego function, symbol structure, treatment* (3rd ed.). Routledge.
Marcus, E. R. (2018). Psychoanalytic meta-theory: A modern ego psychology view. *Psychodynamic Psychiatry*, *46*(2), 220–239.
Marcus, E. R. (2020). Modern ego psychology and human sexual experience: Fetish, fetish enactments, and perversion. *The Canadian Journal of Psychoanalysis*, *28*(2), 226–246.
Rangell, L. (1965). The scope of Heinz Hartmann. Some selected comments on his essays on ego psychology: An appreciative survey on his 70th birthday. *International Journal of Psychoanalysis*, *46*, 5–30.
Rangell, L. (1988). The future of psychoanalysis: Scientific crossroads. *Psychoanalytic Quarterly*, *57*(3), 313–340.
Richards, A. D., & Lynch, A. A. (1998). From ego psychology to contemporary conflict theory: An historical overview. In C. S. Ellman, S. Grand, M. Silvan, & S. J. Ellman (Eds.), *The modern Freudians: Contemporary psychoanalytic technique* (pp. 3–24). Jason Aronson.
Schafer, R. (1968). *Aspects of internalization*. International Universities Press.
Solms, M. (2019). A neuropsychoanalytic perspective. *Psychoanalytic Inquiry*, *39*(8), 607–624.
Waelder, R. (1936). The principle of multiple function: Observations on over-determinism. *Psychoanalytic Quarterly*, *5*(1), 45–62.
Wallerstein, R. S. (2002). The growth and transformation of American ego psychology. *Journal of the American Psychoanalytic Association*, *50*(1), 135–168.
Wurmser, L. (2007). *Torment me, but don't abandon me: Psychoanalysis of the severe neuroses in a new key*. Rowman & Littlefield.

Chapter 11

Sándor Ferenczi, the Budapest School of Psychoanalysis, and the Ferenczi Tradition: The Bridge Between the "One-Person" and "Two-Person" Psychology

Judit Mészáros

Ferenczi and the Historical Setting of the Budapest School

What is the Budapest school? Whom can we list among its members? The school represents the group that formed around the spirit of Sándor Ferenczi, and its members reflect the perspective of this intellectual community. Many of them contributed significantly to modern theoretical and therapeutic approaches to psychoanalysis, promoted the development of training, and laid the groundwork for the application of understandings drawn from psychoanalysis in a broader social context. It is important to place the Budapest school within the context of the psychoanalytic movement and the historical processes of the 20th century and to highlight the influential personality of Sándor Ferenczi (1873–1933).

Ferenczi was born to a large assimilated Jewish family in Hungary in the Austro-Hungarian Empire. He spoke Hungarian and German as his native languages. Ferenczi studied medicine in Vienna and began his medical career in Budapest.

When Ferenczi first met Freud in 1908, he was a young physician with a great interest in processes of the unconscious and psychological phenomena. He was a forensic medicine specialist with nearly 100 publications to his name in medical and literary journals (Mészáros, 1999). Ferenczi became a member of the Wednesday Society in 1908, which was Freud's inner circle. He had a significant impact on creating and developing the international psychoanalytic movement. Despite emotional strains, Freud and Ferenczi cultivated a strong, lifelong professional relationship and friendship (see their correspondence between 1908 and 1933).

Open to modernization, Ferenczi used every possible forum in Budapest to advocate for psychoanalysis from 1908 whether through medical or literary journals or public lectures. He formed the Hungarian Psychoanalytical

DOI: 10.4324/9781003027768-12

Society in 1913. The various professions represented by the founding members reflected the early interdisciplinarity of Hungary's psychoanalytic movement. Ferenczi's cultural background and liberal spirit drew interest in psychoanalysis from those in the social sciences and the arts, specifically, anthropology, pedagogy, and literature. Psychoanalysis became rapidly embedded in the thinking of the young avant-garde intelligentsia and permeated the Budapest culture. During the First World War, Ferenczi served as an army physician and, based on his experiences with traumatized soldiers, elaborated upon psychoanalytic theories that explained the etiology of war neuroses. Ferenczi was elected president of the IPA at the 5th International Psychoanalytical Congress, which was held in Budapest in 1918, where the primary topic was war neuroses. The congress was held at the Hungarian Academy of Sciences and the event opened by the mayor. It was the last time Freud would attend an IPA congress. Presentations on war neuroses convinced Austro-Hungarian senior officers there to recommend psychoanalysis at military hospitals that treated war trauma. This was the first time in its history that psychoanalysis had managed to move beyond individual psychoanalysts' offices and serve the broader society. Unfortunately, this construction could not be realized due to the collapse of the Austro-Hungarian Empire at the end of the war.

Ferenczi held lectures on psychoanalysis for the Galileo Circle, which had been established by university students who were open to new ideas. This influenced medical students to promote the inclusion of psychoanalysis in their training. The conservative university senate rejected their proposal in 1918, but at the beginning of the country's 133-day Soviet Republic period in 1919, a time of revolutionary innovations, the proposal was approved. It was in Budapest that an independent department of psychoanalysis was established as part of the medical training at the Medical Faculty of the Budapest University (1919). Ferenczi was appointed the first professor of psychoanalysis, "a success not dreamt before," as Freud wrote to Jones (Paskauskas, 1993, p. 349). This demonstrated that psychoanalysis was capable of establishing itself among the academic disciplines. Ferenczi and the powerful Budapest psychoanalytic community—of which Jones was also a member in 1918—as well as a general acceptance of psychoanalysis in society prompted Freud to write in a letter to Karl Abraham before the 5th IPA congress: "Budapest will now become the headquarters of our movement" (Falzeder, 2002, p. 382). This intellectual congruence was greatly aided during the congress by a major donation from philanthropist Antal Freund/Anton von Freund to create a psychoanalytic publishing house and outpatient clinic in Budapest.

However, in the turbulence of the revolutions and various forms of government that followed the collapse of Austria-Hungary (1918–1920), the psychoanalytic department and Ferenczi's appointment were terminated by the regime that followed (Erős, 2019; Mészáros, 2010a). Political retribution and the flames of anti-Semitism prompted two waves of emigration from

Hungary (1919–1921 and 1938–1941). What was called the *numerus clausus* ("closed number" law) squeezed Jewish students out of universities in the 1920s, and the anti-Jewish legislation passed by Hungary's Parliament in the late 1930s also took its toll. One-third of the psychoanalytical society left the country in the first exile, including Sándor Radó, Melanie Klein, and Sándor Loránd. Young émigrés, such as Mihály Bálint/Michael Balint, Alice Bálint/Balint, Margaret Mahler, and Franz Alexander, started their training in Vienna or Berlin. Only a very few returned to Budapest as of the mid-1920s during a ten-year period of consolidation, such as Alice and Michael Balint and Edith Gyömrői, but in the late 1930s the anti-Jewish laws forced them to leave the country permanently (Mészáros, 2014).

The first wave of emigration might well have halted the development of the Budapest school, since it was accompanied by so many personal, professional, and financial losses. Ferenczi lost his professorship, and psychoanalysis was unable to take root in medical training. At the international level, Ferenczi was forced to resign from the IPA presidency at Jones's insistence. The tiny Hungarian society suffered significant setbacks in the permanent loss of its secretary, Radó/Rado, as well as other talented members and ambitious novices. Due to inflation in Hungary, Antal Freund's generous offer had to be used to establish the International Psychoanalytic Publishing House in Vienna instead. The winds of anti-Semitism and terror swept through the country.

> After the unbearable "Red Terror," which lay heavy on one's spirit like a nightmare, we now have the White one … . It will very soon become evident how one can live and work here. It is naturally the best thing for Ψα. to continue working in complete withdrawal and without noise. Personally, one will have to take this trauma as an occasion to abandon certain prejudices brought along from the nursery and to come to terms with the bitter truth of being, as a Jew, *really* without a country.
>
> (Ferenczi to Freud, 28 August 1919)
> (Falzeder & Brabant, 1996, pp. 365–366)

It is no exaggeration that it was the commitment to psychoanalysis exhibited by Ferenczi and the small group surrounding him that made it possible to develop the Budapest school.

The Contribution of the Budapest School to Modern Psychoanalysis

Reflective Relationships: The "Two-Person" Psychology

Ferenczi saw credible, reflective communication and the building of trust as the pillars of the optimal relationship between child and adult as well as between therapist and patient. In 1908, he urged parents to avoid the falseness of omnipotence, which later becomes a source of disappointment for children. He saw the optimal child-rearing principle as no more repression than necessary (Ferenczi, 1908/1980a). Parents can thus provide optimal freedom for the child's development. This spirit can be found in the ideas of Mahler on the optimal individuation and separation process, in Winnicott's aptly termed "the good enough mother," and in Balint's "the basic fault," in which he prioritizes the significance of a sense of safety in the early relationship.

Ferenczi saw it as essential to an appropriate therapeutic relationship that the therapist's actions be emotionally credible as well. This is why he suggested involving countertransference in the therapeutic process (Ferenczi, 1919/1980b). This happened almost a decade after Freud had underscored that the emergence of countertransference should be avoided in psychoanalysis (Freud, 1910). Ferenczi observed that "intellectual help," as Freud wrote about the psychoanalytic process in the context of countertransference, is not enough. He realized that cool, emotionally reserved behavior paralyzes the patient and limits the deepening of analysis. He said, "this would retard the experience of the transference, the pre-condition of every successful psycho-analysis, or make it altogether impossible .... This ... could be characterised as the phase of resistance against counter-transference" (Ferenczi, 1919/1980b, p. 188). Ferenczi saw psychoanalysis as a joint effort between analyst and analysand both intellectually and emotionally. Ferenczi's positive thinking on countertransference represented a fundamental shift in the psychoanalytic relationship (Borgogno, 2019; Ferenczi, 1919/1980b; Haynal, 1988; Martín Cabré, 1998).

Ferenczi also drew attention to narcissistic countertransference, which was pleasing to the analyst (Ferenczi & Rank, 1924). He is also associated with "what nowadays is called the technique of countertransference interpretations" (Balint, 1979, p. 126).

The Budapest psychoanalysts incorporated countertransference into the healing process from the late 1920s. Alice and Michael Balint were convinced "the analytical situation is the result of an interplay between the patient's transference and the analyst's countertransference" (Balint & Balint, 1939, p. 228). From the early 1940s, Therese Benedek was the first at the Chicago Institute to teach how to look at countertransference instead of giving technical advice in supervision. Paul Roazen aptly noted that Hungarians were aware that psychoanalysis was a two-way street. Only a few dealt with countertransference then. Helene Deutsch introduced the notions of concordant and complementary (Deutsch, 1926). Edward Glover differentiated between positive and negative countertransference and underlined resistance in countertransference (Glover, 1927), but countertransference as a useful technique had been accepted in the mainstream of psychoanalysis from the 1950s.

Psychoanalysis became a system of multi-directional processes of intrapsychic and interpersonal dimensions between patient and analyst. In the acceptance of countertransference, a new discourse developed. Communication which had stressed interpretation was replaced with the need for emotional awareness and a relationship reflective of the unconscious processes of oneself and others, while focusing on the patient's current affective and cognitive capacities. Ferenczi became the "founder of all relationship-based psychoanalysis" (Haynal, 2002, p. xi). Psychoanalysis changed from a "one-person" to a "two-person" dimension. Many relational analysts see Ferenczi as the first analyst to have an impact on relational theory (Aron, 1991).

"Right Down to the Mothers": The Early Object Relationship

In his *Clinical Diary*, Ferenczi urged that the level of the mother-child relationship be reached in psychoanalysis, that is, "right down to the mothers" (1932/1988, p. 74). A psychodynamic approach focused on the Oedipus complex expanded borders. Disorders borne of a deficit were added to conflict-based ones.

In an optimal case, after birth, an infant's environment satisfies its needs and offers a substitute "to the child for the intrauterine happiness lost after birth" (A. Bálint, 1933/1993, p. 31). Ferenczi called this state passive object love. Alice and Michael Balint referred to it as the archaic relationship, or primary love, and specified it as primary object love. At this early stage, the baby can receive love unconditionally: "I shall be loved and satisfied, without being under any obligation to give anything in return" (M. Balint, 1949, p. 269).

Ferenczi was referring to the problem of a deficit in the early relationship in his discussion of the "unwelcome child" (Ferenczi, 1929/1980d, p. 104). He noted that adult circulatory disorders and asthmatic diseases stem from the mother's early rejection of the infant—whether prenatal or postpartum:

> Children who are received in a harsh and unloving way die easily and willingly. Either they use one of the many proffered organic possibilities for a quick exit, or if they escape this fate, they retain a streak of pessimism and aversion to life.
>
> (1929/1980d, p. 105)

Winnicott later made a similar observation: "A baby can be fed without love, but loveless or impersonal management cannot succeed in producing a new, autonomous human child" (1971, p. 108). As Brett puts it, "Numerous contemporary psychotherapeutic authors … regard Ferenczi as Winnicott's spiritual precursor in many respects" (2016, p. 215).

In Ferenczi's and the Balints' understanding, the infant operates via object relations:

> In all these instances we are faced with active behaviour on the part of the infant, even with an activity directed towards an object. The fact must also be noted that, contrary to common parlance, the child is not suckled; indeed, it sucks actively.
>
> (Balint, 1949, p. 269)

Beyond Ferenczi and the Balints, Imre Hermann was another Budapest representative of the early relationship. He stressed the primary mother-infant relationship as a mother-child unit or a dual unity borne of an instinctual desire for physical contact, or, as he termed it, the clinging instinct. He had noticed that primate infants spend a few months clinging to their mother and that human infants suffer from being separated too early after birth from the mother-child unit. Here we also observe the Moro reflex as the very early grasping reflex of the baby in this phenomenon.

The common denominator among the Budapest analysts was that they recognized the importance of the early mother-infant relationship (Bowlby, 1958). From the outset, Ferenczi and the Balints viewed it in terms of object relations, while Hermann said it was based on drive: the infant only comes in contact with his or her environment later. The two approaches lead to different psychopathological conclusions, such as with the question of primary and secondary narcissism. According to Ferenczi and the Balints, narcissism is a consequence of the unsatisfied mother-infant/mother-child relationship; that is, "if I am not loved sufficiently by the world, not given enough gratification, I must love and gratify myself. The clinically observable narcissism is, therefore, always a protection against the bad or only reluctant object" (Balint, 1949, p. 269). They therefore reject primary narcissism, "according to which all emotional interest was centred originally on oneself, and only later experiences forced or enticed the individual to detach some of his love from himself and turn it towards part of his environment" (Balint, 1987, p. 66).

René A. Spitz, who had heard Ferenczi's lectures in Budapest, drew attention to the serious consequences of a deficit in early object relations. He emigrated from Hungary in 1919, was later forced to leave Paris, and finally settled in America. He described hospitalization syndrome (Spitz, 1945) and anaclitic depression after his observations in various institutions (Spitz & Wolf, 1946). Spitz made documentaries based on his research, which changed the protocol at American hospitals: the parent was now allowed to be present with the child.

After she had left Budapest, Benedek made her very early mother-infant observations in a hospital in the 1920s. She concluded that a powerful affective—we would now say reflective—relationship developed between them, specifically, that infants show their mother's symptoms. According to attachment theories, mothers and infants form an affective communication system from the beginning of life.

What about Melanie Klein within the context of the Budapest school? How does her object relations theory fit into the system of thinking espoused by the Budapest school—or not? In 1912, Klein turned to Ferenczi for help with her depression and marital difficulties and saw him for analysis between 1914 and 1919. It was Ferenczi who suggested child observation to her and recommended that she treat children with psychoanalysis. She became a member of the Hungarian Psychoanalytical Society after presenting her paper "The Development of the Child" in 1919 (Klein, 1923). It was also Ferenczi who introduced her to Karl Abraham, and she emigrated to Berlin in 1921. Later, Klein continued her analysis with Abraham for eight months.

As regards the early mother-baby relationship, Ferenczi's and the Balints' early mother-child relationship was absolutely different from Klein's approach. Ferenczi and the Balints supported "the theory ... of *primary object relations or primary love*, which maintains that a healthy child and a healthy mother are so well adapted to each other that the same action inevitably brings gratification to both" (Balint, 1987, p. 65). According to the Budapest group, a baby demonstrates pathological reactions as a consequence of inappropriate treatment. The Kleinian starting point is the opposite: the newborn must overcome the tension between the life and death instinct, in which "sadistic instinctual impulses may arise ... without the influence of the external world, as the manifestations of the death instinct turned outside" (Balint, 1949, p. 266).

Paradigm Shift in Trauma Theory

Ferenczi and Rank realized that, in the safety of the therapeutic relationship, reliving instead of merely remembering traumatic events is a key element of therapeutic effectiveness (Ferenczi & Rank, 1924). A new atmosphere develops in the analytic situation based on authentic, reflective communication (Ferenczi, 1928/1980c; Hoffer, 1996). Ferenczi arrived at a paradigm shift in trauma theory in the early 1930s: a combination of the intrapsychic model with interpersonal object relations approaches (Mészáros, 2010b). Elements of his trauma theory can be found in a study which is both his most cited today and his last, *Confusion of Tongues between Adults and the Child* (Ferenczi, 1933/1980e). Although it is based on sexual abuse of children at the hands of adults, its observations apply to a broad spectrum of trauma.

Ferenczi highlights that trauma is a real event. In contrast to Freud's second trauma theory, it is not fantasy that causes trauma. A traumatic experience is subjective. The analyst accepts the subjective truth of experiences—as psychic reality—and does not question their truth content. When an adult abuses a child's need for tenderness, it is not only the sexual abuse that causes the trauma, but also the loss of trust. The child is most commonly unable to turn to his or her environment for help because he or she will only experience rejection or blame. Ferenczi recognized that the presence or lack of a trusted person is a decisive factor in processing the trauma later, whether the traumatization occurred in a family or a religious, school or sports community or, more broadly, on a societal level. These recognitions can be applied to such phenomena as PTSD and transgenerational trauma.

Reading Ferenczi, it becomes clear that trauma is a process that shows signs of a system of object relations. In his last paper, Balint calls the aggressor the "traumatogenic object" (Balint, 1969, p. 431). Ferenczi made a—still—very important recognition in differentiating between the victim's and the aggressor's ego defense mechanisms: he pointed to denial, minimization, and projection on the aggressor's side and, on the victim's, dissociation and identification with the aggressor. This last mechanism was a major discovery for Ferenczi. When there is no chance to escape,

> Anxiety ... if it reaches a certain maximum, compels [the victims] to subordinate themselves like automata to the will of the aggressor ... Through identification ... [the aggressor] disappears as part of external reality, and becomes intra- instead of extra-psychic.
>
> (Ferenczi, 1933/1980e, p. 162)

Unfortunately, identification with the aggressor has another long-term dark side: it allows the possibility of repetition and creates the illusion that the aggressor has been tamed. Later, identification with the aggressor became well-known as Stockholm Syndrome (1973).

It was certainly Ferenczi who first noted the resilient child phenomenon. Using the metaphor of the "wise baby," he described the traumatized child who grows up and is suddenly mature, more mature than any of his or her peers or even the adults who have traumatized him or her. Ferenczi describes a "*traumatic progression*, ... a *precocious maturity* ... It is not only emotionally that the trauma can bring a part of the person to maturity but also *intellectually*" (Ferenczi, 1933/1980e, p. 165). One can view traumatic progression as a keyword in the development of resilience. Later, the term resilience appeared sporadically in the literature from the late 1940s until we find it with increasing frequency in Bowlby's studies. However, systematic research of resilient children only came out after the late 1980s. Ferenczi's concept of trauma led to new approaches that would later emerge in the complex system of modern trauma theory and therapy.

Psychoanalytic Psychosomatics

Psychoanalytic psychosomatics developed in Budapest through the activity of Ferenczi, Lajos Lévy, and Michael Balint. Ferenczi saw the body as a surface for the manifestation of unconscious phenomena. His friend Georg Groddeck in Baden Baden emphasized that disease itself is a secret confession. Ferenczi was convinced that knowledge of psychoanalysis was crucial for family physicians. Invited by the Košice Medical Society (in present-day Slovakia), he gave a lecture in the early 1920s entitled "Psychoanalysis in the Service of the Practicing Physician" (Ferenczi, 1923/2007). This approach piqued Balint's interest, resulting in "Psychoanalysis and Internal Medicine" (Bálint, 1926). Lévy, a charismatic internist, aptly said that "We must get to know the physical and psychological personality of the patient. After all, the physician's task is to cure the patient, not the illness" (Lévy, 1933/1993, p. 301). In London, Balint developed the method of training-cum-research seminars for general practitioners, which became known as the Balint method or Balint group, and published his findings in his book, *The Doctor, the Patient and the Illness* (Balint, 1957).

In Chicago, Alexander developed psychoanalytic psychosomatics from the 1930s and put it in the focus at the Chicago Institute he had established.

Psychoanalytic Anthropology

Géza Róheim, the ethnographer and psychoanalyst, created a new interdisciplinary field in the 1920s: psychoanalytic anthropology. Freud awarded him a prize in 1921 for the best paper in applied analysis for his study on Australian totemism. After his forced emigration to America, Roheim continued his research with Native Americans. Roheim was strongly linked to the views of the Budapest school and thus to the overarching significance of the mother-child relationship in every culture. He demonstrated the universality of the Oedipus complex and the general validity of Freud's dream theory through his expeditions. His last book, *The Gates of the Dream*, explores the relationship between culture and dreams (Roheim, 1952).

Supervision, Psychoanalytic Institutions, and Training Programs

Ferenczi emphasized the necessity of analysts undergoing more analysis than their patients—a notion that was far from contemporary practice—so that their own pathology would not thwart their work with their patients. This is what motivated him, when, at Elizabeth Severn's prodding during a stalled phase of the analysis, he agreed to experiment with mutual analysis. This produced two results. Ferenczi experienced that mutual analysis does not work, but he also understood that analysis must reach the level of the mother-child relationship. He thus called for a better didactic analysis. It was his student, Vilma Kovács, who wrote about "training and control analysis" (1933/1936). What made control analysis unique was that when "the analysand was developed enough to start a first analysis, [she] proposed to include supervision in the analytic process" (Kovács, 1933/1936, p. 351). This became known as the Hungarian method. The aim was to better distinguish the analyst's own inner processes in working with patients. At that time, it was a sensible recommendation, which drew a great deal of criticism later.

The Budapest psychoanalysts shared their accumulated knowledge in founding institutions, teaching in training programs, and serving as presidents of psychoanalytic societies in Europe, America, and Australia. Mention should be made in particular of Sandor Rado, who established the Columbia University Center for Psychoanalytic Training and Research (1945), and Franz Alexander, who founded the Chicago Institute for Psychoanalysis (1932). David Rapaport also had an enormous impact on clinical psychology research, and Clara Lazar Geroe established the Melbourne Institute for Psychoanalysis (1941).

Elected presidents of the New York Psychoanalytic Society were: Sandor Lorand (1947–1948), Robert Bak (1957–1959), and Endre Peto (1975–1977). Michael Balint (1968–1970) served as president of the British Psychoanalytic Society.

From Microphenomena to Macrostructures

As we have seen, members of the Budapest school contributed to the formation of modern theoretical, therapeutic, and educational systems and had an impact on modern psychoanalysis on many continents.

A sensitive observer of intrapsychic and interpersonal processes, Ferenczi established—or contributed his perspective to—institutional structures that have remained significant to the present day. Beyond establishing the Hungarian Psychoanalytical Society as the cradle of the Budapest school, Ferenczi also expanded the psychoanalytic movement internationally. He conceived of the idea of forming the IPA in 1910. He later said, "Of course, I still see my most enduring creation as the International Psychoanalytic Association, to which I gave life" (Ferenczi, 1928/2006, p. 206). He founded the *International Journal of Psychoanalysis* in 1920. These two basic forums for the international psychoanalytic community have been active for over 100 years. Despite the short life of the department of psychoanalysis, he showed that psychoanalysis has a rightful place in academia generally and in the medical curriculum in particular. When Ferenczi spent eight months in the United States (1926–1927) by invitation of the New School for Social Research, he influenced psychoanalysts there, such as Harry Stack Sullivan. In New York, Ferenczi supported lay analysis, drawing no small resistance. In addition, he became influential through his American analysands who visited him in Budapest, including Clara Thompson, Izette de Forest, and Elizabeth Severn. He also carried out supervision with de Forest and Lewis Hill. Thompson and Sullivan went on to become founding members of the still-active William Alanson White Institute in New York.

Finally, it is important to note that a Ferenczi Renaissance over the past 40 years has enabled the Budapest school to take its rightful place in the history of psychoanalysis. Further, Ernest Jones's rivalry with Ferenczi and the conflict between Freud and Ferenczi in Ferenczi's final years paved the way for Jones's successful whisper campaign against Ferenczi after his unexpected death from pernicious anemia in 1933. Jones's false rumor about Ferenczi's madness undermined the credibility of Ferenczi's later writings. This was only intensified by Jones's decades-long powerful influence in the psychoanalytic movement as the president of the British society and the IPA in addition to being Freud's biographer. The spread of fascism and World War II shook the entire psychoanalytic community and distracted attention from Ferenczi. It was thus difficult to hear the sporadic denials of the rumor from Roheim, Balint, and Erich Fromm. Fascism and the subsequent influence of Soviet ideology then annihilated the Eastern European psychoanalytic societies.

The missing link to Ferenczi has been noticed again by peers from the 1980s. The Freud–Ferenczi, Ferenczi–Groddeck, and Ferenczi–Jones correspondences were published, as were theretofore missing Ferenczi publications, such as the *Clinical Diary*. Thanks to four decades of research by generations of the Ferenczi Renaissance, tens of thousands of articles and books published in a number of languages have shed light on the legacy of Ferenczi and the Budapest school.

11. Sándor Ferenczi, the Budapest School of Psychoanalysis, and the Ferenczi Tradition	
Main, general underlying assumptions	1 The early mother-infant/child relationship. Having developed as object relations, this communication system is in operation from the beginning of life. The mother plays a vital interactive role in modulating the infant's affective states. This is one of the basic concepts of attachment theory. 2 The transference-countertransference dynamic. It has become a basic process in all dynamic psychotherapies; it reflects and represents the patient's basic object relations in his/her past. 3 Ferenczi's trauma concept. It opened the door to understanding the role of the ego defense mechanisms of the victim and the aggressor in trauma, from the individual to the societal level, including transgenerational processes. He described the phenomenon of traumatic progression that could be the precursor to resilience.
Specific theoretical assumptions	
psychic structure	Early object relations, as the Budapest school pointed out from the mid-1920s, influence psychic development structurally. Non-appropriate early object relations lie in the background of narcissistic disorders.

(*Continued*)

energy	An unsatisfactory early mother-infant relationship, unwelcome child position, or early separation can diminish the energy necessary for maintaining life/survival.
relationships	The Budapest school (Ferenczi and the Balints) was formed by non-instinct-driven object relations, but Hermann described the primary mother-infant relationship as a dual unity borne of an instinctive desire for physical contact: the clinging instinct. A reflective attitude on the part of the analyst has created a two-person psychology in the psychoanalytic process. Two-person psychology: Integrating countertransference into the psychoanalytic process changed the interpersonal relationship during analysis. A reflective attitude on the part of the analyst strengthened the trust in the patient to be able to reach the emotional level of traumatic events, which is the basic ingredient for change. This lies at the heart of relationship-based psychotherapies.
developmental stages	N/A
body	The body is a reflective surface of the inner psychic process. Psychoanalytic psychosomatics: the physician's task is to cure the patient, not the illness.
anxieties/instincts and defenses	Ferenczi's trauma theory recognized the different ego defense mechanisms of the victim and the aggressor. A new defense mechanism was discovered: identification with the aggressor (seen later as Stockholm syndrome).
Assumptions concerning etiology	An inappropriate mother-infant, or, in a broader sense, infant-environment, relationship has a long-term effect. Therefore, a narcissistic personality disorder is a consequence (secondary narcissism), not a starting point (primary narcissism). An emotional deficit in the early infant-mother/caretaker relationship influences personality development and leads to psychic disorders. (See later attachment theories.) The consequence of a longer separation of a child during the first two-and-a-half years could result in anaclitic depression, hospitalization syndrome, psychosomatic illness, and even death. The emotional rejection of a child forms the background for psychosomatic illnesses and apathy in adulthood. The basic fault constitutes part of the etiology of personality disorders and borderline syndromes.

(*Continued*)

Implications for technique	Ferenczi's experimentation with techniques for a more effective healing process included the active technique and mutual analysis, both of which he discarded. Countertransference has become an indispensable technique. A reflective attitude on the part of the analyst has created a two-person psychology in the psychoanalytic process. Supervision has become part of the process. This so-called Hungarian method has also generated welcome debate.
Subsequent developments of the core concept	Sándor Ferenczi and the Budapest school of psychoanalysis had a great influence on psychoanalysis, including theory, practice, education, and the movement as a whole. Innovations put in place by members of the school have been integrated into modern psychoanalysis and, more generally speaking, into all dynamic psychotherapies. Psychoanalytic anthropology: Principles of the psychoanalytic approach include the universality of the Oedipus complex, early mother-child object relations, and dream interpretation.

References

Aron, L. (1991). The patient's experience of the analyst's subjectivity. *Psychoanalytic Dialogue*, *1*(1), 29–51.

Bálint, A. (1993). A szeretet fejlődése és a valóságérzék [The development of love and a sense of reality]. (Reprint) Párbeszéd Kiadó, T-Twins Kiadó, 30–40. (Original work published 1933.)

Balint, A., & Balint, M. (1939). On transference and counter-transference. *International Journal of Psychoanalysis*, *2*, 223–230.

Bálint, M. (1926). Psychoanalysis és belgyógyászat [Psychoanalysis and internal medicine]. *Gyógyászat*, *66*(19), 439–445.

Balint, M. (1949). Early developmental states of the ego: Primary object love. *International Journal of Psychoanalysis*, *30*, 265–273.

Balint, M. (1957). *The doctor, his patient and the illness*. Pitman Medical.

Balint, M. (1969). Trauma and object relationship. *International Journal of Psychoanalysis*, *50*, 429–435.

Balint, M. (1979). *The basic fault*. Tavistock Publications.

Balint, M. (1987). *Thrills and regressions*. Karnac.

Borgogno, F. (2019). Sándor Ferenczi, a classical and contemporary psychoanalyst. *American Journal of Psychoanalysis*, *79*(4), 453–467.

Bowlby, J. (1958). The nature of the child's tie to his mother. *International Journal of Psychoanalysis*, *39*, 350–373.

Brett, K. (2016). *Tea with Winnicott*. Karnac.

Deutsch, H. (1926). Okkulte Vorgänge während der Psychoanalyse [Occult processes in psychoanalysis]. *Imago*, *12*, 418–433.

Erős, F. (2019). Sándor Ferenczi, Géza Róheim and the University of Budapest, 1918–19. *Psychoanalysis and History*, *21*(1), 5–22.

Falzeder, E. (Ed.) (2002). *The complete correspondence of Sigmund Freud and Karl Abraham 1907–1925*. Karnac.

Falzeder, E., & Brabant, E. (Eds.) (1996). *The correspondence of Sigmund Freud and Sándor Ferenczi. Volume 2, 1914–1919*. Harvard University Press.

Ferenczi, S. (1980a). Psychoanalysis and education. In M. Balint (Ed.), *Final contributions to the problems and methods of psycho-analysis* (pp. 280–290). Maresfield Reprints. (Original work published 1908.)

Ferenczi, S. (1980b). On the technique of psycho-analysis. In M. Balint (Ed.), *Further contributions to the theory and technique of psycho-analysis* (pp. 177–189). Maresfield Reprints. (Original work published 1919.)

Ferenczi, S. (1980c). The elasticity of psycho-analytic technique. In M. Balint (Ed.), *Final contributions to the problems and methods of psycho-analysis* (pp. 87–101). Maresfield Reprints. (Original work published 1928.)

Ferenczi, S. (1980d). The unwelcome child and his death instinct. In M. Balint (Ed.), *Final contributions to the problems and methods of psycho-analysis* (pp. 102–107). Maresfield Reprints. (Original work published 1929.)

Ferenczi, S. (1980e). Confusion of tongues between adults and the child. In M. Balint (Ed.), *Final contributions to the problems and methods of psycho-analysis* (pp. 156–167). Maresfield Reprints. (Original work published 1933.)

Ferenczi, S. (1988). *The clinical diary*. (Ed. J. Dupont). Harvard University Press. (Original work published 1932.)

Ferenczi, S. (2006). A szerelem végső titkai [The ultimate secrets of love]. *Thalassa*, *17*(2–3), 203–206. (Original work published 1928.)

Ferenczi, S. (2007). A pszichoanalízis a gyakorló orvos szolgálatában [Psychoanalysis in the service of the practicing physician]. *Thalassa*, *1*, 107–117. (Original work published 1923.)

Ferenczi, S., & Rank, O. (1924). *Entwicklungsziele der Psychoanalyse. Zur Wechselbeziehung von Theorie und Praxis [The developmental aims of psychoanalysis: On the interrelationship between theory and practice]*. Internationaler Psychoanalytischer Verlag.

Freud, S. (1910). The future prospects of psycho-analytic therapy. In J. Strachey (Ed. and Trans.), *The standard edition of the complete works of Sigmund Freud* (Vol. 11, pp. 139–152). Hogarth Press.

Glover, E. (1927). Lectures on technique in psycho-analysis. *International Journal of Psychoanalysis*, *8*, 504–520.

Haynal, A. (1988). *The technique at issue: Controversies in psychoanalysis from Freud and Ferenczi to Michael Balint*. Karnac.

Haynal, A. (2002). *Disappearing and reviving: Sándor Ferenczi in the history of psychoanalysis*. Karnac.

Hoffer, A. (1996). Asymmetry and mutuality in the analytic relationship: Contemporary lessons from the Freud-Ferenczi dialogue. In P. L. Rudnytsky, A. Bókay, & P. Giampieri-Deutsch (Eds.), *Ferenczi's turn in psychoanalysis* (pp. 107–119). New York University Press.

Kovács, V. (1936). Training- and control-analysis. *International Journal of Psycho-Analysis*, *17*, 346–354. (Original work published 1933.)
Klein, M. (1923). The development of a child. *International Journal of Psycho-Analysis*, *4*, 419–474.
Lévy, L. (1993). Mire figyeljünk szívbetegek anamnézisében? [What should we watch for in a cardiac patient's anamnesis?] In *Lélekelemzési tanulmányok* [Psychoanalytic Studies]. (pp. 297–311). Párbeszéd Kiadó, T-Twins Kiadó. (Original work published 1933.)
Martín Cabré, L. J. (1998). Ferenczi's contribution to the concept of counter-transference. *International Forum of Psychoanalysis*, *7*, 247–255.
Mészáros, J. (Ed.). (1999). *Ferenczi Sándor a pszichoanalízis felé. Fiatalkori írások 1897–1908 [Sándor Ferenczi before psychoanalysis: Early writings 1897–1908]*. Osiris.
Mészáros, J. (2010a). Progress and persecution in the psychoanalytic heartland: Antisemitism, communism and the fate of Hungarian psychoanalysis. *Psychoanalytic Dialogues*, *20*(5), 600–622.
Mészáros, J. (2010b). Building blocks toward contemporary trauma theory: Ferenczi's paradigm shift. *American Journal of Psychoanalysis*, *70*(4), 328–340.
Mészáros, J. (2014). *Ferenczi and beyond: Exile of the Budapest school and solidarity in the psychoanalytic movement during the Nazi years*. Karnac.
Paskauskas, R. A. (Ed.). (1993). *The complete correspondence of Sigmund Freud and Ernest Jones 1908–1939*. Belknap Press of Harvard University Press.
Roheim, G. (1952). *The gates of the dream*. International Universities Press.
Spitz, R. A. (1945). Hospitalism: An inquiry into the genesis of psychiatric conditions in early childhood. *Psychoanalytic Study of the Child*, *1*, 53–74.
Spitz, R. A., & Wolf, K. M. (1946). Anaclitic depression: An inquiry into the genesis of psychiatric conditions in childhood. *Psychoanalytic Study of the Child*, *2*, 313–342.
Winnicott, D. W. (1971). *Playing and reality*. Tavistock Publications.

Chapter 12

Interpersonal Psychoanalysis

Miri Abramis

Interpersonal psychoanalysis refers to the school of psychoanalysis that emerged from the eclectic group of thinkers known as the neo-Freudian or cultural school (see chapter by Roger Frie, this volume). The William Alanson White Institute became the home of interpersonal psychoanalysis, founded by Harry Stack Sullivan, Erich Fromm, Clara Thompson, Frieda Fromm-Reichman, and Janet and David Rioch in New York in 1943. This became the first organized attempt to move away from Freud's drive/structural model and provide a comprehensive psychoanalytic theory of its own, based on interpersonal relations and field theory (Greenberg & Mitchell, 1983).

Fromm's theorizing impediments to human potential imposed by social and economic forces made him a major influence in interpersonal thinking. Similarly, Thompson's early recognition of male privilege and the impact of gender-related expectations of the female psyche were essential to interpersonal theorizing, as was her integration of countertransference data in the "here and now." It is Harry Stack Sullivan, nonetheless, who is generally considered the "primordial father" of the interpersonal school (Levenson, 1992/2018a). Sullivan referred to his work as "interpersonal psychiatry," and unlike all other founders, was never formally trained in psychoanalysis. Sullivan began his work in the 1920s, using Freudian ideas with inpatients described as suffering from schizophrenia, patients not considered amenable to classical analysis, and later developed his thinking with patients struggling with problems of character. Sullivan's colleagues were most responsible for turning his "interpersonal psychiatry" into psychoanalysis. Sullivan died early in 1949 without having compiled his work into a complete text. His followers collated his many presentations and famous personal notebooks into several volumes; tragically, his posthumously written works reflect exacting detail and often tortured prose making them a difficult read. Sullivan's brilliant integration of social systems thinking with psychiatry, however, has lived on in the interpersonal tradition, and an unacknowledged background of much contemporary psychoanalysis.

Despite theoretical and personal differences, the founders of the interpersonal school were united in their opposition to a classical Freudian

DOI: 10.4324/9781003027768-13

theory that emphasized the primacy of endogenous libidinal and aggressive drives and defenses against these drives. This eclectic group of colleagues worked to present a corrective to a psychoanalysis that did not fully recognize the exogenous experience. They thought libido theory was fundamentally wrong in understanding human motivation, the unconscious, and the nature of experience, and therefore misleading in psychoanalytic theorizing and clinical technique (Greenberg & Mitchell, 1983, p. 80). They shared a common belief that interpersonal relations from the beginning of life, lived out in social and cultural context, *must* be integrated into a psychoanalytic theory to account for the origins, development, and "warping" of the personality. The pioneers of interpersonal theory rejected determinist and mechanistic understanding of psychic structure, each adding her own perspective on culture and our fundamental relational existence. They were deeply skeptical of universal and formulaic explanations for the development of personality. Sullivan rejected Freud's theoretical abstractions (i.e., id, ego, superego) in favor of what could be operationalized. Whereas Freud's model focused on the need to tame sexuality and aggression to fit the social, Sullivan's model highlighted the influence of the social on the personality, and our ability to live and get along in society. Sexuality was one among many human motivations; its individual expression formed in the context of relations with key others and in the culture and society at large. Destructive emotions develop in response to anger engendered with significant others, and the social world. Fantasy, per se, did not particularly interest Sullivan. Instead, rather than as the *source* of pathology, fantasy is considered an imaginative construction, a highly personalized creative ability to grapple with real problems with significant others (Bromberg, 2008; Tauber & Green, 1959/2006).

The theorizing behind interpersonal psychoanalysis reflected a fundamental shift in the Western intellectual zeitgeist, an altered frame of reference from the deterministic, mechanistic machine model of Freud's time to a communication paradigm for the information age (Levenson, 1983/2005). This new frame of reference was directly brought into clinical work and practice by Sullivan who was a voracious reader and autodidact who openly acknowledges the many "tributaries" to his ideas. He integrated vast works from 20th-century psychiatry, psychoanalysis, and the American philosophical school of pragmatism at the University of Chicago, especially the work on symbolic interaction in sociology (George Herbert Mead and C. H. Cooley) and the study of communication and linguistics (Edward Sapir). Sullivan also openly acknowledges the important influence of cultural perspectivism in anthropology (Ruth Benedict). From these varied threads, Sullivan wove a psychiatry that looked at what people do with one another, how we communicate through word and gesture, how we come into being, develop capacities for interaction and create symbolic worlds that shape lived experience and behavior. The result is a two-person psychology, which speaks to development as much as to problems of living and a therapeutic method for their amelioration.

For the purposes of this chapter, I will not be able to describe in depth the numerous threads woven into interpersonal psychoanalysis for there is no monolithic interpersonal psychoanalysis, but I will discuss the major assumptions and work that link contemporary interpersonal psychoanalysis to the transforming ideas of its founders. Contemporary interpersonal psychoanalytic praxis largely reflects Edgar Levenson's invaluable critique and extension of Sullivan, compiled in his writings from the 1960s until 2018 (Hirsch, 1992). Levenson, more than any other thinker, has grappled with Sullivan and the founders. He has more fully articulated interpersonalism as the "communication-field theory paradigm," adding his incisive observations and reflections, clarifying, and vitalizing interpersonal thought.

Main Assumptions of Interpersonal Psychoanalysis

Embedded in Communal Existence

The human can only be understood as embedded in interpersonal social systems, beginning with infant and caregiver, family, school, community, and country. Life depends on maintaining constant exchange with the necessary environment. Sullivan argued that it is not our physical being or instinctual drives that make us distinctly human, rather it is our unique capacities for awareness and organization of interpersonal experience, for symbolism, language, and culture.

Communication Is Fundamental to Communal Existence

How we communicate, verbally and nonverbally, shapes our subjective experience of self and other. In the communication-field paradigm, speech is only one part of the extensive semiotic, nonverbal coded cuing that allows individuals to be understood, characterizing the complex communication between individuals and in the consulting room. Interpersonal communication requires learning complex cognitive and social skills, as each social system has its own culture with rules, roles, and meanings, communicated implicitly and explicitly. All human interaction can only be understood in the unique cultural and social context in which complex communication occurs.

Awareness and Subjectivity are Rooted in the Sensorimotor Organization of Interpersonal Experience

Sullivan conceptualizes our animal being as *becoming* human through active engagement with others from the beginning of life. It is what we *do* with one another that provides the foundations for our developing sense of self with other, self-esteem and inner life, and the functioning of our minds. The growing human organism is sensing, learning, and creating, working to make sense of experience. Sullivan recognized that in the early months of life, the infant's cognitive sensorimotor capacities mature, especially perception, recall, and foresight. Awareness expands, subjectivity evolves, and the infant begins to organize and anticipate what he calls "me-you" patterns of interaction. With further maturation, language emerges from relational experience and is used to communicate (or obscure) and master social experience.

Pathology is Rooted in Disruptions in Communication or the "Mystification" of Experience

In Sullivan's theorizing, beginning at birth, the collaborative integration of infant and caregiver needs is disrupted *solely* by the transmission of anxiety from the "mothering one." When the mother is anxious, the caregiver's tenderness and competence at meeting infant needs are replaced by what Sullivan calls vaguely an "unempathic" presence. The nursing infant may have an experience of a "bad nipple," for example, not because the nipple is bad, but because through sensorimotor experience such as subtleties of voice or muscle tone, the mother's anxiety is conveyed through "empathic connection" to her infant. As the infant matures, and the experience becomes more organized and can be anticipated, physical actions of the mothering one become signs of impending anxiety. With anxiety transmission, the infant's communicative bids bring no satisfying integrations of infant and maternal needs. On the contrary, the mothering one is unable to communicate tenderly, unable to soothe, and instead, may exacerbate infant distress, fear, detachment, or disorganization. These disintegrating tendencies (as opposed to collaborative integrating tendencies) break down relatedness, impinging on the growing child's way of relating to the outside world. With repetition, these experiences create vulnerability to pathology and, in Sullivan's thinking, are the basis of what brings patients to treatment.

Sullivan gave a prominent role in his theorizing of an idiosyncratic understanding of anxiety in the organization of human experience. It is caregiver anxiety that *causes* the disruption of experience. As part of its sensorimotor engagement, through what Sullivan calls the "self-system," the growing infant/child is hypervigilant to caregiver anxiety, and threats to self esteem. The child seeks to avoid the threats and anxietyatall costs. Psychic organization requires tender integration of needs *and* the related maintenance of self-esteem. Levenson (1992/2018a) has criticized and altered Sullivan's conceptualization of anxiety. He argues instead that anxiety and overwhelm are caused by a significant disruption in communication in the sensorimotor interpersonal field; further, the growing child's need to avoid parental anxiety is tantamount to a drive in his theorizing and unnecessary in a pure communication paradigm. Rather than a self-system, Levenson suggests that self is better conceptualized as a human emergent property exploring its own potential for learning and creating (Levenson, 1984/2017). Even with these caveats, sensitivity to anxiety in others and the disorganizing impact of felt anxiety on the organization of experience plays a central role in interpersonal theorizing about pathology and treatment.

Utilizing Levenson's clarification of the communication-field theory paradigm, if the caregiver does not appropriately perceive communicative cues and intention, the infant experience is confused or mystified. Such disruptions may include incoherent or conflicting messages. These disturbances in communication may reflect an overwhelming interpersonal mismatch that cannot be comprehended, grossly inhibiting recall and foresight. Such disruptions cause disorganizing anxiety that cannot be psychically integrated, resulting in alterations in awareness and subjective experience. The organism responds by initiating various adaptive measures, "security operations" in behavior and later reflected in language, as a means of altering awareness of the confusion and felt aversive experience. The infant/child may change state, for example, shifting into what Sullivan called "somnolent detachment," a sleep-like dissociation. The child may also alter experience with cognitive distortion or what Sullivan called "parataxic" distortion, or the infant's attempts to grapple with confusing experience. In the quest to figure out what is going on, in uniquely personal ways (i.e., fantasy or distortion) the child grapples with real experience, which helps to predict the situations that previously caused the disturbance. Such parataxic distortions may serve to protect the person in the present, but later will lead to misreading of semiotic cues and intention, and prove highly resistant to new learning.

The "classic" security operation for Sullivan is "selective inattention" as a means of altering awareness and maintaining self-esteem. Selective inattention refers to not remembering, not wanting to know what one obviously perceives, yet may elicit anxiety and discomfort in needed others and the self. More extreme, if interpersonal disruption is catastrophic, the organism can just not see, rather she becomes overwhelmed and may dissociate. This experience that cannot be integrated becomes "not me." Sullivan is reengaging the traumatic experience that Freud left behind. Dissociation is a response to traumatic experience, and the unawareness is total. Such experience may escalate into terror, what Sullivan likened to a "blow to the head," overwhelming the mind and derailing interpersonal collaboration. In later life, such trauma is haunting and can illicit revived "uncanny" overwhelming emotional experience.

Development

The interpersonal theory of development comprises the unfolding of relational life and the organization of experience. Sullivan's developmental approach draws a thread from infancy to adulthood (Sullivan, 1953). He focuses on attempts to get needs met through our engagement with others and the development of patterns of interaction, which may allow for flexibility, growth, and more mature forms of intimacy, or alternatively, foster rigidity and psychic/social isolation. If based on non-reciprocal "disintegration" of needs, these "me-you" patterns are recreated in later interaction and close off the opportunities for reintegration of positive experience. These patterns also manifest themselves in subjective experience of self: "good-me" (positive appraisals), "bad-me" (negative or anxiety-causing appraisals), and "not-me" (dissociated experience).

Each developmental era in Sullivan's model reflects the organization of embodied experience in interaction with needed others, the unfolding of physical, social, and cognitive competencies and changing needs of the growing child and social surround, and the adjustment to culturally shaped values and opportunities in the social world. For psychoanalysis, Sullivan's developmental model was new in emphasizing learning and growth beyond the family, and the possibility of reworking early disruptions of experience in later relations, rather than development set in stone. Sullivan's model reflects an early appreciation of an infant prewired for social experience and learning, requiring the integration of caregiver interactions for ongoing development. Satisfying capacity to live among others depends on interpersonal learning and honing social cognition during development, especially the ability to appropriately read social cues and communicate one's needs. Sullivan also pays special attention to the influence of acculturation and socialization in development, first through caregivers and families as conscious and unconscious transmitters of culture, and with schooling, teachers, and peers offering essential learning opportunities about the functioning of social groups and new experiences and appraisals of the self. Sullivan's emphasizes that while pathology is linked to confusion in early intraction, societal oppression (i.e. racisim, antisemitism, or other hatreds) also warp human expereince and self-esteem Sullivan acknowledges that his theory is limited and openly calls for greater delineation and correction with the availability of new knowledge and ideas.

The Therapist Is Part of the Field She Studies

Despite our conscious referent and subjective sense of "I," we are always embedded in an interpersonal, social/cultural context. For this reason, Sullivan borrowed the anthropological term "participant-observer" to describe the role of the therapist. Based on his theory and the little clinical material Sullivan left, the therapist makes inferences about the patient's characteristic patterns of living (rather than intrapsychic dynamics) according to the therapist's observations of patient distortion in the "here and now" with the therapist, and on the detailed inquiry into the patient's relations with others. The essential question for the interpersonalist is not "what does this mean," but rather, "what's going on around here?" (Levenson, 1983/2005). What is the patient doing with the therapist? Through inquiry, Sullivan attended to the emergence of holes in the narrative, believed to reflect sources of interpersonal anxiety and threats to self-esteem that shut down awareness. Sullivan seemed to believe the therapist could remain the "expert" in interpersonal relations and take the impact of his own subjectivity out of the mix. Despite his theoretical claims to our being embedded in the social matrix, Levenson challenges Sullivan's conceptualization and his apparent disregard for the unique personality of the therapist. Instead, Levenson argues that despite our understanding or intention, the patient speaks and engages in her way in the analysis, and the therapist, from her own subjectivity and resonance, cannot help but selectively hear and decide what to respond to in the fundamental intersubjective matrix. Levenson transformed Sullivan's participant-observer to give equal attention to the analyst's inevitable, unconscious participation in the patient-therapist dyad (Stern, 2005, pp. v–xvi). Patient distortions based on earlier patterns of experience and exquisite attention to the analyst's needs and anxiety, make the analyst's intentions secondary. The meaning of a word or deed lies in its consequences, and how communication is experienced by the other. Countertransference from the interpersonal perspective is not simply the analyst's emotional reactions, but selective inattention, what she fails to notice, what she does not ask.

Enactment is Pervasive and an Essential Part of Analytic Work

The analyst as participant-observer has become subjective-participant-observer in an intersubjective field (Hirsch, 1996). The enactment in interpersonal clinical work is not an "error" to be minimized, but inevitable and essential. This is a seminal contribution of Levenson's extension of Sullivan's communication paradigm central to interpersonal praxis and has been integrated by relational psychoanalysts. As much as possible, the subjective analyst uses her participation (embodied experience in affect, thought, and action) to reflect upon and facilitate the patient elaboration of experience with the patient in the here and now, as well as an inquiry into idiosyncratic patterns of relating in all aspects of the patient's life. Levenson's incorporation of Sullivan's sensorimotor-rooted communications paradigm, and close attention to the "doing" of language and patterns of interaction in the patient-therapist matrix, led to his brilliant observation of a dialectical interaction between what is said in the analysis and what is done. Form recapitulates content. In the semiotic discourse, the language of speech and the language of action will replicate one another. The patterns of interaction revealed by what is said in language must also be *shown* in a genuine, authentic here-and-now engagement between patient and analyst (Levenson, 2009/2018b).

The Goal of Treatment Is the Expansion of Awareness

Sullivan's original goal of the analysis is the patient's seeing herself the way she is seen by others. The implication is the elaboration of experience and awareness, putting unformulated experience into words that are understandable to another person. The therapist facilitates the unpacking of the data through inquiry, especially into what does not quite make sense or what has been left out of the narrative, asking about the details of experience in relationships historically and in the present. Levenson adds that detailed inquiry gives the patient a nudge to deconstruct her own thoughts, thereby expanding her awareness and embodied experience of self. Through detailed inquiry, and the clarification of mutual influence in the here and now, the analyst will confront resistance, understood not as a defense against intrapsychic conflict or fantasy, but as a holding fast to patterns of experience, and deep loyalty to the family of origin that has become part of the self. In the pressure of the analytic communication field, the stuck dynamic is also experienced by the analyst, as she cannot help but become the unwitting participant in the relational configurations of the patient's life. Rigorous self-reflection into whom the analyst has become (what am I doing with this patient, in myself, and in the patient's history) may expand awareness, automatically facilitating an internal shift in the way the analyst engages the patient. The analyst may also invite the patient's perception of the analyst. Each contributes to the expansion of awareness through association and exploration of the fundamental interpersonal question, "What's going on around here?"

12. Interpersonal Psychoanalysis	
Main, general underlying assumptions	1 The human animal is embedded in communal existence. 2 Communication is fundamental to communal existence (includes explicit and implicit, verbal, and nonverbal, semiotic clues). 3 Awareness and subjectivity are rooted in the sensorimotor organization of interpersonal experience. 4 Pathology is rooted in disruptions in communication resulting in anxiety and threats to self-esteem.
Specific theoretical assumptions	
psychic structure	Rejection of reified structures of internal experience, in favor of process: learned patterns of relating played out in the analytic field, in dreams, fantasies, and out of the consulting room.

(Continued)

energy	• Sullivan's work was criticized by Levenson for making avoidance of anxiety and loneliness a motivational/energy source. Instead, Levenson argues for a pure communication paradigm that is more parsimonious and operational. • Sullivan's integration of a biological systems perspective allows for the essential principle of living systems: continuous impetus for coherence and complexity.
relationship	• Interpersonal relations from the beginning of life, lived out in social and cultural context, are integrated into psychoanalytic theory to account for the origins, development, and "warping" of the personality. • Exploring experience of patient and analyst in the room is central to contemporary interpersonal thought with the goal of expanding patient awareness of experience.
development stages and the body	• Epigenetic model of development: infancy, childhood, juvenile, pre-adolescence, adolescence and adulthood or maturity. Each era reflects the organization of embodied experience based on needed interactions with others, new capacities, and culturally shaped opportunities in the social world. • Need for intimacy and avoiding loneliness/ostracism is a constant.
anxieties/instincts and defenses	• Focus not on instinct but interpersonal relations. • In Sullivan, "security operations" (not defenses) are engendered to protect self and others from the experience of communicated anxiety. Levenson reinterpreted this as anxiety *caused by* an interpersonal experience that cannot be integrated into the psyche. • Anxiety and overwhelm lead to shutting down awareness of interpersonal experience ("selective inattention") and/or dissociation to maintain self-esteem and protect the relationship with needed others.
Assumptions concerning etiology	Pathology caused by disrupted and uncomprehended interpersonal experience that cannot be psychically integrated or put into words. Such disruption forecloses learning from experience.

(*Continued*)

Implications for technique	• Detailed inquiry and deconstruction of experience. • Explore intersubjective ongoing enactment of patient-therapist relationship with therapist attention to becoming part of patient's patterns of experience (what is going on around here?). • Observation and focus on process over the interpretation of content. • Goal of analysis as expansion of awareness of experience, facilitating the patient's inherent growth potential.
Subsequent developments of the core concept	• Edgar Levenson primary contributor to correction and extension of Sullivan's thinking. • Philip Bromberg's furthering of Sullivan's ideas about dissociation and trauma. • Jay Greenberg's integration of interpersonal thought into Freudian theory. • Steven Mitchell shifted focus from the communications paradigm to the integration of interpersonal thought with British object relations theory. • Don Stern's philosophical elaboration of unformulated experience

References

Bromberg, P. M. (2008). "Grown-up" words: An interpersonal/relational perspective on unconscious fantasy. *Psychoanalytic Inquiry*, *28*, 131–150.

Greenberg, J., & Mitchell, S. (1983). *Object relations in psychoanalytic theory*. Harvard University Press.

Hirsch, I. (1992). Extending Sullivan's interpersonalism. *Contemporary Psychoanalysis*, *28*, 732–747.

Hirsch, I. (1996). Observing participation, mutual enactment, and the new classical models. *Contemporary Psychoanalysis*, *32*, 359–383.

Levenson, E. (2005). *The fallacy of understanding (1972) and The ambiguity of change (1983)*. The Analytic Press.

Levenson, E. (2017). Harry Stack Sullivan. In A. Slomowitz (Ed.), *The purloined self: Interpersonal perspectives in psychoanalysis*. Routledge. (Original work published 1984).

Levenson, E. (2018a). Harry Stack Sullivan: From interpersonal psychiatry to interpersonal psychoanalysis. In A. Slomowitz (Ed.), *Interpersonal psychoanalysis and the enigma of consciousness*. Routledge. (Original work published 1992).

Levenson, E. (2018b). The enigma of transference. In A. Slomowitz (Ed.), *Interpersonal psychoanalysis and the enigma of consciousness*. Routledge. (Original work published 2009).

Stern, D. (2005). Introduction to the fallacy of understanding and the ambiguity of change. In E. Levenson (Ed.), *The fallacy of understanding (1972) and The ambiguity of change (1983)* (pp. 7–11). The Analytic Press.
Sullivan, H. S. (1953). *The interpersonal theory of psychiatry*. W. W. Norton.
Tauber, E., & Green, M. (2006). *Prelogical experience: An inquiry into dreams and other creative processes*. Analytic Press. (Original work published 1959).

Chapter 13

The Neo-Freudians

Roger Frie

Main Assumptions

Who Were the Neo-Freudians?

The term "neo-Freudian" is most often associated with psychoanalysts who sought to account for the primacy of social and cultural factors in human development. As a group, these psychoanalysts traced the etiology of neuroses to social and cultural experience, rather than biology, which distinguished them from Freud and the psychoanalytic mainstream. Erich Fromm, Frieda Fromm-Reichmann, Karen Horney, Abram Kardiner, Harry Stack Sullivan, and Clara Thompson are most often identified with neo-Freudianism, though there are many differences between them.

Fromm, Fromm-Reichmann, and Horney arrived in New York City from Germany in the early 1930s and worked with their American colleagues to establish institutes outside of the psychoanalytic mainstream. Fromm, Fromm-Reichman, Sullivan, and Thompson established the William Alanson White Institute of Psychiatry, Psychoanalysis and Psychology in 1943, which became the home of interpersonal psychoanalysis. Horney founded the American Institute of Psychoanalysis in 1941 and the Karen Horney Clinic was created in 1955 after her death. Abram Kardiner co-founded the Psychoanalytic and Psychosomatic Clinic for Training and Research in the Department of Psychiatry at Columbia University in New York in 1945. In what follows I will focus chiefly on the three main representatives of neo-Freudianism, Sullivan (1892–1949), Fromm (1900–1980), and Horney (1885–1952).

Cross-Disciplinary Outlook

The cross-disciplinary outlook developed by Sullivan, Fromm, and Horney during the 1930s helps explain their refashioning of many of Freud's basic assumptions. Sullivan was an American psychiatrist from New York State who received his medical degree from the Chicago College of Medicine and Surgery in 1917. He was steeped in the ideas of the American pragmatic

DOI: 10.4324/9781003027768-14

philosophers, and more specifically in the Chicago School of Sociology. Sullivan had a profound interest in understanding human experience in its social and cultural surround and focused on the role of interpersonal relationships in the etiology of neurosis and the formation of the personality. Beginning in 1938, he edited the innovative and radical journal, *Psychiatry: Journal of the Biology and Pathology of Interpersonal Relations*, which bridged the work of psychoanalytic psychiatry, social science, and the humanities. This cross-disciplinary outlook brought him into contact with Fromm and Horney.

Born in Frankfurt in 1900, Fromm completed his doctorate in sociology in Heidelberg in 1922 and subsequently became interested in psychoanalysis. He entered into an analytic treatment with Frieda Reichmann, which ended soon thereafter when they got married. Both were co-founders of the Southwest German Psychoanalytic Institute in Frankfurt in 1927. Fromm completed his psychoanalytic training at the Berlin Psychoanalytic Institute, where he was analyzed by Hanns Sachs, a disciple of Freud. In Berlin, Fromm met Karen Horney, a founding member of the Berlin Institute, who was also analyzed by Sachs. Horney completed her medical degree at the University of Berlin in 1913, one of the very few women to do so at the time. Horney's growing disagreements with Freud, together with changes in her personal life, led her to leave for the United States in 1932. She went first to Chicago, on the invitation of Franz Alexander, and then moved to New York in 1934, where she would meet Sullivan and be reunited with Fromm, who arrived in the city the same year.

Fromm's departure from Nazi Germany was initiated not by his differences with Freud, which were considerable, but by the fact that he was Jewish. During the years leading up to his departure, Fromm wrote about the changes in German society, particularly about authoritarian proclivities in the working class. A lecture he gave in Frankfurt on "Psychoanalysis and Sociology" was an attempt to create a convergence between Freud and Marx and brought him to the attention of the director of the Institute for Social Research, Max Horkheimer. Fromm was invited by him to join the Institute and was an early contributor to the social theory for which the Institute became known. By the time Horney and Fromm arrived in the United States, their questioning of the primacy of the intrapsychic realm and their left-wing political views set them apart from the American psychoanalytic mainstream. Increasingly isolated, they found a kindred spirit in Sullivan and together set out to develop a psychoanalytic alternative to the mainstream.

Psychoanalytic Anthropology

While neo-Freudian is the term that is often used to describe the combined work of Sullivan, Fromm, and Horney, a better description is the "cultural school of psychoanalysis" (Frie, 2014). Together, Sullivan, Fromm, and

Horney engaged in what might best be described as a "psychoanalytic anthropology" of human experience. Yet the pairing of psychoanalysis and anthropology was not easy. Psychoanalysis examined the individual mind and emphasized the universality of experience. Anthropologists, by contrast, were more likely to concern themselves with the social process of enculturation and cultural difference. In order to overcome these different perspectives, the cultural school of psychoanalysis focused on the interaction *between* the individual and culture, creating what became known as an "integrationist" approach.

The work of American psychoanalyst and anthropologist, Abram Kardiner (1891–1981), provided an early pathway for the cultural school. Kardiner was an analysand of Freud and a member of A. A. Brill's circle of American psychoanalysis during the 1920s. He had studied under Franz Boas, the founder of modern anthropology. Kardiner questioned the universality of drives and maintained that the impact of culture on human experience was always in evidence. Beginning in 1933, he organized an interdisciplinary seminar at the New York Psychoanalytic Institute and later at Columbia University, in which he worked with well-known anthropologists such as Ruth Benedict to develop a psycho-cultural model for personality formation in different societies. Along with Kardiner and Benedict, two other noted anthropologists, Margaret Mead and Edward Sapir, each sought to develop an interdisciplinary bridge with psychoanalysis. All were students of Boas at Columbia University and shared an interest in understanding how humans acquire culture and in the developmental interaction between the individual personality and culture.

Specific Assumptions

Psychic Structure

As a group, the neo-Freudians were interested in the social and cultural constitution of the individual, and did not engage in developing an intrapsychic model of the mind.

Energy

Neo-Freudians explained human experience in terms of society and culture, not in terms of biology and drives. In conjunction with Edward Sapir and the Culture and Personality Seminar at Yale University, Sullivan delimited biological drives and emphasized the importance of culture for interpersonal relations. In describing his interpersonal approach, Sullivan stated: "this is the antithesis of any document of human instincts" (Sullivan, 1950, p. 302). Sullivan presented human experience as an unfolding interaction between interpersonal, environmental influences, and a personal meaning system that shapes perception and responses. Sullivan wanted to know what a particular experience meant to a person, in addition to being interested in his patient's history and pattern of interpersonal experiences. The way in which a person experiences an event is determined by how the person comes to know the world, through the formulation of a set of ideas, assumptions, and imaginations, based on their development *and* environment.

Relationship

The notion of the relationship is central to the work of the neo-Freudians. Sullivan rejected the intrapsychic theory of mind and maintained that the individual person is fundamentally shaped by his or her interactions with other people. As Sullivan states:

> It makes no sense to think of ourselves as "individual," "separate," capable of anything like definitive description in isolation, that the notion is just beside the point .... The field of observation is what people do with each other, what they can communicate to each other about what they do with each other. When that is done, no such thing as a durable, unique, individual personality is ever clearly justified. For all I know every human being has as many personalities as he has interpersonal relations.
>
> (Sullivan, 1964, pp. 220–221)

For Sullivan, the self-process was located squarely in the interpersonal field, which included two-person interactions as well as the wider sociocultural sphere. Under the influence of Sapir, Sullivan noted the pervasive impact of culture on the formation of all psychological experiences. For Sullivan it was precisely the:

> Vast amounts of culture, of socially meaningful, rather than biologically meaningful, entities, which exert very powerful influence .... Human beings are human animals that have been filled with culture—socialized, if you like the word—in which process they move from the biological realm into the world of people.
>
> (Sullivan, 1964, p. 210)

Thus, we might say that Sullivan grants culture the same kind of primacy that Freud gave to biology.

Fromm likewise positioned the person within social and political relations, revealing their inalterable effect upon us. Fromm was interested in how unconscious social structures and forces shape the person. He posited a primary social relatedness that precedes the emergence of the individual. Fromm maintained that the intrapsychic realm was secondary to the interpersonal dimension, and that the interpersonal dimension was itself subordinate to the wider sociocultural context of all experience. For Fromm, society was always at work in the person, so that the person exists as a fundamentally social being. In a work from 1937, entitled *Man's Impulse Structure and Its Relation to Culture*, Fromm writes:

> Society and the individual are not "opposite" to each other. *Society is nothing but living, concrete individuals, and the individual exists only as a social human being.* His individual life practice is necessarily determined by the life practice of his society or class and, in the last analysis, by the manner of production of his society, that is, how this society produces, how it is organized to satisfy the needs of its members. The differences in the manner of production and life of various societies or classes lead to the development of different character structures typical of the particular society. Various societies differ from each other not only in differences in manner of production and social and political organization but also in that their people exhibit a typical character structure despite all individual differences. We shall call this "*the socially typical character*."
>
> (1937/2010, p. 58)

According to Fromm, the way in which a person participated in society revealed specific modes of being that were characteristic of that society. In other words, Fromm was concerned with demonstrating how society produced persons who were adapted to specific roles, which he called "social character types."

Fromm's early study of social character culminated in his first major book, *Escape from Freedom* (1941), in which he examined the nature of the "authoritarian character" of Germans who supported the rise of Nazism. According to Fromm, societies are structured in such a way that individuals take on the roles which their particular society requires of them. He was particularly interested in demonstrating how society produces persons who unconsciously adapt to meet society's economic needs even though these may conflict with our own emotional well-being. As Fromm would famously remark in a later work:

> It is the function of social character to shape the energies of the members of society in such a way that their behavior is not left to conscious decisions whether or not to follow the social pattern but that *people want to act as they have to act* (1949, p. 5).

In a manner akin to Sullivan, Fromm (1941) asserts that the person is best understood in terms of interpersonal processes. One of the clearest position statements of the neo-Freudian or cultural school perspective can be found in the Appendix of *Escape from Freedom*:

> The fundamental approach to human personality is the understanding of the human being's relationship to the world, to others, to nature, and to him or herself. We believe that the human being is primarily a social being, and not, as Freud assumes, primarily self-sufficient and only secondarily in need of others in order to satisfy his or her instinctual needs. In this sense, we believe that individual psychology is fundamentally social psychology, or in Sullivan's terms, the psychology of interpersonal relationships (p. 290).

Developmental Stages

For the neo-Freudians, human development is explained interpersonally and in the broader contexts of society and culture. The neo-Freudians all talk about development to varying degrees. Sullivan delineated what was perhaps the clearest account of distinct stages, beginning with infancy and moving through childhood, the juvenile era, pre-adolescence, adolescence, and adulthood. What is noteworthy is that each stage is shaped by interpersonal processes and reflects the larger social and cultural contexts in which it occurs. For instance, an infant is born into a primary group that consists of two people, an infant and a mother, and the interactions between them. In childhood, the child's personality is shaped by sociocultural factors through the acquisition of language. In the juvenile era, the child interacts with people beyond his or her immediate family members, such as teachers and classmates in school, so that others come to carry more importance. In preadolescence, the egocentric character of the child's sociality changes with the emergence of the need for an intimate playmate of similar age, a so-called chum. In adolescence, the need for an intimate interpersonal relation is directed toward another person. The achievement of stable relations involving another person heralds entry into adulthood.

Body

For Freud, human sexuality was a universal, biological force that shaped the course of development across cultures. For Sullivan, Fromm, and Horney, by contrast, Freud's biological assumptions resulted in a neglect of society's role, particularly in the construction of gender and women's experiences of their own bodies, which could differ across cultures. Horney's concern with culture's constitutive effects was most evident in her focus on gender and what she called "feminine psychology." Throughout the late 1920s and 1930s, Horney wrote a series of papers and lectures (published posthumously as a collection entitled *Feminine Psychology* in 1967), in which she took Freud to task for his misogyny and for presenting women as castrated creatures whose development was determined by their need to compensate for the lack of a penis.

Horney soundly rejected Freud's anti-feminist bias. In a 1926 paper, *Inhibited Femininity: Psychoanalytic Contributions to the Problem of Frigidity*, she argued that the "disadvantage under which women labor in social life" is all but ignored in male-dominated psychoanalytic theory (quoted in Paris, 2000, p. 6). According to Horney, "a girl is exposed from birth onward to the suggestion—inevitable, whether conveyed brutally or delicately—of her inferiority, an experience that constantly stimulates her masculinity complex" (Horney, 1967, p. 69). Horney's espousal of the notion of womb-envy led her to argue, in effect, that men's envy of the ability to bear children played a powerful role in their need to subordinate women. Horney also took issue with the Oedipus complex, suggesting that the idea that the child was envious of one parent while clinging to another was more likely the result of a disturbance in the parent-child relationship, thus pointing to the influence of the immediate environment as well as the broader social and cultural forces that shape the development and understanding of gender.

Horney's conviction that cultural factors could exert influence on conceptions of gender was radical for her time and stood out within the male-dominated psychoanalytic movement and the medical establishment. Pointing to the powerful cultural biases at work in society, Horney wrote: "The view that women are infantile and emotional creatures and as such incapable of responsibility and independence is the work of the masculine tendency to lower women's self-respect" (Horney, 1967, p. 146). In other words, Freud's biological emphasis not only became a means of rationalizing patriarchy, it failed to account for the way in which the family structure was itself a product of a specific social and cultural constellation.

Anxiety

Neo-Freudians avoided the term "pathology," preferring instead to talk about "problems in living," which could be traced back to negative environmental conditions imposed on the individual by society and culture. Anxiety played a central role in this process, ultimately determining how individuals came to shape their experience and their interaction with other people. Individuals engage in security operations that establish patterns of interaction that can be difficult to change over time. Thus, according to Horney, the object of analysis:

> Is not to help the patient gain mastery over his instincts but to lessen his anxiety to such an extent that he can dispense with his "safety devices." Beyond this aim there looms a new therapeutic goal, which is to restore the individual to himself, to help him regain his spontaneity and find his center of gravity in himself.
>
> (quoted in Paris, 2000, p. 167)

Sullivan was less concerned with the individual per se, than with how the person relates to others in their social and cultural contexts. In a lecture given to students of the Washington School of Psychiatry in 1948, one year before he died, Sullivan explained the centrality of anxiety in his entire account of psychology:

> Anxiety is the problem, but the unnumbered operations which human skill has devised—your patients' skill and experience have devised—to avoid and minimize anxiety, are what you have to struggle with in getting to the problem .... When you have become fairly clear on the specific and particular vulnerabilities to anxiety which are irrational from the standpoint of the broader culture or the particular world in which a person is living or is to live, you have come to that which can be cured, that to which psychotherapeutic technique can apply (1949, p. 328).

Implications for Technique

The neo-Freudians viewed psychoanalysis as a vehicle for improving patients' relationships with the world, with others and with themselves. In order to understand the patient, it was necessary to examine what happened between people and the sociocultural contexts in which they lived. The analytic setting could shed light on how the patient relates to others and on the implicit patterns of interaction that guide a person's way of relating.

The emphasis that Sullivan, Fromm, and Horney placed on the formative role of relationships was reflected in their evolving view of therapeutic interaction. From a therapeutic perspective, they were interested in how formative relationships within and outside of the family can shape the patient's approach to living. They carried out an analysis of patients without relying on such concepts as drives or infantile sexuality. For example, Horney saw neurosis as a product of culture and the dynamics of the family, not of libidinal development. She and Fromm both suggest that a culture oriented towards competition and success can create individuals who seek dominance in their economic and personal lives, thereby neglecting their emotional well-being. In a similar sense, Sullivan saw problems in living as social and interpersonal rather than as individual and intrapsychic.

To varying degrees, Sullivan, Fromm, and Horney all emphasized the importance of genuineness and openness in the therapeutic relationship. Although Fromm and Horney were classically trained psychoanalysts, over time they did away with the strictures of orthodox technique. Sullivan's therapeutic approach was influenced by his work with schizophrenics and by his close interaction with Clara Thompson, who had undergone a training analysis with Sandor Ferenczi in Budapest in the early 1930s. All of the neo-Freudians emphasized the presence and irreducibility of the analyst in the therapeutic encounter. They acknowledged the importance of the therapeutic interaction between the patient and analyst—what Fromm came to call "direct therapy," by which he referred to the analyst's immediacy and presence with the patient. For Sullivan, the psychiatrist, or analyst, takes the position of participant-observer, helping the patient recognize implicit patterns of interaction which can play out in their lives and in the therapeutic setting. As a group, the neo-Freudians enabled the emergence of a "two-person psychology" that came to define modern interpersonal, intersubjective, and relational psychoanalytic schools. Their approach made talk of transference and countertransference possible. But although Sullivan, Fromm, and Horney acknowledge the analyst's role, they don't yet account for the full influence of his or her subjectivity on the therapeutic process, or for the co-construction of meaning in the analytic setting.

Subsequent Developments

Sullivan, Fromm, and Horney set the foundation for explaining psychological experience *within* culture and society, rather than seeing culture and society as separate or apart from the psychoanalytic process. Today, their viewpoint finds expression in psychoanalytic schools that take as their starting point our unconscious embeddedness in social and cultural worlds that are laden with values and norms that often remain implicit or unconscious. This applies to such issues as race and racism as well as gender and patriarchy, which were long neglected by the psychoanalytic mainstream. Once psychoanalysts recognize that they exist in contexts of shared understandings, made possible by specific sociocultural frameworks, it becomes possible to examine how psychoanalytic theory and the analytic process are shaped by social systems. The more psychoanalysts can be aware of their own social and cultural embeddedness, the better they can understand their role in the therapeutic process and its impact on their work with patients.

13. The Neo-Freudians	
Main, general underlying assumptions	An overall focus on the primacy of social and cultural factors in human development. The etiology of neuroses is traced to social and cultural experience, rather than biology, which distinguishes this approach from Freud and the mainstream.
Specific theoretical assumptions	
psychic structure	Neo-Freudians were interested in the social and cultural constitution of the individual, not in the psychic structure within the mind.

(Continued)

energy	Biological drives are delimited and the importance of social relations and of cultural structures is emphasized.
relationships	Interpersonal relations are a central developmental concept, according to which individuals are fundamentally shaped by their interactions with other people.
developmental stages	Sullivan has the clearest account of distinct developmental stages. Each stage is shaped by interpersonal processes that reflect the larger social and cultural contexts in which they occur.
body	Society's role in the construction of gender and embodied experience, which can vary across cultures, is emphasized. Horney's focus on gender fundamentally challenges Freud's conceptualization of female psychology.
anxieties/instincts and defenses	Anxiety determines how individuals shape their experience and their interaction with other people. Sullivan introduces the notion of "security operations," which create patterns of interaction that can be difficult to change.
Assumptions concerning etiology	The etiology of neuroses is traced to social and cultural experience, rather than biology.
Implications for technique	The formative role of relationships gives way to an evolving view of therapeutic interaction. Importance is placed on genuineness and openness in the therapeutic relationship. Fromm uses the term "direct therapy" to refer to the analyst's immediacy and presence with the patient. Sullivan prefers the term "participant observer."
Subsequent developments of the core concept	As a group, they enable the emergence of a two-person psychology, with an emphasis on countertransference and the subjectivity of the analyst. They open up space to explain psychic experience within society and culture and to examine our unconscious embeddedness in social and cultural systems that shape what we see, know, and do as psychoanalysts. This is especially relevant when it comes to the exploration of systemic racism and gender bias and its effects.

References

Frie, R. (2014). What is cultural psychoanalysis: Psychoanalytic anthropology and the interpersonal tradition. *Contemporary Psychoanalysis*, *50*, 371–394.
Fromm, E. (1941). *Escape from freedom*. Ferrar and Rinehart.
Fromm, E. (1949). Psychoanalytic characterology and its application to the understanding of culture. In S. S. Sargent & M. W. Smith (Eds.), *Culture and personality* (pp. 1–12). Viking Press.
Fromm, E. (2010). Man's impulse structure and its relation to culture. In R. Funk (Ed.) & A. Schreiber (Trans.), *Beyond Freud: From individual to social psychology* (pp. 17–74). American Mental Health Foundation. (Original work published 1937).
Horney, K. (1967). *Feminine psychology*. W. W. Norton.
Paris, B. J. (2000). *The unknown Karen Horney: Essays on gender, culture, and psychoanalysis*. Yale University Press.
Sullivan, H. S. (1949). The study of psychiatry: 1948 orienting lectures. *Psychiatry: Journal for the Operational Statement of Interpersonal Relations*, *12*, 325–337.
Sullivan, H. S. (1950). Tensions interpersonal and international. In H. Cantril (Ed.), *Tensions that cause war* (pp. 79–138). University of Illinois Press.
Sullivan, H. S. (1964). The illusion of personal individuality. In H. S. Sullivan (Ed.), *The fusion of psychiatry and social science* (pp. 198–226). W. W. Norton. (Original work published 1950).

Chapter 14

Self Psychology, Kohut, and the Kohutian Perspective

Allen Siegel

Main, General Underlying Assumptions

Assumption 1: Psychoanalysis as a Science

Heinz Kohut considered psychoanalysis to be a science. He asserted that its proper field of study is the complex emotional states of humankind. Affect, the data of psychoanalysis, is collected through the human information-collecting instrument of empathy. Corollary to Kohut's primary assumption is that psychoanalysis, as a science, has an obligation to adhere to the epistemological requirements of the scientific method.

While basic assumptions underlie each of the many psychoanalytic theories, I believe that Dr. Kohut would have taken issue with a basic assumption asserted here, that psychoanalysis was founded in "the willingness to accept something as true, without question or proof. Basic assumptions usually involve a set of rules a person may hold about themselves, others, and the world. These rules are seen as unquestionably right" (B. Huppertz, personal communication, 2020).

In fact, Dr. Kohut was so distressed by the unquestioning nature of psychoanalysis that, as early as 1959 (1959/1978), he raised a question about Freud's core assumption, namely that "drives" are the primary motivators of Freud's System Unconscious. Freud's conceptualization of an unconscious mind was his major contribution, however, he faced a problem in his need to identify the motivating "contents" of his reified concept of the System Unconscious. He turned to Charles Darwin to help him with that task.

Freud believed he had found an answer to his "unconscious contents" quandary in Darwin's seminal work, *On the Origin of the Species by Means of Natural Selection* (1859). In that biological work, Darwin observed two existential instincts. One, an aggressive instinct assured the survival of the individual. The other, a sexual instinct, assured the survival of the species.

Freud speculated that Darwin's observations were universal across all living organisms and, in the absence of his own direct observations, Freud

DOI: 10.4324/9781003027768-15

imported Darwin's work about the dual instincts into psychoanalytic theory. Freud then speculated that Darwin's sexual and aggressive instincts were the unconscious contents of the mind.

Freud, with this single link to biology, solved two essential problems. He had answered his motivating "contents" of the unconscious question while, at the same time, he found legitimacy for his own embryonic science through its link to biology. Nonetheless, this seemingly fortuitous link created a problem that Freud did not recognize. Contrary to the scientific method, he had anchored his new science in a speculation rather than upon the solid foundation of scientific observation.

This was a curious epistemological mistake since Freud, a physician, neurologist, and scientist, was familiar with the scientific method. In fact, Freud even wrote about the relationship between observation and speculation in the formation of scientific theory in his paper "On Narcissism: An Introduction," where he wrote:

> For these ideas [speculations] are not the foundation of science, upon which everything rests: *that foundation is observation alone* [emphasis added]. They [speculations] are not the bottom but the top of the whole structure, and they [speculations] can be replaced and discarded without damaging it (1914).

Despite Freud's awareness that speculation did not occupy the same vaunted place within the scientific method as did observation he nonetheless built his idea of unconscious "contents" entirely upon the speculation, he gleaned from Darwin's biology. Blinded by need, Freud and his followers treated Freud's speculations as though they were the foundational "bottom" of the structure rather than the speculative top. Tragically, Freud's speculation evolved into an idealized, seemingly unerring lens. For Freud and his followers, all unconscious phenomena were viewed through that speculative lens. From a place within that idealized speculation, any questioning of Freud's speculative notion was treated by Freud and his followers as heresy.

It was this endemic, unquestioning assumption that motivated Heinz Kohut to write his epistemological paper, "Introspection, Empathy and Psychoanalysis: An Examination of the Relationship between Mode of Observation and Theory" (1959/1978). In that 1959 paper, Kohut implied that Freud had created a cognitive "experience-distant" theory that was founded on unquestioning faith in biological speculations. This was in direct contrast to Kohut's idea of psychoanalysis as that science that studied the complex emotional states of humankind with affect, collected empathically, as its primary data. Kohut asserted that a convincing theory about the human condition could only evolve from "experience-near" theorizing.

Assumption 2: An Unconscious Mind is the Foundation of Psychoanalysis

The basic assumption of self-psychology is the same as that for all of psychoanalysis. It assumes the influence of a non-conscious mind that influenced human thought, feeling, and behavior. The various psychoanalytic theories differed from each other in their understanding of what motivated the unconscious mind. For example, for Freud the drives and their associated conflicts were the primary concerns of his conception of a reified unconscious mind. Kohut differed, and based upon his "experience-near" clinical observations, concluded that a variety of narcissistic forms and their associated needs contributed to the foundational non-conscious issues.

Assumption 3: Kohut's New Developmental Line of Narcissism

Kohut conceptualized an experience-near, developmental line of narcissistic development that initially he considered being an addition to Freud's object-libidinal line of development. In Freud's developmental line, narcissism was relinquished in favor of object-love. Kohut's conceptions, drawn from clinical observations of his patients' current affective experiences and from the reconstructions he was able to form of his patients' early development suggested, however, that narcissism never was relinquished.

Kohut suggested that in his new developmental line, narcissism began in a primary state of infantile bliss. This was similar to Freud's idea of primary narcissism. In Kohut's speculation, as in Freud's as well, that bliss was inevitably disrupted. The baby became hungry and didn't get fed immediately, got wet and wasn't changed in a timely way, or was lonely and didn't get held. At that point in development, Kohut added something new. He speculated that the infant, in an inchoate form, "attempted" to restore its previous blissful state. In that attempt at restoration, only two avenues were available. One avenue sought to find an idealized other that, in its perfection, had the ability to restore what had been lost. The other route turned toward the inchoate self as the new source of perfection. It's with these two speculations that Kohut conceptualized a second line of narcissistic development.

In this new line Kohut described three basic routes of narcissistic development. Each route consisted of specific unconscious needs that were narcissistic in origin. For Kohut, these unconscious narcissistic needs, wishes, and yearnings were the contents of a non-conscious part of the mind.

They were:

1 A need for an idealized other that Kohut called **an idealizing need**.
2 A need for an affirmation of one's grandeur and existence that Kohut called **a mirroring need**.
3 A need to belong to a group of like-minded others that Kohut called **a kinship need**.

All these nascent narcissistic needs originated in infancy and transformed, over time, into mature forms of narcissism. What follows below are brief descriptions of these narcissistic needs and, since Kohut's theory is "experience-near," I will describe the feeling experiences that are associated with each of these unconscious needs.

Idealizing Narcissism

According to Kohut's speculation this form of narcissism began with the unavoidable disruption of the infant's bliss. The infant, in some inchoate form, then responded with attempts to restore its lost bliss by assigning perfection, omniscience, and omnipotence to an idealized other. This idealized person, by virtue of its attachment to the infant, restored the infant's previous bliss. Kohut called this idealized other an idealized selfobject. In Kohut's creation of his term selfobject as a single word, he recognized that the idealized selfobject, in serving its sustaining psychological function, was experienced by the idealizing person as being part of the person's self.

Developmentally, the baby's experience of being picked up and held securely by her idealized parent created a memory of security that was provided by an attachment to a powerful other. This experience became a lifelong template for feeling secure and evolved into a continuous unconscious search for an attachment to an idealized selfobject in order to avoid the anxiety of emotional disintegration.

When the secure bond with this idealized selfobject was disrupted, the selfobject lost his/her healing perfection. This loss occurred as a result of the experience of a variety of disappointments. An example might be when the child told her first lie and didn't get caught. A similar loss occurred when the idealized parent was physically or emotionally removed or when, at any time, the idealized selfobject failed in its narcissistic function.

The idealizing form of narcissism contained the feeling:

> **"You are great and when I am with you, I feel that I am a part of you and therefore I feel whole, safe, and even powerful."**

Mirroring Narcissism

This second form of narcissism carried the unconscious feeling of greatness and grandeur. The experience of "greatness," however, felt hollow without an echo from a valued witness that affirmed one's emotional existence and sustained one's feelings of self-confidence and well-being.

The person or entity that provided the narcissistic affirmation is further experienced as being part of the self. Analogous to the situation with the idealized selfobject, Kohut called this affirming person or entity a mirroring selfobject.

The feeling associated with this form of Mirroring Narcissism is:

"I am great, but I need you to affirm my greatness or else I feel empty."

The mirroring form of narcissism described a developmental course that began in early infancy. It embraced an unconscious sense of grandeur, boundless expansiveness, and omnipotence. This sense of internal wonder and greatness, however, was fragile and readily changeable, as seen in a little girl who wanted the world to witness her perfect pirouette. She was delighted when she had her witness and deflated when her witness was distracted. The mood associated with this experience of grandeur can be fun-filled and joyful when the need for a witness was affirmed. It can become demanding and terrorizing, however, when that echo was missing. When we see expressions of the immature state of grandiosity in a child, we understand both the child's "boastful" nature as well as the child's fragility. However, in the adult, people find immature forms of mirror narcissism obnoxious. Even psychoanalytic therapists tend to respond negatively to immature narcissism, forgetting that it was developmental in nature. Unfortunately, this aversive response cast a negative shadow over narcissism in general.

When things go well in a child's early development, narcissism can evolve into its mature forms. As that fortunate person develops, the self-aggrandizing narcissism transforms into a modulated, contained form of narcissism that eventually moves into healthy self-esteem. For example, let's assume the young pirouetting girl goes on to become a recognized ballerina who dances for many years and is justifiably proud of her talents and accomplishments. In her later years, when she no longer can dance, she opens a studio that becomes well-known and, as a result, she feels healthy pride in what she has built. She is not boastful and no one thinks of her as "too full of herself." As her physical powers diminish with age, she accepts the fact that her "star" time as both dancer and teacher has come to its end. She is able to retire without too much angst and lives with few regrets until her death. In such fortunate people, the maturation of grandiosity develops in later life into an acceptance of one's mortality. This realization is accompanied by a sad, but comfortable, acceptance of one's transience. Kohut asserted that acceptance of one's transience is probably the single most important psychological accomplishment of one's life.

Kinship Narcissism

This third form of unconscious narcissism is the need to be connected to a group into which one "fits" and with whom one shares a set of values. It counters the potential for feeling alone and isolated in the world. The feeling of belonging in this way enhances the sense of one's self-worth. Its feeling quality is:

"I belong. I am not alone and lost in this uncertain world."

According to Kohut, these three forms of unconscious narcissism are neither good nor bad in themselves. They are ever-present, and exert powerful influences on human thought, feeling, and behavior. When the unconscious needs associated with these forms are fulfilled, a feeling of well-being and emotional balance develops. When they are not fulfilled the experience is one of disappointment, insult, annihilation anxiety, and a disruption of a person's emotional sense of wholeness and balance.

Assumption 4: The Co-Created Interactive Dyad, in Which Neutrality is Not Possible, is the Locus of Therapeutic Work

Humans are intensely interactive and relational throughout life. While we are born with innate elements of personality, our affects from infancy forward are contextually determined. Freud, writing 109 years ago, was not yet unaware of this contextual reality. In fact, in 1912 he wrote, "I cannot advise my colleagues too urgently to model themselves during psychoanalytic treatment on the surgeon who puts aside all his feelings, even his human sympathy, and concentrates his mental forces on the single aim of performing the operation as skillfully as possible." In the same paper he also wrote, "The doctor should be opaque to his patients and, like a mirror, should show them nothing but what is shown to him" (Freud, 1912).

Deeply influenced by his medical background, Freud conceived of the unconscious mind as an isolated, self-contained specimen, neither impacted by, nor interactive with, its environment. With this medical orientation it follows that Freud would conceive of treatment as existing in an antiseptic field in which the analyst/surgeon retains the pristine purity of the passive subject.

Over many years, our field has moved beyond the constraint of medical bounds and now listens to the dynamic, co-constructed, and interactive nature of the therapeutic dyad. Change in our field, however, is slow and spotty. When I teach in countries where psychoanalytic thinking is a relatively new import, I hear rumbly remnants of Freud's "neutrality" beneath the surface. New therapists, in particular, who have been taught by an older generation, give it voice when they present their work to me.

In truth, the idea of neutrality and its misunderstood non-responsive analytic distance creates an ambiance that often repeats the unintended, parentally inflicted, traumas of childhood. Meant to be helpful, but depriving ambiance actually is rude, hurtful, and definitely not neutral. It inflicts iatrogenic injuries. Ironically it distorts the transferences it was meant to enhance.

In reality the therapist is never neutral and opaque. She has an office designed a certain way, she dresses a certain way, she has a changeable composure, posture, and demeanor that varies day to day, and she has biases and personal values that inadvertently express themselves. Our patients observe all this and draw their conclusions. We definitely impact our patients and when we overlook the interactive, relational bi-directionality of our relationships we actually diminish the possibility for useful transferences to emerge.

Finally, the Freudian and other analytic therapist's distant and opaque mindset deprives the therapist of the affective data that Kohut suggests is the core of psychoanalytic inquiry and understanding. Again, it interferes with the natural flow of the treatment.

Specific Theoretical Assumptions

Assumptions about the Nature of Psychic Structure

The psychic structure is an idea that stems originally from Freud's structural model and later from ego psychology's focus on the ego as a structure. Theory in self-psychology does not conceptualize reified structures, although it does conceptualize narcissistic needs and dynamic transferences, not as structures. Kohut, a post-modern thinker, assiduously avoided defining "self" for fear that it would become reified, encased, or considered to be a structure, as had Freud's concept of the unconscious, and would become eventually dogmatized as happens to so many analytic concepts.

Assumptions about the Sources and Nature of Energy

Psychic energy is another concept that stems from Freud's speculative theorizing. In this case it is the hydrodynamic, physics-based models of the mind that Freud conceptualized. In those models, energy, libido, flows freely and energizes human thought, feeling, and behavior unless that flow is inhibited due to an unconscious conflict. Self-psychology theory eschews reifications and conceptualizes neither libidinal energy nor Freud's unconscious. Instead it theorizes functionally in terms of emotional vitality, emotional balance, optimal functioning, and an unconscious part of the mind. It also conceptualizes the converse, emotional deadness brought about by arrests in emotional development and/or by impending emotional fragmentation.

Assumptions about the Nature of Relationships

Relationships, especially early formative relationships with childhood caretakers in which adults respond to the child's developmental needs, are central to theory in the psychology of the self and to the cure as well, since the current theory of treatment is that it occurs in an interactive, dynamic dyad.

Assumptions about Developmental Stages

Please see Assumption 3: Narcissism as a New Developmental Line.

Assumptions about the Body

From my perspective, a weakness is present in self-psychology theory in relation to body issues. It has not adequately addressed issues of the body beyond the uses of body for enlivening self-stimulation.

Assumptions about Anxieties/Instincts and Defenses

In the psychology of the self theory, the deepest anxiety is primarily annihilation anxiety, which means the experiential obliteration of a self that has previously been in emotional balance. Another way to think about this is the experience of "falling apart."

In the psychology of the self theory, anxiety is considered within a context. The self-psychological approach to anxiety is always the exploration of possible contextual origins of that anxiety. The theory does not recognize unconscious biological instincts per se so there are no assumptions about instinctual anxiety.

Defenses are conceived of as protections the mind creates against overwhelming anxieties and traumatic experiences. They are not resistances against the treatment nor against anything else. Instead of defenses, an idea that stems from Freud's war-like analogies, the psychology of the self understands protections in a positive light rather than from a negative perspective, as the best a child, now adult, could do to protect itself earlier from toxic, traumatizing situations.

Assumptions Concerning Etiology

Please see Assumption 3: Narcissism as a New Developmental Line.

Implications for Technique

Kohut's theory of cure differs significantly from Freud's. It begins with the therapist's awareness that the three forms of narcissism exist, each with its associated unconscious needs. In a suffering person the unmet narcissistic needs became buried deeply within an unconscious mind until that person found a healing milieu. In such a milieu the revival of the buried, immature forms of narcissism and their associated needs expressed themselves in the form of new specific narcissistic transferences. As these transferences form in the treatment they are identified and then lived through in a therapeutic process where they carry the opportunity for a rebirth of stalled psychological development. With that renewed growth and development comes the repair of a broken self.

Subsequent Developments of the Core Concept

Much of what I have already written describes the history and amplification of the core concepts of Kohut's self-psychology and its deviation from ego psychology, its predecessor.

Theorists in self-psychology after Kohut's premature death, at the age of 67, have not taken great issue with his core concepts. The most notable change in the theory has been the addition of a relational component, initiated by Robert Stolorow who spoke of the intersubjective perspective. This idea is captured in Assumption 4 which speaks about the co-constructed, interactive dyad as the locus of the therapeutic work. The two theories, Kohut's self psychology and the relational-intersubjectivist theorists' ideas, work well together in a treatment.

Kohut's ideas provide a developmental perspective on the evolving forms and transformations of narcissism that exist within an individual. These ideas about narcissism in health and in distress serve as guides for the therapist's accurate empathy which is essential to the treatment. The relational-intersubjective position shines a light on the more technical matter of co-creating an active field in which the forms of narcissism emerge and can be explored.

14. Self Psychology, Kohut, and Kohutians	
Main, general underlying assumptions	1 Psychoanalysis as a science 2 An unconscious mind is the foundation of psychoanalysis 3 Narcissism as a new developmental line 4 The co-created interactive dyad, in which neutrality is not possible, is the locus of the therapeutic work
Specific theoretical assumptions	
psychic structure	N/A
energy	N/A
relationships	Bond with emotionally sustaining others is essential for a sense of wholeness and balance of the self
developmental stages	New developmental line of narcissism
body	N/A

(Continued)

anxieties/instincts and defenses	Disruption of sustaining selfobject bond creates experience of fragmenting
Assumptions concerning etiology	New developmental line of narcissism
Implications for technique	Mobilization of unconscious narcissistic transferences and renewal of arrested development
Subsequent developments of the core concept	Self-psychology's awareness of unconscious narcissistic dynamics works well with the intersubjective-relational view of the dyad as the technical focus of treatment.

References

Darwin, C. (1859). *On the origin of the species by means of natural selection.* John Murray, Albemarle Street.

Freud, S. (1912). Recommendations to physicians practicing psychoanalysis. In J. Strachey (Ed. and Trans.), *The standard edition of the complete works of Sigmund Freud* (Vol. 12, pp. 7–121). Hogarth Press.

Freud, S. (1914). On narcissism: An introduction. In J. Strachey (Ed. and Trans.), *The standard edition of the complete works of Sigmund Freud* (Vol. 14, pp. 67–102). Hogarth Press.

Kohut, H. (1978). Introspection, empathy, and psychoanalysis: An examination of the relationship between mode of observation and theory. In P. Ornstein (Ed.), *The search for the self* (Vol. 1, pp. 205–232). International Universities Press. (Original work published 1959).

Chapter 15

Post-Kohutian Self Psychology[1]

Amanda Kottler

From its Freudian beginning, psychoanalytic theory has been "in a state of continuous organic development" (Sandler, 1983, p. 35). Many assumptions have been preserved by stretching them to encompass new ideas. However, radically different concepts have ruptured any connections with previous ideas and necessitated the formation of new psychoanalytic schools. Kohut's self psychology (KSP) and post-Kohutian self psychology (PKSP) evolved this way, although more acrimony was involved in the first than the second evolution. This may explain why it might be hard to distinguish the new iterations from their antecedents. I hope to clarify this by introducing a historical perspective on the main assumptions of the PKSP.

Main Underlying Assumptions

The kind of therapeutic transformation the PKSP school envisions for its patients cannot occur without empathy, selfobject experiences, and the idea of a two-person bi-directional process, involving what Kohut (1985) referred to as various selves.[2] Each assumption is implicit in the PKSP perspectives included in this chapter, namely: Bacal's (2011) *Specificity Theory*, Brandchaft's (2007) *Pathological Accommodation*, Togashi and Kottler's (2015) *Psychology of Being Human* and Tolpin's (2002) *Forward Edge*.

Empathy

Kohut (1959) suggested that empathy was the only way analysts[3] could understand their patients' struggles. Elaborating, he referred to "vicarious introspection" that involves attempts to "think and feel oneself into the inner life of another person" (1984, p. 82). This is nearly impossible as the subjective experience of another cannot be directly observed. However, approximations are possible (and necessary) given this school's focus on the subjective experiences of patients.

DOI: 10.4324/9781003027768-16

Kohut developed his ideas about empathy after experiencing recurrent experiences of clinical ruptures[4] while using the classical psychoanalytic framework. The ruptures led him to believe that the unreflective emphasis psychoanalysts put on their theories compromises their capacity to listen effectively to their patients' subjective experiences and needs.[5] This *experience-near* emphasis remains central to PKSP and constitutes a fundamental difference between it and many other psychoanalytic frameworks.

When Kohut (1959) first posited his idea of empathy, he was a prestigious leader in the international field of classical psychoanalytic theory. However, this idea was too radical and not favorably received. It prompted Kohut's painful expulsion from the Freudian psychoanalytic community and the development of KSP. Kohut's unresolved need for acceptance of his theories by his peers motivated his ongoing attempt to disguise and compromise his ideas. But three days before he died, he frustratingly returned to clarify the concept of empathy (Kohut, 1981/2010). His attempt only muddied the waters. His death left questions that post-Kohutian theorists have addressed and developed. Empathy is considered the foundation of all authentic human relationships and its elaborated manifestations remain crucial for the deeply effective transformation that PKSP analysts seek for their patients. The elaborations have generated diverse perspectives about what analysts should *do* with their empathic understanding (see implications for technique below).

Selfobject Experiences

The elaborated idea of selfobject experience is as fundamental as empathy in this school and, like empathy, selfobject experiences cannot be externally observed. An analyst cannot provide a selfobject experience by applying a technique, and the experience can only be felt subjectively.

Kohut (1971) described these experiences as "transference like" needs that he called "narcissistic transferences" (p. 25). However, the more he was shunned by the classical psychoanalytic world, the more Kohut began to create new concepts. Narcissistic transferences became self-object transferences which became self-object experiences. Finally, he dropped the hyphen between the words *self* and *object,* positing the idea that selfobject experiences are developmentally crucial for establishing a cohesive self. If these experiences have not occurred in our patients' or our own lives, all is not lost. Later relationships have the potential to transform a person's sense of self by generating a restructuring of the self that mutates into a more balanced (Seigel, personal communication) and resilient (Doctors, 2020) way of being in the world.

Kohut identified the twinship/alter-ego, mirroring, and idealizing selfobject experiences as essential. They provide, for example, the experience-near comfort of feeling calmed when excessively anxious, relief when understood, pleasure when sharing an emotional experience or a creative task with others, joy when a respected person appreciates one's uniqueness, and revitalized following affirmation by an admired person. Each experience energizes the self by enhancing self-esteem and creativity. Each nurtures personal and relational growth and development.

Prior to his elaboration of selfobject needs, Kohut considered resistant behaviors as defensively concealing a hidden "truth"[6] that analysts would unmask. But he learned from pejoratively labeled "narcissistic" patients like Miss F., considered untreatable within the classical framework, that this model did not work. Kohut's empathic stance led him to reconsider[7] the classical assumptions about who was not treatable and why. He now understood the apparently self-defeating, "untreatable" behaviors as manifestations of healthy attempts to redress earlier experiences with significant others whose capacity to contain and nurture was emotionally deficient.

The idea of selfobject needs shifted Kohut to a deficit model in which he conceptualized the development of a cohesive self as a direct consequence of the experiences provided by significant others. Understanding this developmental need led Kohut to argue that throughout life there is a need for selfobject experiences, particularly at times of change and crisis.

Magid et al. (2021) argue that selfobject experiences only derive from a person. Orange (1995) introduces the idea of secondary selfobject relatedness drawn from healthy activities shared with others, which later provide the same calming or energizing selfobject experience without the presence of the person. Examples include music, art, baking, carpentry, and exercise.

In contrast, Ulman and Paul (2006, p. xix) describe selfobject-like effects of *ersatz* selfobject experiences that do not derive from any kind of relationship with another person. This substitute experience is often gained, for example, from uncontrolled recreational use of substances that alter states of consciousness. In these altered states, there is relief from what Kohut called states of "fragmentation" that occur as a consequence of traumatic experiences. The relief is short-lived and usually followed by intense feelings of shame and self-loathing. However, the temporary sense of feeling calmed or energized compels people to repeat this behavior that, viewed from an experience-distant perspective, seems self-destructive. Such substance-induced experiences with no link to another person[8] are understood as fake substitutes that will not result in transformation.

Therapeutic Transformation Occurs in a Two-Person Space of Mutual Influence

Kohut's recognition of the transformative significance of selfobject experiences shifted his idea of a one-person analytic process towards an understanding that something more is involved. His (1984) posthumous elevation of the twinship/alter-ego selfobject experience to the most significant, and his redefinition of it as an experience of "being human among other human beings,"[9,10] (p. 200) speaks to this idea.

The significance Kohut gave to the selfobject experience inspired the PKSP shift to the assumption of a two-person, non-linear, dynamic system in which internal and external influences interact continuously (Magid et al., 2021). This idea embraces the belief that the analyst's subjectivity and everything about their way of being in the room profoundly influences the relationship. The effect, never pathologized, will differ from patient to patient, and from moment to moment in an ever-changing analytic field that depends on each patient's particular relational deficits and traumatic experiences. Transformation occurs within this complex, contextual, intersubjective, and relational space in which analyst and patient reciprocally and mutually affect each other. This idea is substantially more complex than was articulated in KSP and warranted the establishment of a separate PKSP school.

Multiple Selves/Self States

KSP focused on the building of a cohesive "self" but never clearly defined the concept. This is not surprising perhaps given the following:

> If we … put our trust in empirical observation, using introspection and empathy as our tools, we will be open to a bewildering increase in the complexity of the relevant phenomena. Instead of the single self of conscious experience … we will encounter a variety of incongruous and inconsistent phenomena. We will see different selves … each experienced as absolute and as the center of the personality, not only in different agencies of the mind but also side by side within the same agency. We see these various selves fighting for ascendancy, one blocking out the other, forming compromises with each other, and acting inconsistently with each other at the same time. In general, we will witness what appears to be an uneasy victory of one self over all the others ….
>
> (Kohut, 1985, p. 33)

This astoundingly prescient postmodern idea was written in 1970 but only published posthumously (1985), clearly indicating that Kohut's empathic stance alerted him to the fact that the self is neither static nor unitary.

Explanations of how this multiplicity appears in the room include conflict between "archaic" and "mature" selfobject experiences (Kohut, 1984, p. 185). The archaic involves old ways of being, developed to avoid unbearably painful feelings in the past. The mature, hoping for new empathically informed experiences, ventures into new ways of being.

Stolorow and Atwood (1996) described unvalidated unconscious self-states operating in the repetitive dimension in opposition to the selfobject dimension of the transference. The repetitive does everything to avoid a dreaded repeat with the therapist of earlier traumatic experiences (Ornstein, 1991). The selfobject dimension involves risking new behaviors and hoping for new ways of being.

Tolpin (2002) also writes about the old and the new. Trailing edge transferences repeat behavior manifesting an unconscious belief in their protective function. The forward edge behaviors signal hope and trust following the analyst's provision of needed selfobject experiences.

The assumption of multiple self-states existing within patient and analyst adds to the complexity of their minute-to-minute way of coming-into-being and going-on-being *with* the other in the analytic process (Kottler, 2018; Togashi & Kottler, 2021). It also speaks to the more specific theoretical assumptions that I address below.

Specific Theoretical Assumptions

Psychic Structure

This school does not conceptualize the self as a static and unitary structure. It comprises patterns of "being" in the world that materialize and shifts over time as a consequence of a person's relational experiences and the historical/cultural context in which these experiences have occurred.

Energy

Selfobject experiences generate energy understood as subjective experiences of, for example, vitality, confidence, and creativity.

Relationship

The quality of the bi-directional, co-created relationship is *the* most significant factor in what is considered an effective therapeutic process. The actual provision of whatever works to provide patients with needed selfobject experiences influences the quality of the developing analytic relationship. How PKSP analysts work towards repairing the inevitable ruptures, misunderstandings, and contextual complexities that arise in the relational process depends on the way each analyst empathically conceptualizes the patient's struggles, how best to work with them, and the quality of the relationship that evolves in the analysis. The choices made depend on the sensibility of the analyst, their capacity to be open to their own and their patient's affective states, and how they and their patients make sense together of what has gone wrong and how best to repair it (Buirski et al., 2020).

Development Stages

Development is not linear and does not follow universal stages. It occurs as a result of early and later selfobject experiences that are necessary throughout life.

Body

The body is not seen as separate from the mind. Body posture and facial expressions inform the analyst's empathic understanding of what is happening affectively in the therapeutic relationship.

Anxieties/Instincts and Defenses

Disintegration anxiety occurs as a result of early absences or deficits in, and later ruptures to, selfobject experiences. Behaviors understood in other schools as instinctual or defensive are recognized as healthy, protective attempts to contain unbearably painful feelings and to restore balance to an anxious and "fragmenting" sense of self.

Etiology

Patients' struggles are caused by early and later relational experiences with significant others whose capacity to provide the necessary selfobject experiences has been emotionally deficient.

Implications for Technique

Within the PKSP school there are many responses to the question of what should become the analytic focus. To think of the diverse foci as differences in "technique" is a stretch too far from the PKSP experience-near way of thinking. It is, however, a useful heading under which to describe the different emphases of some PKSP perspectives and their implications for treatment. Each is influenced by their particular empathic understanding of a patient's developmental deficits, their influence on what is happening in the analytic relationship, and the best way to respond.

Bacal's (2011) *Specificity Theory* maintains that the:

> sine qua non of psychoanalytic therapy is not empathy culminating in verbal interpretation … but the entire process that includes understanding the complex mental states of another and discerning responses that may be therapeutic for that patient, and possible for that analyst, in the uniqueness of their unfolding process (p. 283).

Tolpin's (2002) view of patients as hopeful and healthy (in Hagman et al., 2019) led her to focus on any forward edge behavior reflecting what she referred to as "tendrils of health." Empathic recognition and affirmation of these tendrils yields powerful transformatory effects.

Togashi and Kottler's (2015, 2019, 2021) psychology of being human model argues that meaningful transformation cannot occur without a twinship/alter-ego selfobject experience. This experience of being human among other human beings cultivates an appreciation of how we are all human beings living in a traumatizing and alienating world, which the model urges analysts to acknowledge. It also calls on analysts to identify their particular vulnerabilities, their own fallibility, the fallibility of the theories they use, and how all of this influences their own patterns of "being" and relating in the room. This internal work includes reflecting on their own capacity to allow for and react authentically to the unknowable and the unpredictability of any phenomena witnessed and experienced in the analytic process. Such an experience enables patients and analysts to empathically find ways of understanding themselves, the context they grew up in and currently inhabit, and the ways they understand the effects of these experiences on their way of "being" and going-on-being in the world. Togashi and Kottler (2019) draw attention to the significance of honesty and authenticity in the relationship, which influences whether the analyst and patient can find themselves in themselves (Kottler, 2018) and in each other (Togashi, 2012). Togashi and Kottler (2021) assert that this internal work influences the capacity that analyst and patient have for an I-Thou dialogue (Buber, 1999) in which they find a mutually respectful and acceptable way of "being" and working together in what needs to become a safe and relational home: safe to drop the need to pathologically accommodate to others (Brandchaft, 2007) and safe enough to discover and reveal their contradictory self-states and differences that have been hidden from themselves and others for so long.

Subsequent Developments of Core Concepts

Core concepts are continually being elaborated by those perspectives included above and others, notably Lichtenberg et al. (2021) motivational systems theory and Geist's (2020) idea that structure building requires the patient and analyst to share a sense of connectedness and permeable boundaries.

15. Post-Kohutian Self Psychology	
Main, general underlying assumptions	Therapeutic transformation requires: 1 Empathic listening, 2 selfobject experiences, and 3 a two-person, intersubjective bidirectional space which is 4 organized by multiple self states of patient and analyst.

(*Continued*)

Specific theoretical assumptions	
psychic structure	The self is not a static and unitary structure.
energy	Selfobject experiences generate subjective feelings conceived of in terms of energy (vitality, etc.).
relationships	The quality of the co-created relationship is the most significant aspect of the therapeutic process.
developmental stages	Development is neither linear nor does it follow universal stages. It occurs as a result of early and later selfobject experiences necessary throughout life.
body	Body and mind are not conceived of as separate entities.
anxieties/instincts and defenses	Early absences or deficits in, and later ruptures to, necessary selfobject experiences cause anxiety. Behaviors understood in other schools as instinctual or defensive are recognized as healthy attempts to contain unbearably painful feelings and restore balance to an anxious "disintegrating/fragmenting" sense of self.
Assumptions concerning etiology	Painful struggles caused by early and later relational experiences with significant others whose emotional capacity to provide the necessary selfobject experiences has been deficient.
Implications for technique	The idea of "technique" is not compatible with PKSP's understanding of treatment. One size does not fit all.
Subsequent developments of the core concept	Core concepts are continually being elaborated by those perspectives included in this chapter and others, notably Lichtenberg et al. (2021) motivational systems theory and Geist's (2020) idea that structure building requires the patient and analyst to share a sense of connectedness and permeable boundaries.

Notes

1 My grateful thanks to Allison Christen-Porter and Kevin Birch for editorial assistance on earlier drafts and to Suzi Naiburg for editorial assistance and commentary on earlier versions and this final draft.

2 I refer to these as multiple self states.

3 I refer to analysts throughout this chapter but the ideas apply equally to psychoanalytic psychotherapists.
4 Enraged, Miss F. said Kohut (1971) was "wrecking her analysis" (p. 412). He was not listening to her and his interpretations were undermining.
5 Hence Kohut's (1984) "if there is one lesson I have learned during my life as an analyst, it is ... that what my patients tell me is likely to be true—that many times when I believed that I was right and my patients were wrong, it turned out, though only after a prolonged search, that my rightness was superficial whereas their rightness was profound" (pp. 93–94).
6 Orange's (2011) hermeneutics of suspicion.
7 Orange's (2011) hermeneutics of trust.
8 This experience is quite different from the guided use of psychedelic drugs in the treatment of trauma, which occurs in the context of supervised clinical and relational settings.
9 Ideas elaborated by Togashi and Kottler (2015, 2021).
10 Kottler (2015) describes this experience as one of "feeling at home" with "a sense of belonging."

References

Bacal, H. A. (2011). Specificity theory: The evolution of a process theory of psychoanalytic treatment. *American Imago*, *68*(2), 267–285.

Brandchaft, B. (2007). Systems of pathological accommodation and change in analysis. *American Psychological Association*, *24*(4), 667–687.

Buber, M. (1999). *Martin Buber on psychology and psychotherapy: Essays, letters, and dialogue*. Syracuse University Press.

Buirski, P., Hagland, P., & Markley, E. (2020). *Making sense together: The intersubjective approach to psychotherapy* (2nd ed.). The Rowman & Littlefield Publishing.

Doctors, S. (2020). The selfobject concept: The heart of Kohut's psychology of health. *Psychoanalysis, Self and Context*, *15*(1), 25–32.

Geist, R. A. (2020). Interpretation as carrier of selfobject functions: Catalyzing inborn potential. *Psychoanalysis, Self and Context*, *15*(4), 338–347.

Hagman, G., Paul, H., & Zimmermann, P. B. (2019). *Intersubjective self psychology: A primer*. Routledge.

Kohut, H. (1959). Introspection, empathy, and psychoanalysis: An examination of the relationship between mode of observation and theory. *Journal of the American Psychoanalytic Association*, *7*, 459–483.

Kohut, H. (1971). *The analysis of the self. A systematic approach to the psychoanalytic treatment of narcissistic personality disorders*. International Universities Press.

Kohut, H. (1984). *How does analysis cure?* The University of Chicago Press.

Kohut. H. (1985). *Self psychology and the humanities: Reflections on a new psychoanalytic approach*. W.W. Norton and Company.

Kohut, H. (2010). On empathy. *International Journal of Psychoanalytic Self Psychology*, *5*(2), 122–131. (Original work published 1981).

Kottler, A. (2015). Feeling at home, belonging and being human: Kohut, self psychology, twinship, and alienation. *International Journal of Psychoanalytic Self Psychology*, *10*(4), 378–389.

Kottler, A. (2018, October). *Multiple selves, intersubjective taboos and alter egos: Creating order out of chaos, the self psychology way*. [Paper presentation] 33rd IAPSP Conference, Vienna, Austria.

Lichtenberg, J. D., Fosshage, J. L., & Lachmann, F. M. (2021). *An experience-based vision of psychoanalytic theory and practice*. Routledge.

Magid, B., Fosshage, J. L., & Shane, E. (2021). The emerging paradigm of relational self psychology: An historical perspective. *Psychoanalysis, Self and Context, 16*(1), 1–23.

Orange, D. M. (1995). *Emotional understanding: Studies in psychoanalytic epistemology*. The Guilford Press.

Orange, D. M. (2011). *The suffering stranger: Hermeneutics for everyday clinical practice*. Routledge.

Ornstein, A. (1991). The dread to repeat: Comments on the working-through process in psychoanalysis. *Journal of the American Psychoanalytic Association, 39*(2), 377–398.

Sandler, J. (1983). Reflections on some relations between psychoanalytic concepts and psychoanalytic practice. *The International Journal of Psychoanalysis, 64*, 35–45.

Stolorow, R. D., & Atwood, G. E. (1996). The intersubjective perspective. *Psychoanalytic Review, 83*, 181–194.

Togashi, K. (2012). Mutual finding of oneself and not-oneself in the other as a twinship experience. *International Journal of Psychoanalytic Self Psychology, 7*(3), 352–368.

Togashi K., & Kottler, A. (2015). *Kohut's twinship across cultures: The psychology of being human*. Routledge.

Togashi, K., & Kottler, A. (2019). Contemporary self psychology and the treatment of traumatized patients. In B. Huppertz (Ed.), *Approaches to psychic trauma: Theory and practice* (pp. 323–332). Roman and Littlefield.

Togashi, K., & Kottler, A. (2021). From a cohesive self to a relational being: The evolution of the psychology of the self to the psychology of being human. *Psychoanalytic Inquiry, 41*(3), 187–198.

Tolpin, M. (2002). Doing psychoanalysis of normal development: Forward edge transferences. In A. Goldberg (Ed.), *Progress in Self Psychology*, (Vol. 18, pp. 167–190). The Analytic Press.

Ulman, R. B., & Paul, H. (2006). *The self psychology of addiction and its treatment: Narcissus in wonderland*. Routledge.

Chapter 16

Relational Psychoanalysis: An Assessment at this Time

Neil Skolnick

In order to address the goals of this volume, which attempts a comparative study of the basic assumptions of the multitude of psychoanalytic schools that populate the realm of psychoanalysis, I have chosen to present a critique of relational theory as it exists today. Relational psychoanalysis, at this juncture in time, has established itself as a major force in psychoanalytic theorizing and practice and is currently traversing its middle age. No longer a neophyte seeking to establish its validity amongst the more established psychoanalytic schools, it has yet to consolidate its mature identification. Will it rise to the gravitas of classical psychoanalysis, or recede into a historical footnote?

To begin, I reiterate what Susan Warshaw and I maintained in the introduction to our 1992 compendium of relational authors, *Relational Perspectives in Psychoanalysis*. Written to commemorate the inauguration of the relational training track at the NYU Postdoctoral Program, we noted that there was no one integrated relational theory. Relational psychoanalysts hale from many diverse camps, from object-relational, self-psychological, interpersonal, intersubjective, infant research, field theory, neurobiological approaches, neo-Kleinian schools, and others. All share the major assumption that the basic building blocks of human development, character formation, motivations, and psychopathology are rooted in human relational configurations rather than the psychosexual drives of classical psychoanalysis.

The situation remains somewhat the same today. While relational psychoanalysts have more clearly delineated some of the important similarities and differences amongst the different schools, each offering a relational perspective, we have yet to produce a unified relational theory. While that was arguably the hope back then, a more unified theory has not materialized. That's not necessarily a bad thing. It is what it is, a group of diverse psychoanalytic approaches that have rejected Freud's meta-psychological drives as the ultimate explanatory bottom line. The meta-psychological drives, rooted in powerful biological imperatives, remain as important variables in relational theories but are thought to be shaped by relational configurations and not the reverse.

DOI: 10.4324/9781003027768-17

I have divided my assessment of current relational theorizing and practice into a few sections below. Some of my criticisms fall under big "C" criticisms, challenging basic assumptions of relational thinking. I also include small "c" criticisms, better thought of as pet peeves. Of note, many additional excellent critiques have been written, in particular, the two edited volumes by Aron et al. (2018a, 2018b).

A Plea for a Measure of Less Hubris

This criticism is not directed solely toward relational psychoanalysts but rather toward all psychoanalysts engaged in this endlessly fascinating though endlessly impossible work. What I refer to as hubris is the basic assumption that a psychoanalytic exploration in general, and a relational exploration in particular, will surface all essential information about a person's suffering, dynamics, and experience. I start with a true story.

A good number of years after I completed my own analysis, my aunt, my father's sister, died. When rifling through her papers we discovered my grandfather's naturalization papers. Listed on it were his children—my father, my aunt, my uncle—and Gertrude. Who the hell was Gertrude? Turns out Gertrude was another child of my grandfather's, born of a previous marriage, prior to his marriage to my grandmother. His first wife (Gertrude's mother) had died. Gertrude was my father's half-sister. So what happened to Gertrude? Turns out she was ejected from the family, my father, with only disgust in his voice, informed us. "Why?" we, of course, demanded to know. He could only respond sullenly and tersely, "She wasn't good enough for the family," and that was the last we ever heard from my father about Gertrude. He refused to say more. He took the secret of Gertrude to his grave. There being no other living relative who could inform us, we were left to our own unsuccessful internet searches and finally just to our speculations and fantasies. We figured she must have had an out-of-wedlock child, and left it at that.

But the discovery fell on my ears and soul with a thunderous resonance. When my father was about 8–10 years or so, his older sister, Gertrude, a teenager (we figured), was thrown out of the house and family, never to be heard of again. While my analysis was successful on many fronts, there was a question that it never answered, and now it turns out, never could have been answered in analysis because I did not know what I did not know. My father, a reasonable, hardworking, and in many ways unpsychologically-minded father of the 1950s, periodically, during my growing up, would disown my sister or me because we, in his mind, had done something unspeakably bad. For example, when my wife and I sent out birth announcements for our first child the announcement read, "Neil Skolnick and Karen Goldberg are thrilled to announce the birth of their daughter …" to which he responded after several months of sulking (sulking and not talking to us being his usual announcement of imminent disownment), "People are going to think you are not married." This, despite the fact we had sent it to his friends who had attended our wedding. So for years I added this periodic disowning to the list of my grievances against my father.

But knowledge of Gertrude changed all that. I now, many years after my analysis ended, appreciated that my father was traumatized as a latency-age young boy. He lost his sister to some unspeakable, shameful sin. My father, like a good latency age boy, reasoned that if you do not adhere to an absolute right, you are unworthy of continued love and deserve to be abandoned, just as his sister was. Years of my resentment toward my father slowly melted away as I began to experience compassion for his plight in a universe that had been interrupted by a trauma that became locked in time, stamping in a hyper-rigid conception of morality that he, averse to self-exploration, held until his death. We never talked about Gertrude; his shame precluded that. My own sadness was overwhelming, but as is often the case with sadness, it proved less imprisoning than the restraining iron bars of resentment. And it led to a continuous diminution in my own sense of worthlessness and shame, which had been significantly reduced in my previous "concluded" analysis, but never to this extent.

I bring up the story of Gertrude in an attempt to make a plea for a measure of humility as we attempt to assess not only a relational theory, but also any set of theories, models, or paradigms that guide us in the study and practice of psychoanalysis. We practice an odd, mostly unstated, version of grandiosity to assume that our particular theory of choice will best uncover, integrate, explain, and synthesize the information we gather about a person, and point us toward successful resolutions in their therapy. There's so much we do not know, nor will ever know, or is kept private by the patient, or has been lost to a secret, or has been forgotten or distorted, or as the existence of my phantom Aunt Gertrude so vividly demonstrated—we do not know what we do not know. To me, this further lends support to what Guntrip (1975) in his landmark paper, *My Experience of Analysis with Fairbairn and Winnicott*, sagaciously stated, "Theory does not seem to me to be the major concern. It is a useful servant but a bad master liable to produce orthodox defenders of every variety of the faith" (p. 145).

I must add that my analysis, while devoid of Gertrude, probably influenced my procedural processing of Gertrude once her existence surfaced. Had I not been analyzed, resentment might have prevailed rather than sadness.

I continue to maintain that relational theories have provided an important correction to the drive-based psychoanalytic canon. From its inception as a formalized "school" at the end of the 20th century, relational psychoanalysis hit the ground running. Many have appreciated a model or paradigm (Skolnick & Warshaw, 1992) of a psychoanalysis based on human connections, rather than quasi-biological explanations.

I'd like to stress that there was not, at its inception, nor is there today, only one unified relational theory. Instead there are a number of theories embracing a relational perspective. Several difficulties have arisen with this broad tent pluralist model of relational psychoanalysis. First and foremost there is a tendency, wish, or hope that by focusing on all brands of the theory that do not maintain the drives as the ultimate bottom line explanations, we will ultimately come up with a unified relational theory of human functioning. I emphatically maintain that the puzzle is too vast, too complicated, and contains too many uncertain moving parts operating in too many uncertain contexts for such a unifying theory to be viable.[1] The assumption of a unified relational theory is untenable.

A subset of the quest for a unified relational theory has spawned a tendency, misguided I hold, by different relational camps, to define the construct "relational" according to the narrow perspective of their own camp. Instead of viewing relational as a large pluralistic tent encompassing a number of theoretical approaches with a relational cast, some approaches have been considered by their adherents to be the sole rightful proprietor of the relational imprimatur. So it has come to pass that some consider relational to mean object-relational, others consider it to encompass only intersubjective theory, others field theory, and so forth and so on. This has been but one problem that arose when we abandoned the large tent approach to embracing multiple theories.

When looking to define relational by elevating a single theoretical camp, i.e., intersubjectivity, to encompass the entire endeavor, we run the risk of creating a Rashomon on steroids. Which one of the multiple particular theoretical paradigms do we choose, and how will that in any way create a more useful understanding? I continue to maintain that relational theory is still a work in progress and that it has room for plurality, a number of differing approaches included under its umbrella. They can usefully be seen as existing in tensions with each other, but none can be held up as the predominant identifying essence of the entire relational project.

A Plea for a Measure of Less Co-Construction

Almost synonymous with a relational approach and seen ubiquitously throughout the relational literature is the assumption that all human thought and affect, conscious and unconscious, and behavior, are co-created. Of the many who write about the universality of co-creation, I find Ogden (1994) to be one of the clearest proponents of this sentiment. Co-creation adheres to the idea that no human thought, action, or creative endeavor can exist apart from the human context within which it occurs.

This idea becomes more complicated in that it is sometimes not clear whether an author is referring to the current context in which something occurs (i.e., a therapy session) or the developmental origin of the particular something being observed. The roots of co-construction can be located in some versions of Sullivanian interpersonal psychoanalysis and have found a comfortable home in post-modern philosophy. I have always taken issue with this assumption, especially when considering the clinical situation in which the observation occurs. When analyzing any moment in a psychoanalytic session, the genesis of that moment might lie with the patient, or with the analyst, or it might be co-created by both. Acknowledging that it is rarely clear from whom any interactive moment arises, is an imperative I believe we all need to entertain, accept, and live with.

Moreover, if we take the confluence of psychoanalysis and temporality seriously, the situation becomes infinitely more complicated. If any moment in the dialogue between a patient and analyst can be considered a melding of past, present, and/or future, the context of the dialogue not only is set by the two participants in the treatment space, but now includes the interaction of each participant, potentially operating in three tenses of temporality (past, present, and future) with the other participant functioning in their three tenses. Given that each participant is possibly functioning in more than one tense at the same time (e.g., past and future) the permutations and combinations of analyst, patient, and temporal tenses of past, present, and future create a virtually unknowable and frankly absurd context for their interactions. A similar conundrum exists when we consider that each actor in an interaction is operating in potentially 3 vertical modes (conscious, preconscious, and unconscious). The conundrum deepens at a geometric rate if we consider horizontal splits, let's say the psychic organizational positions as defined by the Kleinians (paranoid/schizoid and depressive). Often thought to exist diametrically (Ogden, 1986), if we consider each person existing in differing organizational positions, one can hardly picture what a co-construction might resemble.

Obviously, I am creating this exercise in absurdity (and overly concrete obsessiveness!) to make a point that to conceive of all clinical interaction as co-constructed is resorting to a limited, most likely unknowable proposition. In the time-unhinged space of subjectivity and intersubjectivity there's room for a spectrum of influencing factors operating in an untold number of temporal directions. We must rely on our knowledge of the patient, ourselves, and the circumstances of each to make our best clinical judgment to determine, in the words of Edgar Levinson, "What's going on around here?" Bottom line, sometimes moments are co-created, and sometimes they are not.

A Plea for a Measure (Literally) of Validity

It is well recognized that psychoanalysis falls at the crossroads of many disciplines and is not just a purely empirical scientific pursuit. It overlaps realms of study including, but not limited to philosophy, social and natural sciences, art, anthropology, gender studies, and developmental and child psychology. All of the above have made useful contributions to a psychoanalytic discipline. As such the construct of "validity" has peppered our papers in a number of different ways. I maintain that we should only apply the concept *vvalidity*when a construct has met the rigorous testing required to denote *scientific* validity. Otherwise, we should use *useful.*

Our psychoanalytic literature is filled with examples of precedence masquerading as scientific validity. Just because a construct has been used repeatedly in the literature does not mean it is valid vis-vis the scientific method. Numerous psychoanalytic constructs, derived from theory (e.g., "the third" or "projective identification") have a long proud history of being clinically useful but have not acquired the status of scientific validity. They enrich the texture and depth of our work but without rigorous testing, they cannot be considered either empirically valid or not. We need to accept that our constructs are not necessarily scientifically valid. Projective identification is often spoken of by some schools contemptuously as not a valid construct, and by other schools as valid because of its ubiquitous usage. Neither side is correct. But it is a *useful* construct.

A Plea for a Measure of Lucidity

> Q: What do you get if you cross a member of the Mafia with a postmodernist?
>
> A: An offer you can't understand.

This joke pokes good-humored fun at the style of writing adopted by many relational analysts who write from a postmodern perspective, with a style of writing that aims to obscure rather than elucidate. They will often attempt to present their ideas by constructing a language that obscures conventional meanings and deconstructs formal rules of language. Verbs become nouns and time-worn jargon is appropriated to express new meanings. I do understand the advantages of postmodern *theory* to tear down encrusted meanings, linkages, attitudes, and beliefs and make space for new constructions, novel arrangements, and orderings of beliefs, attitudes, and even truths. But I struggle to find the usefulness of mangling language to make a point. The confusion it creates does not elucidate. It merely confuses.

I think it is a mistake for relational psychoanalysts to overuse this style of writing. In that it can serve to obscure rather than elucidate clearly what an author is attempting to say, it can be overly confusing to a reader not schooled in the principles of postmodernism. This would include many psychoanalysts from other orientations and probably a fair number of relational psychoanalysts as well. If we are attempting to reach out to a wider and wider audience who could potentially benefit from our craft, it does not serve our purposes to represent our discipline in cumbersome, difficult to comprehend, obscuring language that has undertones of elitism, if not intellectual discrimination. If we want to keep psychoanalysis alive as a viable alternative for people in need of relief from their pain, suffering, and self-defeating patterns, we need to be clear, and write clearly, about what we do.

A Quick Look Toward the Future

Relational psychoanalysis continues to be influential theoretically and clinically. Witness the large number of psychologists holding memberships in divisions and sections of the American Psychological Association concerned with relational perspectives, as well as the large national and international membership of the International Association for Relational Psychoanalysis and Psychotherapy (IARPP). Relational journals such as *Psychoanalytic Dialogues: The International Journal of Relational Perspectives* continue to be well subscribed. I think I am safe in making the prediction that relational psychoanalysis is here to stay for the foreseeable future, but I do think it is in need of an infusion of new ideas and energy to keep it vital. I list for the reader's perusal and criticisms, several suggestions for future direction:

We need to promote younger members in our ranks and not discriminate or exclude them. We need to celebrate their creativity.

We need to include more peripheral disciplines under the relational tent, rather than treating them as the hated "other." We could revisit theories long ago scorned.

We need to put renewed focus on the integration of biology, development, and evolution. (Kandel, 2012). Our understanding of the links between the study of evolution and development has undergone an interesting trajectory over the course of the last century. Hofer points out in his (2014) seminal article, exciting new recent discoveries have promoted a rapprochement between the long diverging studies of development and evolutionary biology in the creation of a new field familiarly referred to as "evo-devo." The advances in evo-devo research (especially at the molecular/genetic level) have brought about radical change, especially with the advent of the burgeoning study of epigenetics, in which the expression of an organism's genetic make-up can be influenced by environmental changes. Not only have animal model studies demonstrated that early changes in mother-infant interaction can have marked effects on an animal's development that persist into adulthood, but the effects can persist into future generations (Skolnick et al., 1980). As Hofer (2014) stated:

> Our new knowledge of the nature and role of genes, and of the *many novel mechanisms for their regulation during development* [emphasis added] has restored our understanding of biology to a position much more supportive of Freud's formulation of psychoanalytic theory than at any time since the end of the nineteenth century" (p. 13).

16. Relational Psychoanalysis	
Main, general underlying assumptions	1 The building blocks of character, motivation, development, and psychopathology are human relationships and not the meta-psychological drives. 2 All interactions are co-constructed
Specific theoretical assumptions	
psychic structure	Relational thinking embraces a number of assumptions about psychic structure, including vertical (i.e., conscious, preconscious, and unconscious) and horizontal (i.e., split) models, temporal models, and dialectically constructed models
energy	Energy considered as an open system
relationships	Relationships are assumed to be the primary building blocks of human psychology
developmental stages	Considered as less lockstep, more non-linear and diametrically constructed
body	Increasingly, relational models are including the body as a crucial component of development, character structure, and pathology.
anxieties/instincts and defenses	Relational thinking generally assumes that anxieties are rooted in interpersonal and intersubjective conflicts
Assumptions concerning etiology	Relational theories typically stress early configurations of parental figures who do not supply the love and connectivity needed by the developing child.
Implications for technique	Relational analysts view the relationship between analyst and patient as the primary locus of change.
Subsequent developments of the core concept	N/A

Note

1 See an interesting conversation between A. Bass and A. Harris in Aron et al. (2018b).

References

Aron, L., Grand, S., & Slochower, J. (Eds.). (2018a). *De-idealizing relational theory: A critique from within*. Routledge.

Aron, L., Grand, S., & Slochower, J. (Eds.). (2018b). *Decentering relational theory: A comparative critique*. Routledge.
Guntrip, H. (1975). My experience of analysis with Fairbairn and Winnicott. *International Review of Psycho-Analysis*, *2*, 145–156.
Hofer, M. A. (2014). The emerging synthesis of development and evolution: A new biology for psychoanalysis. *Neuropsychoanalysis*, *16*, 3–22.
Kandel, E. R. (2012). Biology and the future of psychoanalysis: A new intellectual framework for psychiatry revisited. *Psychoanalytic Review*, *99*, 607–644.
Ogden, T. H. (1986). *The matrix of the mind*. Aronson.
Ogden, T. H. (1994). The analytic third: Working with intersubjective clinical facts. *International Journal of Psycho-Analysis*, *72*, 593–605.
Skolnick, N. J., Ackerman, S. H., Hofer, M. A., & Weiner, H. (1980). Vertical transmission of acquired ulcer susceptibility in the rat. *Science*, *208*, 1161–1163.
Skolnick, N. J., & Warshaw, S. C. (1992). *Relational perspectives in psychoanalysis*. The Analytic Press.

Chapter 17

Intersubjectivity: Intersubjective Systems Theory

Joshua R. Burg

Main, General Underlying Assumptions

Beginning with the work of Atwood and Stolorow (1979), intersubjective systems theory[1] has grown to include the contributions of many psychoanalytic thinkers. While each individual has added something of their own perspective, in this chapter I focus on three core underlying assumptions. Specifically, how intersubjectivity's theoretical foundation is built upon ideas related to an attitude of fallibilism, the organization of subjectivity, and the primacy of affect in human experiencing. As this chapter delves into the topics of psychic structure, development, and body, it is my hope that an appreciation may be gained regarding how these underlying assumptions shape the conclusions intersubjectivity makes about treatment. While these are not an exhaustive list of underlying assumptions, they are the three I speak most of as I think about and teach this theory.

Before moving into these ideas though, we must establish a common understanding of some key terminology. First, the word intersubjective itself can have a variety of meanings across psychoanalytic perspectives. For our purposes, the term refers to the constitutional unit of two subjectivities and their interactions. This literal *inter*-subjective field provides the precondition for the development and elaboration of all human experience. As Stolorow et al. (2002) put it, psychological phenomena do not arise from "isolated intrapsychic mechanisms" but rather from the "interface of reciprocally interacting worlds of experience" and this interaction "constitutes the domain of psychoanalytic inquiry" (p. 102). "A person's self-experience is at all times determined by and dependent upon the specific intersubjective contexts in which it takes shape" (Hagman et al., 2019, p. 7), and this contextually oriented focus is at the heart of what it means to think and practice intersubjectively.

Second, I will reference organizing principles, patterns, themes, and structure using these phrases interchangeably. Generally, organizing principle is the more theory-specific term, but each of these phrases refers to a sort of unconscious affective-cognitive schema; an emotional conviction formed through relational experiences that serves to shape and organize

DOI: 10.4324/9781003027768-18

one's subjectivity. Though they cannot always be captured in this way, for illustrative purposes it can be helpful to think of these organizational structures in an "if this, then that" format:[2] "If no one is there for me when I need them, then why bother forming relationships," or "If I am not the best, then I am nothing." We all have many of these structures operating outside of awareness and altogether they shape our experience of self, other, and world. Illuminating these principles through the treatment process is another core component of intersubjective practice.

With this mutual understanding, let us now return to the underlying assumptions that provide intersubjectivity's foundation. As a "phenomenological contextualist perspective" (Stolorow & Atwood, 2019, p. 57), intersubjectivity assumes a fundamental characteristic of human beings is the effort we make toward organizing and making meaning out of our experiences (Atwood & Stolorow, 2014). The intersubjective sensibility builds from a foundation of fallibilism[3] (Burg, 2018) and also rejects the motivational primacy of instinctual drives in human life, replacing them with affect, or subjective emotional experience, as the central motivating force (Buirski et al., 2020; Stolorow, 2013).

Starting with fallibilism, this concept helps us to *subjectify* rather than *objectify* our patients. Engaging others with a fallibilistic attitude means acknowledging the limitations of our own subjectivity and holding onto the notion that our ideas and perceptions may be wrong. We must be willing to loosen the grip of our own organizations of experience and dwell within the subjectivity of our patients. Fallibilism leads us to a recognition that an experience-near inquiry into our patients' subjectivities is essential for understanding and transforming their lives; if I might be wrong, then let me understand the rightness of their world and work from that vantage.

As the intersubjectivist grounds themselves in this form of therapeutic engagement, the primacy of subjective organizing activity transforms into an underlying assumption, theoretical concept, and technical guide all wrapped together as one: believing in the importance of subjective organizing activity leads to theoretical ideas that hold such activity at the heart of their functioning, e.g., organizing principles. This then informs technique, as the intersubjectivist seeks to illuminate these organizational structures by orienting themselves toward the elaboration of how these principles pattern our patients' worlds.

Of course, with all the use of the term organizing, it raises the question of *what* exactly is being organized. From this sensibility, one of the central answers to this question of "what?" is emotional experience. The intersubjectivist finds that with an attuned engagement towards illuminating the organizing patterns of our patients, these patterns often act as governing rules for what our patients can or cannot experience emotionally. Recognition of the central role affect plays in organizing subjectivity moves us away from instinctual drives and towards the individual's unique constellation of affects, which become organized into their experience of self. The focus on emotional experience has even helped develop intersubjectivity's understanding of the selfobject concept, as we believe that "selfobject functions pertain fundamentally to the integration of affect into the evolving organization of self-experience" (Stolorow et al., 1995, p. 86). Fallibilism leads to subjective experience, subjective experience leads us to organizing patterns, and organizational patterns lead us to the centrality of affect.

Psychic Structure, Affective Experience, and Development

This seems like the appropriate place to speak more directly to affective experiences, as well as how they relate to psychic structure and development. As mentioned, in the place of Freudian drives, intersubjectivity recognizes affect at the heart of personality development. Within intersubjective contexts, affect is attuned or misattuned to and through repetitive interactions over the course of life; these responses are organized into thematic meaning structures. Over time, the specific constellation of organizing principles that one develops largely come to constitute what we label the patient's personality and sense of self. In this theory, emotional experience lies at the core of development and the establishment of psychic structure. Focusing on affect also reinforces intersubjectivity's contextual emphasis and contrasts it with theories that assume instinctual drive energies at the heart of psychic functioning. As Stolorow and Atwood (2019) explain, affect, unlike drives, are:

> Something that from birth onward is co-constituted within ongoing relational systems ... and ... is inseparable from the intersubjective contexts of attunement and malattunement in which it is felt. Therefore, locating affect at [intersubjectivity's] motivational center automatically entails a radical contextualization of virtually all aspects of human psychological life. (p. 59)

Affects and the intersubjective contexts in which they occur become the foundation upon which our psychic structure is built, and subsequently through which our sense of self is established.

Regarding psychic structure, two main concepts are the unconscious and organizing principles. While I have previously addressed organizing principles, we have yet to explore how they are integrally related to the formulation of the unconscious. Intersubjectivity breaks the unconscious down into the dynamic, prereflective, and unvalidated unconscious (Orange et al., 1997, pp. 7–8). The dynamic unconscious consists of emotional experiences once known that have been "sequestered or forgotten because [they] created conflict" (Orange et al., 1997, p. 7). This is achieved through repression, which intersubjectivity conceptualizes as a "negative organizing principle" that excludes from awareness the organizational configurations of self and other that are associated with "emotional conflict and subjective danger" (Atwood & Stolorow, 2014, p. 29). When certain feelings, memories, or ideas threaten the stability of one's established organizing principles, repression and defensive processes come into play to protect the ongoing cohesion of one's subjectivity.

Then there is the prereflective unconscious which is viewed as the home of one's organizing principles. The prereflective unconscious is not unconscious via repressive processes, but rather in the sense that it is outside of awareness. It is described as prereflective to capture how one's awareness can be directed, over time, to the very organizing patterns that structure one's experiential world. Illuminating a patient's organizing principles and helping them achieve a more reflective and flexible relationship with these emotional convictions is an important aspect of psychological growth within intersubjective practice.

Finally, intersubjectivity posits an unvalidated unconscious as home to all the "aspects of subjective life that could never fully become experience because they never found a validating response in the emotional environment" (Orange et al., 1997, p. 8). If you use the metaphor of a person as a house, Stolorow and Atwood (1992) aptly describe the contents of the unvalidated unconscious as all the unused construction materials remaining in the house. This unused lumber, tile, and sheetrock lies in wait; something that could have been but never was and will remain unconscious as long as the "requisite validation" (p. 35) it requires to be integrated into consciousness remains absent.

Moving to ideas on development, intersubjective theory does not focus on the universality of specific psychological phases, but rather keeps the emphasis on the process of organizing subjective experience. As Atwood and Stolorow (2014) note:

> Every stage in a child's development is best conceptualized psychoanalytically in terms of the unique, continuously changing psychological field constituted by the intersection of the child's evolving subjective universe with those of caretakers. This observational stance brings into sharpened focus the specific intersubjective contexts that shape the developmental process and that facilitate or obstruct the child's negotiation of developmental tasks and passage through developmental phases (p. 66).

This grounds intersubjectivity in a process and systems viewpoint, allowing for the unique complexity of each individual patient to emerge. Rather than postulating universal developmental concepts that the patient *must* be fit into or that the treatment *must* address, the intersubjective approach focuses on the ways in which the developmental system functions in the service of helping the child establish and maintain an organization of their subjectivity throughout different life phases. Psychoanalytic concepts may then be utilized as they become an emergent property of the dyad with a revised focus on the processes and development of the patient's organization of their experiential world.

This focus on subjectivity frees up the therapist to respond more individually to the patient's needs. For the intersubjectivist, while the language of the oedipal phase, object constancy, or rapprochement might act as an aid for our own sense of "knowing" with the patient, when we approach them with an experience-near focus on their subjectivity, we can often develop co-created language for the negotiation of developmental tasks, rather than predetermined psychological jargon. Neither I nor my patient needs language from the literature on separation-individuation to make sense of and deeply feel what it is like to let go of one edge of the pool, tread into deeper waters, and be unable to see the other edge we were hoping to grasp onto. The therapeutic task here is not about intellectual understanding, as helpful as that can be at times, but about affective integration of these developmental experiences into the patient's sense of self. The more I stay close to my patient's experience, the more these evocative images emerge, and the more meaningful it is when we come to the point where we can acknowledge together that they have learned to swim, found the other side of the pool, or some combination of both. The felt experience within the intersubjective field is what allows for emotional integration and structural development.

Body

When addressing the ideas intersubjectivity has about the body, we must look to some philosophical roots and discuss René Descartes. While a more comprehensive discussion of Cartesian thinking[4] is beyond the scope of this chapter, I would like to briefly mention the myth of the isolated mind (Stolorow & Atwood, 1992). This manifestation of Cartesian thinking views minds as self-enclosed entities separate from external reality (Stolorow et al., 2002). It splits apart our minds and bodies, ultimately serving to shield us from the vulnerability of being embedded in our bodies and the intersubjective field. An illustrative caricature of this would be the image of two isolated minds acting on one another in the room; one reified thinking thing effecting change on the other, much in the way comic heroes utilize telepathic powers to influence the psyches of others. In this caricature, the bodies are irrelevant and the telepath (i.e., therapist) experiences little psychic threat from the non-telepath (i.e., patient) as they use their psychic powers on them!

Intersubjectivity's response is to reject Cartesian thinking and dispel the illusion that there is any separation between mind and body. We are not simply thinking things, but complexly developed beings with mind, body, and context all forming an indissoluble whole. As I (Burg, 2018) and others have written (Jaenicke, 2008, 2015), a challenge for the intersubjective practitioner is the vulnerability that comes from removing the psychological armor granted through Cartesian thinking. Not only can we more readily be changed without this Cartesian armor, but our treatment relationship often demands we *must* be changed in the service of our patients' growth (Jaenicke, 2011; Slavin & Kriegman, 1998).

Defense, Resistance, and Transference

Given all that we have covered, I would like to now turn to the clinical situation and briefly address how these underlying ideas influence intersubjectivity's understanding of defense, resistance, and transference. Starting with defense and resistance, intersubjectivity's conviction of the need to organize and make meaning out of subjective experience leads to an idea summarized with the phrase "striving for health" (Buirski et al., 2020). Resistance and defense are not understood as pathology but are taken within their emergent contexts as the patient's best efforts to maintain a sense of "personal agency and self-cohesion" (Buirski et al., 2020, p. 157). To paraphrase Bernard Brandchaft, resistance is the attitude exhibited by heroes in the face of oppression (Brandchaft et al., 2010). This phrase embodies intersubjectivity and I repeat it to supervisees when they describe their patients as acting borderline or engaging in irrational thinking. This helps them see how the sentiments they have just expressed are often indications they have fallen out of an empathic listening stance and felt their own organizations of experience threatened in some way by their patient. Preserving our subjective organization may help alleviate our own anxieties, but if left unexamined, it is rarely of benefit to more deeply understanding our patients.

This brings me to intersubjectivity's views on transference. Seen as "neither a regression to nor a displacement from the past, but rather an expression of the *continuing influence* of organizing principles ... that crystalized out of the patient's early formative experiences," (Stolorow et al., 1995, p. 36, italics in original) transference, at its most basic level is conceptualized as ongoing organizing activity. This general conceptualization allows space for the varying dimensions of the transference to become a point of focus as needed, though intersubjectivity attends most frequently to the shifting figure-ground relationship between developmental and repetitive dimensions of the transference. For the intersubjective practitioner, the developmental dimension of the transference is home to the patient's selfobject longings and strivings towards the development of their self-experience, while the repetitive dimension is home to the anticipations of retraumatization and the desires for an antidote to painful experiences that are already present (Brandchaft et al., 2010; Burg, 2018; Hagman et al., 2019).

Conclusion

While much more could be said, it is my hope that even in this overview form, readers can understand the foundational importance to intersubjectivity of a fallibilistic attitude, focus on subjective organizations of experience, and the primacy of affect in motivating human life. I shall end with a description of a moment with my patient David, highlighting how these assumptions are deeply embedded in an intersubjective practice.

David has a long history of absent boundaries, traumatic intrusions, and usurpations of his sense of self. During one session, we break a prolonged silence with his revelation that he feared our eye contact would lead to me crossing the room and kissing him. This challenges my own perceptions of the silence and I must consciously reorient myself towards David's reality and experience of the intersubjective field (engaging my fallibilistic attitude and orienting myself towards his subjective organization of the moment).

As he continues, I reflect and articulate the organizing theme he communicates with an emphasis on its emotional core (the centrality of affect): when David allows himself to seek connection, he feels violated and overpowered by the other, leaving him with the choice of maintaining connection at the cost of submitting himself or choosing disconnection leading to an overwhelming loneliness that ends in suicidal despair. David feels understood and there is an ease to our remaining conversation.

In intersubjective language, we focused our efforts on an experience-near understanding of his subjectivity, leading us to the appreciation of an important organizing principle born out of repeated experiences of misattunement within David's early emotional milieu. Simultaneously, through our connection, we helped to begin establishing a different organizing principle, one in which David's crushing loneliness and longing for connection could be shared, attuned to, and held without the kinds of overwhelming mergers and subjective annihilations he experienced as a child. Repetition and further illumination will help establish new ways of being and connecting for David, while older ways can exist more consistently in the background.

17. Intersubjectivity	
Main, general underlying assumptions	Intersubjectivity builds from a foundational, fallibilistic epistemology. It assumes human experience can only be understood contextually and that a fundamental characteristic of humanity is our effort to organize and make meaning of subjective experience. Intersubjectivity assumes that affect is the primary motivational force in the development of self-experience.

(Continued)

Specific theoretical assumptions	
psychic structure	The basic unit of psychic structure is the organizing principle. There are also three different levels of unconscious to understand—the dynamic, prereflective, and unvalidated unconscious.
energy	Intersubjectivity has moved away from instinctual drives to affect as the primary source of energy and motivation in life.
relationships	All experience is only understandable within the intersubjective contexts in which it emerges. Relational, i.e., intersubjective experiences are the precondition for human development and understanding.
developmental stages	Intersubjectivity moves away from universalizing specific developmental concepts and instead focuses on the intersubjective field created between the child and caregiver, as well as the patient and therapist. By focusing theory more on the process of development, it makes room for any needed developmental concept to be utilized as it becomes an emergent property of the therapeutic dyad.
body	Intersubjectivity eschews Cartesian mind/body duality and views mind, body, and context as inseparable and reciprocally influencing.
anxieties/instincts and defenses	Anxieties and defenses are understood as emergent experiences within an intersubjective field that occurs as the patient (or therapist) attempts to maintain and manage the established organizational structure of their self-experience.
Assumptions concerning etiology	Psychological structure, growth, or pathology arise from the repetitive experiences of attuned or malattuned interactions throughout the lifespan.
Implications for technique	Intersubjectivity leads to technique that emphasizes an empathic listening-stance, affective attunement, illumination of organizing principles, and an appreciation of the context dependent nature of all psychological phenomena.
Subsequent developments of the core concept	Intersubjectivity's main concepts have been further developed by various authors, often applied to specific clinical presentations such as psychosis, addiction, supervision, couples work, etc. Additionally, intersubjective concepts have been integrated into self psychology and other relational theories.

Notes

1 I use the terms intersubjective systems theory, intersubjective sensibility, and intersubjectivity synonymously to refer to the theory developed from the ideas of George Atwood and Robert Stolorow.
2 I am indebted to Shelley Doctors for this language and helpful way to teach the concept of organizing principles.
3 While fallibilism is an integral part of intersubjectivity, Donna Orange is most responsible for explicitly introducing the term and has written much about this idea.
4 For a more comprehensive discussion of Cartesian thinking see Chapter 2 in Stolorow et al. (2002).

References

Atwood, G., & Stolorow, R. (1979). *Faces in a cloud: Intersubjectivity in personality theory*. Aronson.

Atwood, G., & Stolorow, R. (2014). *Structures of subjectivity: Explorations in psychoanalytic phenomenology and contextualism* (2nd ed.). Routledge.

Brandchaft, B., Doctors, S., & Sorter, D. (2010). *Toward an emancipatory psychoanalysis: Brandchaft's intersubjective vision*. Routledge.

Buirski, P., Haglund, P., & Markley, E. (2020). *Making sense together: The intersubjective approach to psychotherapy* (2nd ed.). Rowman & Littlefield.

Burg, J. (2018). A therapist's fallibilism and the hermeneutics of trust. *Psychoanalysis, Self and Context*, *13*(3), 272–287.

Hagman, G., Paul, H., & Zimmermann, P. (Eds.). (2019). *Intersubjective self psychology: A primer*. Routledge.

Jaenicke, C. (2008). *The risk of relatedness: Intersubjectivity theory in clinical practice*. Aronson.

Jaenicke, C. (2011). *Change in psychoanalysis: An analyst's reflections on the therapeutic relationship*. Routledge.

Jaenicke, C. (2015). *The search for a relational home: An intersubjective view of therapeutic action*. Routledge.

Orange, D., Atwood, G., & Stolorow, R. (1997). *Working intersubjectively: Contextualism in psychoanalytic practice*. Routledge.

Slavin, M., & Kriegman, D. (1998). Why the analyst needs to change: Toward a theory of conflict, negotiation, and mutual influence in the therapeutic process. *Psychoanalytic Dialogues*, *8*(2), 247–284.

Stolorow, R. (2013). Intersubjective-systems theory: A phenomenological-contextualist psychoanalytic perspective. *Psychoanalytic Dialogues*, *23*, 383–389.

Stolorow, R., & Atwood, G. (1992). *Contexts of being: The intersubjective foundations of psychological life*. Routledge.

Stolorow, R., & Atwood, G. (2019). *The power of phenomenology: Psychoanalytic and philosophical perspectives*. Routledge.

Stolorow, R., Atwood, G., & Orange, D. (2002). *Worlds of experience: Interweaving philosophical and clinical dimensions in psychoanalysis*. Basic Books.

Stolorow, R., Brandchaft, B., & Atwood, G. (1995). *Psychoanalytic treatment: An intersubjective approach*. Routledge.

Chapter 18

American Object Relations: The Assumptions of American Object Relations Theories

Frank Summers

Main, General Underlying Assumptions

The phenomenology of Edmund Husserl (1913) showed that all experience is the experience *of* something. This translates at the dynamic level to the fact that every self-state has a corresponding object. The self-state and object are connected by an affect, and it is this unit of self-affect-object that constitutes an object relationship (e.g., Kernberg, 1976). The fundamental assumption of this school is that object relationships constitute the basic unit of the human personality. The object is the other pole of the self-state, and therefore is embedded in all human experience.

There is no single object relationship theory; there are a variety of ways of thinking about and conceptualizing object relationships and the role they play in emotional life and in the analytic process. Theorists as diverse as Fairbairn (1952), Melanie Klein (1957/1975), Winnicott (1965), Michael Balint (1968), Thomas Ogden (1983), Kohut (1984), and Kernberg (1976), and many others fall under the umbrella of object relationship theories because they see personality growth and emotional life as a function of the way others are seen and encoded. These often contrasting theories share a type of "middle position" between classical psychoanalysis and the interpersonal tradition. According to classical analysis, drives and their psychological expression as wishes are the fundamental units of human motivation. For the interpersonal school, originating in Harry Stack Sullivan's work (1954), human experience is between two or more people. By contrast, for object relations theory, the object may exist at any ontological level: a person, a fantasy, an illusion, or even a hallucination, and even when it is another person, the emphasis is on the meaning of that person to the self. The object relationship is different from interpersonal relating; it is the template for the way the self forms such relationships. That distinction is the decisive difference between object relations theories and any interpersonal theory.

DOI: 10.4324/9781003027768-19

Assumptions about Psychic Structure

Object relations theories can be divided by the aggressive drive into two broad categories. On one side are Kleinian (1957/1975) and neo-Kleinian theorists, such as Kernberg (1976), who view health and pathology as primarily a matter of the aggressive drive. On the other side are theorists such as Fairbairn (1952), Winnicott (1965), and many others who see the self at the center of human motivation.

This second group has become the foundation for a distinctively American object relations paradigm, sometimes called "the American Middle School" (Spezzano, 1995). This broad viewpoint encompasses prominent English theorists as well as the relational school. The latter emphasizes the "relational matrix" that forms between patient and analyst, and the inevitability of the analyst's participation in their interaction. Given our definition of object relationships, the relational viewpoint fits as one particularly American form of object relations theory.

The overriding principle of relational sensibility is that the analyst inevitably participates in the relational configurations that develop between the patient and the analyst. Enactments between patient and analyst are not pathological, nor healthy, but they are inevitable. While this is an approach that includes the person of the analyst in all that happens, it is an object relations model because the analytic relationship is understood to lie in the templates of early relationships of both participants. In brief, the relational model adds the analyst's object relationships to the understanding of the analytic relationship.

To qualify for the appellation "object relations," a theory must emphasize the development of the individual as a product of those early relationships and their enactment in later life. The templates formed from those early relationships create a pattern of object relationships that strongly influence later relationships and the analytic process. Object relations means the patient is understood in terms of the pattern of perceiving others. It is the need for and influence of others on the self that is the hallmark of an object relations viewpoint.

Assumptions Concerning Etiology: Development and Relationship Formation

We now turn to the assumptions on which this paradigm is based. The primary assumption is that the child seeks object relationships at the very beginning of life (Fairbairn, 1952) and needs a responsive environment to reflect back her affective states (Beebe & Lachmann, 2002; Benjamin, 1995). The assumption that the child is born with affects is backed by solid evidence (Tomkins, 1962) although the number of such inborn affects may be disputed.

The results of different research groups show that the child does not just possess affects from birth, but actively seeks response to their affective states from caretakers or anyone with whom they interact (Beebe & Lachmann, 2002; Stern, 1985). The child develops patterns of interaction with the caretaker in the first days of life. Those patterns and their subsequent development lay down the template for the child's ways of relating to others. The patterns that evolve in this way are the object relationships that form the foundation of the child's ways of relating to others, and that, in turn, is the basis of the child's growing personality. Who the child becomes cannot be separated from the child's relationships with others, and, most importantly, the patterns of those relationships are reenacted throughout life. The assumption is that templates for interaction are laid down in the formative years and continue to determine the way the child relates to others and himself throughout the life cycle.

It should be underscored that these templates are not only ways of relating to others but also are equally determinative of the way one relates to oneself. The child treats himself as he was treated by the caretaker (Bollas, 1987). Self-perception is largely an internalization of the early object relationships. That is to say, the self-image reflects the nature of the early object relationships. What the child experienced in those early object relationships lives on not only in the way the adult treats others but in the way the adult treats himself.

This is not to say that the early relationships are wholly determinative of all later relationships and the self-image. There are other influences. It is assumed that we are all born with a biological makeup that is a major factor in development, and of course there are a variety of environmental influences beyond those early relationships. Later relationships, especially in adolescence, influence the nature of the child's object relationships, and other experiences, traumatic or otherwise, must be factored in. So, object relationships are not necessarily determinative of later relationships, but they are the most emotionally powerful factors in the way later relationships are constituted. The ultimate form relationships take includes a variety of other factors.

Assumptions about Motivation and Defense: Without Instinct

This concept of development implies that there is an inborn motivation to utilize inherent capacities. These include cognitive, emotional, motoric, as well as other human capabilities. One can see this motivation in the newborn as early as the first days and weeks of life as the infant uses what capabilities it has to look, observe, emit sounds, and soon makes the effort to move, touch, and manipulate objects. This is what Winnicott (1965) called the "spontaneous gesture." The assumption is that the natural state of the human being is to utilize and exercise capabilities for the very purpose of developing them

(Tomkins, 1978). They need no external push, the desire to develop potential is inborn and will occur unless impinged upon by some other force.

The implication of this assumption is that the patient has an inborn motivation to develop and utilize her or his potential, and the pathological patterns are a product of the derailment of this process. So, the patient enters the consulting room with her pathological patterns resulting from early trauma or impingement that has not allowed the potential to become realized in one or more areas of the self. The assumption is made that each patient suffers from a truncated self resulting in the pathological patterns the analyst finds and attempts to ameliorate. Therefore, the assumption is that beneath or even embedded in the object relationships with which the patient presents is a need and desire to realize buried potential.

For the object relations theorist operating on this model, it is assumed that there is an indomitable drive to realize and express all aspects of the self, analogous to the "return of the repressed" at the center of classical theory. But the energy concept and instinct theory have no role here. The assumption is that it is possible to work through the patient's defenses and presenting pathological patterns to reach the drive for self-realization that motivates the patient and fuels her self-expression. The pathological object relations patterns constitute a distorted expression of the indomitable push within the patient to become who he or she can potentially be.

From a self-psychological viewpoint, Tolpin (2002) called this the "forward edge" of the patient's pathology. While only self-psychologists use this term, the concept on which it is based is a standard assumption of all American object relations theories. It is assumed that there is a healthy striving embedded in the patient's pathological patterns that can be uncovered through the analytic work. The success of the analysis hinges on the discovery and articulation of the part or parts of the self that continues to strive for realization and expression despite their distortion into the defensive and pathological patterns the analyst sees when the patient appears for help.

Assumptions Concerning Clinical Technique: The Psychoanalytic Process

From this viewpoint, the analytic process makes some of the same assumptions about the process of analysis as any other model. First, the assumption is that the source of the psychopathology is to be found at an unconscious level. So, critical to the analysis is the uncovering of unconscious meaning and motivation. The assumption is that this unconscious level must be made conscious before any changes of analytic significance can take place. This is not to say that making what is unconscious conscious is the whole of therapeutic action. In fact, the assumption is that more than interpretation is necessary but rarely sufficient to achieve analytic goals.

Several assumptions are made about the analytic process that differs from most other models of analysis. The assumption that interpretation alone is rarely sufficient means that another dimension must be added to the interpretive process in the therapeutic action of analysis. While this "something more" differs among theorists, it is assumed that there must be analytic input that goes beyond interpretation.

Even more fundamentally, the relational movement, a branch of American object relations theory, sees analytic treatment as a "two person" process. The assumption of the "relational matrix" means that the analyst is involved just as the patient is and because the analyst is embedded in this matrix, he or she has no place to observe the process (Greenberg & Mitchell, 1983). The analyst is in it, and cannot extricate himself to observe what is going on for the patient and in the analytic relationship. This viewpoint undermines any notion of analytic "objectivity." The assumption is that any perceptions or understanding of the patient is relative to the context of the analyst's perspective and cannot be regarded as "objective knowledge." The assumption here is that the analyst participates in all that goes on, whether wittingly or not, so that one cannot make a statement about the patient apart from the influence of the analyst, and the analyst is inevitably influenced by the patient. This assumption marks the very essence of the relational viewpoint.

The second major assumption on which the relational movement is based is that because of the analyst's involvement in all that happens the analyst is drawn into enactments that repeat the patient's interpersonal patterns. The assumption is that the analyst is drawn into the patient's dynamics and participates in their enactment in the analysis, however unwittingly. This is not good or bad, it is inevitable. The analyst and patient will repeat the patterns of the patient's developmental process.

Not all American object relations theorists subscribe to this concept of the analytic process in just the way I have depicted it. Those known as members of the relational group, such as Mitchell (1988), Aron (1990, 1996), Davies (1994), Stern (2010), Hoffman (1998), and others all make the "relational matrix" assumption. But others not so firmly ensconced in the relational paradigm do not share the assumption of the "relational matrix" such that the analyst cannot make valid observations of the patient and the process from within the analytic dyad. This second group, represented by theorists such as Ogden (1983), Grotstein (1985), Spezzano (1995), and Summers (1999, 2013), among others, share the assumption that one can never eliminate the analyst from what the patient says and does in analysis, but they do not believe that implies a relational matrix that the analyst cannot see out of. Similarly, they do not assume that enactments between patient and analyst are inevitable. The assumption here is that despite the analyst's involvement in all that happens in the analytic dyad, the analyst can see his own involvement with the patient, the influence he has on the patient, and make observations of the patient's dynamics.

Epistemology

This last point leads the discussion to epistemology. While the relational group seems to hold a relativistic position, other object relations theorists do not share the extreme version of what the analyst can see and do. Now it is true that relationalists such as Hoffman (1998) have addended the name of their epistemological stance to differentiate it from what they call "radical relativism." However, there is no elucidation of how their viewpoint is "not radical" or how it differs from "radical relativism." The name change does not change the epistemological position. Their logic is that the involvement of the analyst in the dyad means that the analyst cannot make any observations not influenced by the relative position of the analyst. So that assumption remains despite the re-naming. The other group of American object relations theorists does not share this epistemological position but does agree the two people in the analytic dyad influence each other.

Further Development of the Core Concept

As we have seen, this model assumes that psychopathology is rooted in a developmental derailment. The reasons vary from patient to patient, but common sources of developmental distortion are overt traumas, as in sexual, physical, or verbal abuse, or neglect, as happens more commonly, when parents do not respond to the child's affects and desire to be heard. Such children are subject to "cumulative trauma" (Khan, 1963/1974). Under the condition of parental neglect, the child will not be able to be aware of or utilize her own affects, leading to a defect in the self. In cases of overt trauma, the child's emotional and/or sensual life is assaulted and does not develop normally. In either case, there is a rupture in normal self-development, so that the evolution of the self is arrested, resulting in one of many forms of pathology. That is to say, the assumption is that any form of psychopathology that is not clearly biological in origin is a product of some form of childhood disturbance resulting in an arrest in self-development. Relations with others become a product of the distorted self, either as a direct product or a defense against awareness of the defect.

So, to summarize, the concept of psychopathology assumes:

1 an arrest in self-development due to environmental impingement of some type;
2 the aspect of the self that is arrested is dissociated or repressed;
3 the resulting split off or repressed part of the self seeks expression and articulation in the world;
4 the form of the expression is the symptom or dysfunction.

Conclusion: Most General Underlying Assumptions

The overriding assumption of American object relations theories is that units consisting of self-affect-object are the fundaments of human experience and are the constituents of which the self is composed. If we unpack the self, we find a variety of object relationships, the templates for how to relate to others. These are the fundamental assumptions of object relations theories. In turn, they lead to a clinical process, and that process will take place according to the way the patient's object relationships play out in the transference and the analytic process as a whole. The crux of therapeutic action, whatever the particulars, will always be about the understanding of the patient's object-relational patterns and their transformation into a healthier template for interpersonal relationships.

18. American Object Relations	
Main, general underlying assumptions	1 There is an indomitable need for each person to realize the potential in every area of human capability. 2 The realization of this potential becomes the self.
Specific theoretical assumptions	
psychic structure	Psychic structure is not relevant to the analytic process.
energy	Energy is not a useful concept for understanding the human process.
relationships	The self is formed from relationships throughout the life cycle, but the early relationships are the most formative. The need and ability to relate to others is inborn.
developmental stages	Developmental stages are real, but they are not definitively demarcated from each other. That is, there is movement back and forth among developmental stages throughout life.
body	The experience of the body is largely a product of how the body is treated by the caretakers during early life and sensuality is one among the many ways the body is experienced.
anxieties/instincts and defenses	Instinct is not a useful concept, but anxiety is formative in that it constitutes a sense of threat to the self.
Assumptions concerning etiology	The adult is formed from biological constitution interacting with the way the caretakers relate to the infant and growing child. The experience with the early caretakers is encoded in the child's mind and that is the most crucial factor in self development.

(Continued)

Implications for technique	The analytic process has to include "something more" than interpretation, but analysts differ on what this "more" is. The patient must develop previously arrested parts of the self in the analytic process.
Subsequent developments of the core concept	People do not internalize "objects," they internalize "object relationships," which means they take in a relationship between self and object, so that means the roles can be and often are reversed. In the analytic process, the patient may enact the self and relate to the analyst as object, or become the self and treat the analyst as the self, that is, as they were treated. Analysis is, in part, a recognition of who the two players are at any given moment and how and why that changes and even reverses. Inevitably, patient and analyst will reverse roles and shift their enactments with each other. This is one critical component of the development of object relations theory.

References

Aron, L. (1990). One person and two person psychologies and the method of psychoanalysis. *Psychoanalytic Psychology*, *7*(4), 475–485.

Aron, L. (1996). *Meeting of minds*. The Analytic Press.

Balint, M. (1968). *The basic fault*. Brunner/Mazel.

Beebe, B., & Lachmann, F. (2002). *Infant research and adult treatment*. The Analytic Press.

Benjamin, J. (1995). *Like subjects, love objects*. Yale University Press.

Bollas, C. (1987). *The shadow of the object*. Columbia University Press.

Davies, J. (1994). Love in the afternoon: A relational reconsideration of desire and dread in the countertransference. *Psychoanalytic Dialogues*, *4*(2), 153–170.

Fairbairn, W. D. R. (1952). *Psychoanalytic studies of the personality*. Routledge.

Greenberg, J., &. Mitchell, S. (1983). *Object relationships in psychoanalytic theory*. Harvard.

Grotstein, J. (1985). *Splitting and projective identification*. Aronson.

Hoffman, I. (1998). *Ritual and spontaneity in psychoanalysis*. The Analytic Press.

Husserl, E. (1913). *Ideas: General introduction to pure phenomenology*. Collier Books.

Kernberg, O. (1976). *Object relations theories and clinical psychoanalysis*. Aronson.

Khan, M. (1974). The concept of cumulative trauma. In *The privacy of the self* (pp. 42–58). International Universities Press. (Original work published 1963).

Klein, M. (1975). Envy and Gratitude. In *Envy and gratitude and other works, 1946–1963* (pp. 176–235). Dell. (Original published 1957).

Kohut, H. (1984). *How does analysis cure?* University of Chicago Press.

Mitchell, S. (1988). *Relational concepts in psychoanalysis*. Harvard University Press.

Ogden, T. (1983). The concept of internal object relationships. *International Journal of Psychoanalysis*, *64*, 227–241.

Spezzano, C. (1995). "Classical" versus contemporary theory—The differences that matter clinically. *Contemporary Psychoanalysis*, *30*, 20–45.
Stern, Da. (1985). *The social world of the infant*. Basic Books.
Stern, Do. (2010). *Partners in thought*. Routledge.
Sullivan, H. S. (1954). *The interpersonal theory of psychiatry*. Norton.
Summers, F. (1999). *Transcending the self: An object relations model of psychoanalytic therapy*. The Analytic Press.
Summers, F. (2013). *The psychoanalytic vision*. Routledge.
Tolpin, M. (2002). Doing psychoanalysis of normal development: Forward edge of transferences. *Progress in Self Psychology*, *18*, 167–190.
Tomkins, S. (1962). *Affects, imagery, and consciousness: Volume I. The positive affect*. Springer.
Tomkins, S. (1978). Script theory: Differential magnification of affects. *Nebraska Symposium on Motivation*, *26*, 201–263.
Winnicott, D. W. (1965). *The Maturational process and the facilitating environment*. International Universities Press.

Chapter 19

Infant Research-Rooted Therapies in the UK

Alejandra Perez

Psychoanalytic work has been informed, to some extent, by research into infants' socio-emotional development, and neuroscience, as well as by investigations into the psychological and biological changes in new parents. Such research has mainly contributed to the emergence of innovative psychoanalytic ways of working, most notably, parent-infant psychotherapy.

The term "infant research-rooted psychotherapies" does not describe a homogenous group. Rather, it includes various forms of psychoanalytic work with adults, children, and parents and infants, influenced by research but also by a range of psychoanalytic theorists; particularly Winnicott, Klein, Anna Freud, and Bion. What these therapies have in common is a general underlying assumption that learning more about early infancy and parenthood—encompassing biological, psychological, and interpsychic as well as intrapsychic processes, and nonverbal forms of communication—can contribute to psychoanalytic clinical work.

Historical Background

Early Psychoanalytic Pioneers

Possibly the earliest pioneers of infant research in psychoanalytic practice were Anna Freud, Winnicott, and Klein, all of whom, in the 1940s, observed and worked with parents, infants, and young children. While Sigmund Freud attached considerable importance to infancy in his theories of the mind, most of his formulations relied on reconstructions from adult analytic patients and their retrospective views of their childhoods. Anna Freud, by closely observing children and documenting these observations, developed a deeper understanding of the changes and defenses that arise in normal childhood at each stage of development. Her "double approach": integrated direct observations and reconstructions and she considered the innate urge for a new experience as strong as the urge to repeat (i.e., transference) (Midgley, 2013). Winnicott, working as a pediatrician and as a psychoanalyst, saw parallels in the analyst-patient and the mother-infant

DOI: 10.4324/9781003027768-20

relationship. His formulation of the relational environment as necessary for the development of the self stems from his understanding of this early relationship between mother and baby. Winnicott also suggested the conditions needed for the scientific study of early infantile processes and the emotional foundation of infant mental health which were greatly debated at the time (Caldwell & Joyce, 2011). Both Anna Freud and Winnicott brought to psychoanalytic thinking their interest in allied professions—education and pediatrics—thereby opening new possible sources of contributions to psychoanalytic theory beyond the analytic consulting room. Klein was also innovative, not only in being one of the first to work psychoanalytically with children but also by working with children with severe psychological disturbances and psychoses. She focused on children's play as a communication of their unconscious, thus expanding psychoanalytic work beyond the realm of verbal communication (that is, free association). These three theorists' work aroused much debate at the time—and perhaps still does today—about the methods of direct observation that they used to arrive at psychoanalytic formulations of early infancy, and its importance for psychic development. They also faced criticism for the ways in which they challenged conceptions of psychoanalytic work and the role of the analyst.

Attachment Theory and Research

The work of Anna Freud and Winnicott indirectly questioned the primacy of the drives in psychoanalytic theory, by recognizing the importance of early relationships and the environment. However, it was Bowlby who more directly questioned the primacy of the drives and unconscious processes, so was seen by many as departing from psychoanalysis (Fonagy, 2001). Bowlby's interest in attachment began early in his clinical career when he worked in a home with boys deemed to be "maladjusted." He began looking into their histories and found that they had all suffered from prolonged separation from their parents in early childhood, and now presented an "affectionless" character (Bowlby, 1944). Together with Robertson and Rosenbluth, he set out to investigate the impact of early separation by recording on film a standard practice at the time: keeping young children in hospital unaccompanied by their parents. What he observed confirmed his understanding of the impact of early separation. Bowlby (1958) described attachment as a function in its own right and not a secondary process designed to obtain physiological gratification (i.e., the drives). The rift between Bowlby and many in the psychoanalytic community meant that he went on to develop his work separately. Bowlby's followers were not psychoanalysts but clinical researchers and developmental psychologists, who went on to further his ideas. Arguably the greatest contribution of attachment theory has been the large body of research demonstrating the importance of the early bond with caregivers, which is then internalized and plays a strong role in all aspects of development and future relationships (Fearon & Roisman, 2017; Fonagy et al., 1991).

Infant Observation

Since 1948, infant observation has been included in the curriculum of various adult and child psychoanalytic trainings. Bick (1964) pioneered this unique psychoanalytic learning experience. Abundant clinical papers on observers' experiences, countertransference reactions, and understanding of mothers and their babies (see, Infant Observation for various examples) have been written since then. These papers have demonstrated the intense emotions and unconscious dynamics that can arise, both between mothers and their infants, and between mothers and observers, informing psychoanalytic work with adults and also with parents and infants. Rustin (2006) has argued that infant observations are not only a method of learning but also a method of research, allowing early relations between baby and caregiver to be observed, and enabling the infant's experience to be explored through the observer's countertransference.

Developmental Research

A growing body of developmental research has, in various ways, demonstrated how the infant is primed from the start, for affective interactions with others, and how the relationship is, "the fundamental unit in which development takes place" (Seligman & Harrison, 2012, p. 339). Several research studies in the 1970s filmed live interactions between parents and babies, allowing accurate measurement of the minute changes in these, demonstrating that they engage in early forms of conversation (see Trevarthen & Aitken, 2001 for an overview) and that these relationships are bidirectional (Cohn & Tronick, 1988). More recently, studies have shown how communication begins and develops in infancy, responding to the interest and feelings of others, and influencing many aspects of a baby's development, such as perception, learning, and self-regulation (Trevarthen & Aitken, 2001). Further to studies on the parent-infant dyad, studies on the quality of early family relationships have found that parents' capacity for triadic relationships, that is to think of themselves as a triad without excluding themselves or their partners for the relationship with their baby, predicted the quality of the child's play (von Klitzing et al., 1999) and their behavioral and representational functioning at preschool age (von Klitzing & Burgin, 2005).

Neuroscientific Research

Neuroscience has confirmed the bi-directionality of parent-infant relationships and the importance of the early years. Our neurophysiology and early brain development play an important part in our behavior and subjective experience (Schore, 2001), and our brain development is impacted by the external environment (McCrory et al., 2019). Furthermore, brain plasticity is greater in the early years.

Neurobiological studies have also helped us to further understand the complex physiological changes that parents undergo in the transition to parenthood. These changes help parents to respond to their infant's needs, by heightening their sensitivity to infants' cues (Rutherford & Mayes, 2011), as postulated by Winnicott (1958) through his concept of "primary maternal preoccupation." However, these neurobiological studies have made possible investigations into how these changes and mental states occur not only in mothers but also in fathers (Feldman et al., 2019), as well as physiological variations in parents diagnosed with depression (Rutherford & Mayes, 2014).

Tensions Between Research and Psychoanalysis

Discussions about the value of infant research—and research more generally—for psychoanalytic theory and practice, have been fraught. Broadly speaking, those seen as representing research argue for its value, while those representing psychoanalysis argue against it (see Blass & Carmeli, 2007; Britton, 2000; Fonagy, 2000; Green, 2000; Stern, 2000; Yovell et al., 2015). Arguments disputing its value have centered around the impossibility of scientific research methods capturing the unconscious, and have claimed that any research study is limited to reporting external, observable behavior, thereby offering little of value to psychoanalysis. The split between psychoanalysis and infant research perhaps has been more pronounced in the UK. However, parent-infant psychotherapy has been one field that has developed from this cross-fertilization.

PPIP

Psychoanalytic Parent-Infant Psychotherapy (PPIP) was developed to address the repetition of unconsciously motivated pathological parenting behaviors and the traumatic experiences these create for babies across generations, as well as to help infants' development (Baradon, & Joyce, 2005). One of its aims is to enable parents to reflect on their infant's different states of mind, and on the different ways in which these states are manifested. Another aim is to facilitate the baby's age-appropriate dependency and a move toward separation, as well as parents' capacity to see their baby as a separate person (see Baradon & Joyce, 2005, for a full list and description of the aims of PPIP work). It is recognized that, while there is a pull toward the repetition of trauma (Fraiberg et al., 1975) parenthood can also be a period of psychic change in which parents are more open to revisiting and working through unconscious conflicts as they live the new experience of being a parent (Joyce, 2005).

PPIP has made use of infant research and developed new ways of working with parents and infants. The parent-infant relationship is the focus of the therapy and video recording of sessions allows the therapist to show parents' (primarily positive) interactions with their baby, helping them understand their baby's individuality and capacity to relate and perceive affective states. Considering the importance of the triad and the father's role in the baby's development, PPIP encourages partners to be part of the therapy and attend sessions. The therapist works with the different family members and their relationships at different levels. The work with parents involves building a therapeutic alliance, by understanding their needs, their struggles, and their unconscious conflicts. The therapist also needs to understand the baby's needs and assess their development. At times, parents may feel threatened by the therapist's attention to their baby and so, the therapist observes the baby with "peripheral vision" and holds both parents' and baby's needs in mind. Baradon et al. (2016) described the importance to help parents "claim their baby."

Interpretations in PPIP are directed at different family members and their relationships at different levels. Some interpretations start by pointing out shared experiences, moving to create separateness, and indicating differences (Perez, 2018). In other interpretations, the therapist speaks and engages with the baby, describing the baby's experience. The therapist becomes a "new developmental object" for the baby, an object who can co-create the meaning of their experience. However, these interpretations are also "speaking" to parents, allowing them to hear the unspoken voice of the baby, communicating a new understanding of the baby, and helping them to recognize and experience the baby differently from what their unconscious conflicts had not allowed them to see. The indirect manner of these interpretations helps parents come to see things that could otherwise feel too threatening if spoken to directly to them. These interpretations, in many ways, facilitate a "third position" (Britton, 2004). The therapist builds and maintains a therapeutic alliance where the parent feels deeply understood and also moves alongside parents, to observe and understand their baby and the relationship, allowing a reflective, thinking "third position" in the therapy (Perez, 2018).

It is apt that psychoanalysis engages in work with infants (and parents) since psychoanalysis was the first field to formulate theories on infants' early experience. Infant research has given us a greater understanding of infants' capacities and perceptions which has, in turn, contributed to techniques used in PPIP to encourage healthier ways of relating between parents and their infant. An important contribution of infant research and of PPIP work to psychoanalytic technique has been further understanding of non-verbal behavior.

Drives

Salomonsson (2012) has postulated on the importance of infantile sexuality and the drives in PPIP work. He explains that Freud's theory of the drives neglected the baby's unconscious experience, and the early representations that might emerge out of it. He postulates that the drive is a messenger that affects both sender and receiver, its meaning emerging once the mother and infant have interpreted it.

Nonverbal Communications

Baradon et al. (2018) investigated the importance of non-verbal communication in PPIP and describe the multimodal, interactive processes that take place within the moment-to-moment exchanges in a session, between parent and baby, parent and therapist, and therapist and baby. A microanalysis of video material from several sessions, as well as therapist's countertransference revealed the verbal and implicit interactional processes involved in the work.

Contributions of Infant Research on Psychoanalytic Theory

Parent-infant research has demonstrated the complexity of early forms of communication, the infant's awareness of the other, and a capacity for emotion, cognition, and sensitivity from the very beginning. Not only does this research challenge the theory of the initial narcissistic stage, and the object as merely a form of drive satisfaction, it also places greater emphasis on interpsychic processes. Winnicott's (1960) statement that "there is no such thing as a baby, only a baby and mother" is central in PPIP work—the environment, how this is experienced, internalized, and played out in relation to unconscious drives/fantasies.

Contributions of Infant Research on Psychoanalytic Practice

Perhaps the greatest contribution of infant research has been the ways in which it has complemented and enhanced psychoanalytic clinical work. In terms of adult work, the move away from a one-person psychology to a two-person psychology is important. There is now greater insight into how meaning and understanding are "created" by analyst and patient, and how the analyst-patient relationship can in itself be transformative, not only via interpretations, or reconstructions of the past. There has also been a greater focus on the non-verbal behavior in the analytic setting and on embodied countertransference and communications between patient and analyst (Boston Change Process Study Group, 2002). Finally, further understanding of the neurobiological and psychological changes that occur in the infant, children, and adolescents has given child analysis of other perspectives from which to consider typical development and age-appropriate defenses and behavior.

19. Infant Research-Rooted UK Therapies	
Main, general underlying assumptions	1 Infants' early experiences and relationships play an important role in their future development. 2 Nonverbal communication (including facial expressions, tone of voice, etc. and the resulting bodily experiences from these communications) play an important role in all aspects of experience and development. 3 The relationship between patient and analyst/therapist (with its nonverbal components) is a key factor for psychic change/therapeutic progress.
Specific theoretical assumptions	
psychic structure	• Psychic structure develops through, and is shaped by, early relationships and experiences (for example, experiences of separation and loss, of being attended to and held in mind or intruded upon). This relates to the relationship between parent and baby but also includes the internalized early experiences of the parent, and how these play out. • While important psychic processes of integration, self-regulation, attachment formation, and internalization are lifelong processes, these are actively negotiated between infant and others from the very beginning.
energy	• The focus of infantile sexuality/drives as primary motivating energy in infant research-rooted therapies takes an equal or secondary position to the need for attachment (caregiver-seeking behavior and safety produced from the caregiver-infant relationship).
relationships	• Infants are receptive, interactive, and searching to form relationships from the beginning of life. • A positive parent-infant relationship plays an important role in the baby's development of a sense of self, self-regulation, and healthy future relationships.
developmental stages	• Development advances in a predominantly continuous and cumulative way with progressions and regressions. • Progression along developmental lines involves the maturational push of innate or biologic characteristics, as well as the interaction between biology and environmental conditions (predominantly, the caregiver-child relationship). • Understanding the complexities of normal development provides a means of understanding the presence or absence of psychopathology at any stage.

(*Continued*)

	• There has been a dominance of Western theorizing about development. Infant research has offered additional cultural perspectives.
body	• Interactions with another become embedded in "body knowledge": in the infant, in the parent/caregiver, and in the analyst/therapist. • Early bodily experiences and interactions allow a particular understanding of some symptom formations in the infant. • These interactions between caregiver and baby entail a complicated mixture of self-preservation function and erotic pleasure (infantile sexuality) which, if conflicting in the caregiver, can be experienced and fantasized as conflicting by the baby.
anxieties/instincts and defenses	• Early anxieties occur within the parent-baby relationship. These are either due to a lack of containment of infant's early unprocessed and intense internal bodily experiences or stimulation from the environment, or due to projections to the baby of mother's unprocessed early experiences. • In instances of overwhelming anxiety, baby resorts to early defenses, such as averting gaze, inhibiting attachment-seeking behavior, precocious capacity to soothe him/herself, or dissociation (i.e., a frozen, unresponsive state).
Assumptions concerning etiology	• Etiology of pathology is assumed to come from a complex interaction of biological, inherent, and environmental factors.
Implications for technique	• A focus on the real relationship with the analyst/therapist (for example, through concepts such as "corrective emotional experience" or "developmental object"). The analyst/therapist helps the patient(s) reflect/mentalize, find the right distance between self and other, and in parent-infant psychotherapy, help the parent recognize the infant as dependent but distinct, and with a developing mind. In parent-infant psychotherapy, the therapist helps the infant by maximizing opportunities for the potential for growth and for the establishment of a "coherent" or "true" self.
Subsequent developments of the core concept	• Technique on the real relationship with the analyst/therapist. • Technique making use of the non-verbal behavior between analyst/therapist and patient.

References

Baradon, T. (2016). Preface. In T. Baradon, M. Biseo, C. Broughton, J. James, & A. Joyce (Eds.), *The practice of psychoanalytic parent-infant psychotherapy: Claiming the baby* (2nd ed., pp. xi–xiv). Routledge.

Baradon, T. (2018). Microanalysis of multimodal communication in therapy: A case of relational trauma in parent-infant psychoanalytic psychotherapy. *Journal of Infant, Child, and Adolescent Psychotherapy*, *17*(1), 1–13.

Baradon, T., & Joyce, A. (2005). The theory of psychoanalytic parent-infant psychotherapy. In T. Baradon, C. Broughton, I. Gibbs, J. James, A. Joyce, & J. Woodhead (Eds.), *The practice of psychoanalytic parent-infant psychotherapy* (pp. 25–40). Routledge.

Bick, E. (1964). Notes on infant observation in psycho-analytic training. *International Journal of Psychoanalysis*, *45*, 558–566.

Blass R. B., & Carmeli, Z. (2007). The case against neuropsychoanalysis. On fallacies underlying psychoanalysis' latest scientific trend and its negative impact on psychoanalytic discourse. *International Journal of Psychoanalysis*, *88*(1), 19–40.

Boston Change Process Study Group (BCPSG), Bruschweiler-Stern, N. Harrison, A. M., Lyons-Ruth, K., Morgan, A., Nahum, J. P., Sander, L. W., Stern, D. N. N., & Tronick, E. Z. (2002). Explicating the implicit: The local level and the microprocess of change in the analytic situation. *International Journal of Psycho-Analysis*, *83*(5), 1051–1062.

Bowlby, J. (1944). Forty-four juvenile thieves: Their characters and home life. *International Journal of Psychoanalysis*, *25*(19–52), 107–127.

Bowlby, J. (1958). The nature of the child's tie to his mother. *International Journal of Psychoanalysis*, *39*, 350–373.

Britton, R. (2000, March 1). *The Nettle* [Paper presentation]. Annual Research Lecture of The British Psychoanalytical Society.

Britton, R. (2004). Subjectivity, objectivity, and triangular space. *Psychoanalytic Quarterly*, *73*, 47–61.

Caldwell, L., & Joyce, A. (2011). *Reading Winnicott*. Routledge.

Cohn, J. F., & Tronick, E. Z. (1988). Mother-infant face-to-face interaction: Influence is bidirectional and unrelated to periodic cycles in either partner's behavior. *Developmental Psychology*, *24*(3), 386–392.

Fearon, R. M. P., & Roisman, G. I. (2017). Attachment theory: Progress and future directions. *Current Opinion Psychology*, *15*, 131–136.

Feldman, R., Braun, K., & Champagne, F. A. (2019). The neural mechanisms and consequences of paternal caregiving. *Nature Reviews Neuroscience*, *20*(4), 205–224.

Fonagy, P. (2000, March 1). *Grasping the nettle: Or why psychoanalytic research is such an irritant* [Paper presentation]. Annual Research Lecture of The British Psycho-Analytical Society.

Fonagy, P. (2001). *Attachment theory and psychoanalysis*. Other Press.

Fonagy, P., Steele, H., & Steele M. (1991). Maternal representations of attachment during pregnancy predict the organization of infant-mother attachment at one year of age. *Child Development*, *62*(5), 891–905.

Fraiberg, S., Adelson, E., & Shapiro, V. (1975). Ghosts in the nursery: A psychoanalytic approach to the problem of impaired infant-mother relationships. *Journal of the American Academy of Child and Adolescent Psychiatry*, *14*(3), 387–421.

Green, A. (2000). Science and science fiction. In J. Sandler, A. M. Sandler, & R. Davies (Eds.), *Clinical and observational psychoanalytic research: Roots of a controversy* (pp. 41–72). International Universities Press.

Joyce, A. (2005). The parent-infant relationship and parent-infant mental health. In T. Baradon, C. Broughton, I. Gibbs, J. James, & J. Woodhead (Eds.), *The practice of psychoanalytic parent-infant psychotherapy* (pp. 5–24). Routledge.

McCrory, E., Ogle, J. R., Gerin, M. I., & Viding, E. (2019). Neurocognitive adaptation and mental health vulnerability following maltreatment: The role of social functioning. *Child Maltreatment*, *24*(4), 435–451.

Midgley, N. (2013). *Reading Anna Freud.* Routledge.

Perez, A. (2018). From pathological merger to a reflective, triangular space: Parent-infant psychotherapy with a mother with borderline personality disorder. *Journal of Infant, Child, and Adolescent Psychotherapy*, *17*(1), 15–27.

Rustin, M. (2006). Infant observation research: What have we learned so far? *Infant Observation*, *9*(1), 35–52.

Rutherford, H. J. V., & Mayes, L. C. (2011). Primary maternal preoccupation: Using neuroimaging techniques to explore the parental brain. *Psyche*, 65, 973–988.

Rutherford, H. J. V., & Mayes, L. C. (2014). Minds shaped through relationships: The emerging neurobiology of parenting. In R. N. Emde & M. Leuzinger-Bohleber (Eds.), *Early parenting and prevention of disorder: Psychoanalytic research at interdisciplinary frontiers* (pp. 50–69). Karnac Books.

Salomonsson, B. (2012). Has infantile sexuality anything to do with infants? *The International Journal of Psychoanalysis*, *93*(3), 631–647.

Schore, A. N. (2001). The effects of early relational trauma on right brain development, affect regulation, and infant mental health. *Infant Mental Health Journal*, *22*(1–2), 201–269.

Seligman, S., & Harrison, A. (2012). Infancy research, infant mental health, and adult psychotherapy: Mutual influences. *Infant Mental Health Journal*, *33*(4), 339–349.

Stern, D. (2000). The relevance of empirical infant research to psychoanalytic theory and practice. In J. Sandler, A. M. Sandler, & R. Davies (Eds.), *Clinical and observational psychoanalytic research: Roots of a controversy* (pp. 73–90). International Universities Press.

Trevarthen, C., & Aitken, K. (2001). Infant intersubjectivity: Research, theory, and clinical applications. *Journal of Child Psychology and Psychiatry*, *42*(1), 3–48.

von Klitzing, K., & Burgin, D. (2005). Parental capacities for triadic relationships during pregnancy: Early predictors of children's behavioral and representational functions at preschool age. *Infant Mental Health Journal*, *26*(1), 19–39.

von Klitzing, K., Simoni, H., & Burgin, D. (1999). Child development and early triadic relationships. *Journal of Psychoanalysis*, *80*, 71–89.

Winnicott, D. W. (1958). Primary maternal preoccupation. In *Collected papers: Through paediatrics to psycho-analysis* (pp. 300–306). Basic Books.

Winnicott, D. W. (1960). The theory of the parent-infant relationship. *International Journal of Psycho-Analysis*, *41*, 585–595.

Yovell, Y., Solms, M., & Fotopoulou, A. (2015). The case for neuropsychoanalysis: Why a dialogue with neuroscience is necessary but not sufficient for psychoanalysis. *International Journal of Psychoanalysis*, *96*(6), 1515–1553.

Chapter 20

Infant Research-Rooted US Therapies: History of Development of Infant Research-Rooted Theories and the Core Concept of a Developmental Theory of Psychoanalysis

Alexandra Harrison and Ed Tronick

Early Baby Watchers

Psychoanalytic observations of babies perhaps began with Freud's "fort-da" descriptions of his grandson's efforts to master the separation experience when his mother left him in the crib. Melanie Klein contributed to this scarce but important literature with her account of the infant watching his mother's face while nursing (Klein, 1952). A major contribution to understanding parent-child relationships—particularly children's responses to parental separation and loss—was made by Anna Freud and Dorothy Burlingham's written descriptions of the children in the war nurseries (Burlingham & Freud, 1942). These psychoanalytic observations of the parent-infant relationship contributed to the foundation of a theory of object relations—the importance of the caregiving relationship in development. The theory of the influence of the caregiving relationship on ego development was elaborated by Kris (1950), Spitz (1959), and especially Erikson (1950).

Contemporaneously, John Bowlby was developing his ideas about the primary motivational factor of security in the caregiving relationship (Bowlby, 1950). He encouraged Esther Bick to introduce infant observation into the Tavistock psychotherapy training in 1948 (Waddell, 2006). The Tavistock method of infant observation is now recognized as a tool to develop the analyst's capacity for observation and self-reflection. In 1954, a group of U.S. psychoanalysts headed by Eleanor Pavenstedt started a longitudinal study of early personality development at Boston University. Drawing on prevailing psychoanalytic thinking, they designed a study to test the hypothesis that healthy development infants depended on the psychological maturity of their mothers, measured by psychological instruments. The group collected detailed observations of 22 infant-mother pairs from birth to 36 months. The results showed no relationship between the measures of the

DOI: 10.4324/9781003027768-21

mother's maturity and the infants' healthy development (L. Sander, personal communication). Unfortunately, these discouraging findings led to the abandonment of the research. Later, Lou Sander acknowledged regret that the study was discontinued, commenting that he should have realized the results signaled a paradigm shift from a linear to a nonlinear model of human development (Sander, 2008, L. Sander, personal communication).

Boston Change Process Study Group

The Boston Change Process Study Group (BPCSG)[1] came together in the late 1990's to study the interface between psychoanalysis and infant research. Sander's seminar work introducing dynamic systems theory into infant research was foundational to the group's explorations of the process of change. The group studied transcripts of adult analyses and applied some of the general principles of dynamic systems theory to the analytic material. The result of these discussions was their 1998 paper (Stern et al., 1998). During the meetings of the group, Tronick discussed his match, mismatch, and repair model (MMR) of infant-parent interaction and began to develop his Dyadic Expansion of Consciousness Model (DSC), positioning the MMR within an overarching metatheory of nonlinear systems theory (Tronick & Cohn, 1989). At the same time, Harrison was experimenting with videotape analysis as a way of exploring the nonverbal processes of change in her child analytic sessions (Harrison & Tronick, 2007). The nonlinear metatheory facilitated her making sense of the variability at the microscopic level of behavioral exchange in time frames smaller than speech can be formed. Core concepts of this model of therapeutic action derive from the Boston Change Process Study Group and discussions bringing infant observation research and psychoanalytic theory and clinical work together in an effort to create an integration of the two perspectives. The evolution of this integrative perspective involved the continued collaboration of these two authors and many others.

Dyadic Expansion of Consciousness Model (DSC)

According to DSC, human beings are living systems that grow and change in a manner consistent with the general principles of non-linear dynamic systems theory. The first principle is that the individual must gain resources to grow in complexity and coherence or, failing that, dissipate. Human development occurs through making meanings in an evolving process of exchange that occurs in multiple simultaneous cognitive processes including the conscious, dynamic unconscious, and nonconscious, as well as neurosomatic bodily processes. A DSC may occur between individuals when they use behavior to exchange intentions, affects, states of mind, and cognitive meanings with each other. This interaction has the potential to co-create new meanings that in turn can then be appropriated by each individual into their own state of consciousness (SOC), their private sense of self. Individuals overcome the limitation of self-organizing meaning-making by engaging in dyadic meaning-making, in that way creating intersubjectivity. When an individual's SOC gains complexity and coherence, the individual undergoes an amplification of self-experience, a sense of emotional and cognitive expansion. Typically this is pleasurable, but not always (Tronick, 2007).

The DSC model appealed to Harrison as a practicing psychoanalyst in that it seemed to offer her the possibility of integrating the new nonlinear model of development she had been learning in the BCPSG with the more linear psychoanalytic theory she had found so useful in her work with patients. The psychoanalytic theory formed the meat in the sandwich—the story of what happened—whereas the nonlinear theory helped acknowledge the evolutionary processes of change such as the creation of mountain ranges (top slice of bread) and of the microscopic exchanges that she was discovering in her videotape microanalysis of analytic sessions (bottom slice of bread) (Harrison, 2014).

Polysemic Meaning-Making

After the group, Harrison and Tronick continued to collaborate in studying processes of change in psychoanalysis and in natural development, working to elaborate some of the theory of the BPCSG and to connect it to clinical material (Harrison & Tronick, 2007, 2011). They emphasized the multiple levels and dimensions of meaning-making occurring simultaneously in the process of growth and referred to this as polysemic meaning-making (Harrison & Tronick, in publication). One of the great benefits of using the general principles of nonlinear systems theory as an overarching framework is that this conceptualization includes hierarchical levels of the organization, in which the personal, private world of the individual is protected as a valuable level of meaning. In addition, because the higher levels of organization of meaning within the system—for example, the level of thoughts and fantasies organized by language—maintain a certain level of linear coherence—or continuity—the lower levels of meaning-making such as behavioral cues or internal neurosomatic processes—are understood as providing a necessary context for the narrative (Harrison & Beebe, 2018). Furthermore, given the multiplicity of meaning-making processes, there is the constant possibility of dynamic conflict of the meanings at different levels.

In the exchange of meanings in an analytic treatment, just as in other relationships, the match, mismatch, and repair process results in new meanings that can then be incorporated into the private inner world of each individual. In this interactive process, a multiplicity of polysemic meanings—the individual's explicit memory, sensory and bodily memory, and dynamic unconscious—are all brought to the exchange in the present moment.

In addition to the language-based meanings about the nature of the world and the individual's place in it, of particular importance is "implicit relational knowing," or an assembly of all the ways the individual has of knowing "how to be" with another person. Although the higher-level meanings that make the individual recognizable as himself may have an outsized role in the new meanings that emerge, there is always a likelihood that an unpredictable new outcome will emerge.

According to this model, the psychic structure is an emergent property of the constantly and messily evolving laminated flow of meanings. The organization that results from this flow creates a sense of continuity in the individual's perceptions of and reactions to the world, and in his sense of himself as a unique individual. In the context articulated above, the psychic structure would be a higher level of meaning. Energy in this model is conceived of as a multiplicity of types of information (meaning) about how an individual feels, what he perceives, desires, thinks, and intends to do. It is through the spontaneous exchange of these bits of "information" within and between individuals that new meanings are created and energy resources are gained. Living systems are required to gain energy in order to maintain life, and psychic structure requires information in order to grow in coherence and complexity. In this model, deficits are conceived in terms of more or less adaptive means of making meaning of life challenges.

Object relations are also central to this theory. Development depends on the exchange of meanings in a relationship. In infancy, meanings created to meet the infant's needs for temperature control, nurturance, and social experience are essential for survival. In older children and adults, as the individual grows in competence and independence, there is a shift in the salience of particular meanings, but the repertoire of meanings continues to include meanings about safety, desire, and intention. Across the lifespan, individuals make meanings in relationships—particularly relationships with "thickness"—ones in which individuals spend a lot of time doing the same activities together—eating, sleeping, sharing the same living spaces, negotiating tasks and activities—creating patterns. These patterns are incorporated into each individual's sense of themselves, creating the unconscious and nonconscious components of transference, the sense of continuity in the individual's perceptions of and reactions to the world, and his sense of himself as a unique individual.

It is important to note that the interactive patterns themselves are taken into an individual, including both roles of the negotiation, and both positions in a conflict. Internal objects are conceptualized as ways of being with another person that has unique characteristics and that can carry along meanings from the—somatosensory as well as cognitive and affective domains. At another level, these patterns participate in the creation of culture.

Relational patterns and their associated meanings—especially those with more "thickness," typically derive from early caregiving relationships.

In this model, development is predictable in a probabilistic sense but is unpredictable in the case of an individual. Infants of a certain age can be predicted to develop the capacity to reach and grasp an object, to share joint attention, or to acquire spoken language and other symbolic functions. However, as noted above, there is no blueprint for human development, and each infant arrives at these developmental accomplishments through intentional engagement with their environment—inanimate and particularly their caregiving environment—and in that sense the exact moment of accomplishment is variable. It is also true that developmental stages have salient features emerging from the child's new competencies and reaction to the environment. The capacity to engage in social exchange is present in the newborn period, compelling the parent and infant to "fall in love" with each other. Emergent symbolic capacity between 2 and 4 years of age allows the magical fantasies of the Oedipal period to flower.

Yet, the multiplicity of resource-enhancing and resource-inhibiting factors influencing an individual's development challenges the prediction of developmental outcomes. A mother with strong nurturing capacities may be compromised in providing her infant's security by the stress of chronic poverty, or an infant born with a cleft palate may associate feeding—even by a competent mother—with stress and frustration. Within the development, there are also sensitive periods within which deprivation of essential resources or harmful stress can have a more deleterious effect than at other times, such as the critical period for neurodevelopment demonstrated by the Bucharest Early Intervention Project demonstrating the irreversible effects of early social deprivation.

The body plays an active role in the meaning-making that creates the individual's sense of themselves. The nervous, motor, endocrine, and sensory organs are involved in constant meaning-making activity, within and among organ systems, in positive and negative feedback loops, creating patterns of perception and response that give meaning to the individual's experience. The premature infant's immature sensory system may be unable to engage with his mother when she simultaneously shows him her expressive face and speaks lovingly, generating for him distressing levels of stimulation. The athlete's sense of power in her arms and legs generates a sense of mastery and confidence in relation to the world. Meanings about gender are central to the meanings an individual makes about their body and vary according to the biology and the social experience of the child. Sexuality is a vital part of body experience. These meanings can continue into adulthood, elaborated in essential ways by meanings generated in relationships—fantasies—meanings about intimacy, dominance and submission, dependence, and nurturance, for example.

Implications for Technique

An important implication for technique in this integration of current developmental theory and psychoanalysis is the acceptance of the notion of polysemic bundles of meaning, or multiple simultaneous meanings to every human act—in other words, in therapeutic formulations and interventions, there is no one correct answer. This assumption underscores the premise of co-creativity and the uniqueness of every individual and of every dyad. It does not mean that at a higher level of conceptualization, there might not be commonly accepted meanings associated with certain life experiences, such as anxiety about commitment to a monogamous relationship, or about competition. It simply means that in any individual case, other meanings might have a more salient or uniquely elaborated, place in the hierarchy of meanings the individual makes. In relation to this assumption, the analyst must take on an attitude of receptivity, interest, and curiosity. The analyst must also entertain the idea that bodily and nonconscious processes may play a prominent role in whatever meaning is being communicated.

Another implication for technique is an emphasis on the connection the analyst makes with the patient. The analyst will pay particular attention to establishing a reciprocal interchange that supports the patient's agency by attending to the patient's communications—bodily as well as verbal—and finding ways of being together with her. The analyst—in or out of awareness—will attempt to create a rhythm of actions (including words) and silences.

As noted above, transference may be seen as the process by which meanings about past relationships are engaged in the meaning-making process through the emergence of a resonance pattern in the analytic relationship. Ubiquitous features of the meanings communicated in the dyad, the result of meanings about past relationships (or other relationships in the present) produce an emergent resonant pattern in the analytic relationship. Implications for technique include the benefit of recognition and often a validation of the pattern as it appears in the analytic relationship, in addition to identifying the pre-existing relational pattern and its original meaning. Often the latter meaning is not possible to retrieve and is not available to reflection by the conscious mind. That acknowledgment can also play an important role in the analytic work. Countertransference in this framework is seen as part of the Transference-Countertransference continuum, or field.

Defense in this framework is conceptualized as stress regulation that becomes organized in patterns of thought and action that are characteristic of an individual. The higher-level stress regulation involves reflective consideration of a threat and comfort from intimate partners (Porges, 2003). These defenses are more flexible and adaptive and are in fact evidence of human evolution. When these higher levels of defensive response to threat are not available, the sympathetic nervous system is engaged in an aggressive reaction or withdrawal. Finally, if that level of defense fails, the primitive vagal system is activated, causing psychological (dissociation) and physiological shut-down. All these neurolo-physiological responses to threat accrue additional associated symbolic meanings in the form of memories, fantasies, etc. Individuals develop recognizable patterns of defensive reaction, but when highly stressed, no individual can maintain a reflective position or openness to comfort from another. Technical implications include being aware that these autonomic nervous system reactions are natural parts of a hierarchical system of stress regulation and these methods of regulation (withdrawal, aggression) in response to threat may be necessary to regain the capacity to reflect. Support in stress regulation—for example, in the form of tolerating some degree of withdrawal or aggression and attention to repair of small ruptures in the connection—is necessary. The acknowledgment of these defenses as legitimate attempts to regulate stress is an important antidote to judgmental reactions to lapses in self-reflection. Finally, deficits in this model can be thought of as constraints to development. If the system does not increase in complexity and coherence, then energy is not gained, and the system will begin to dissipate. However, adaptation is a complicated process, and deficits in one area of function can be compensated for by emergent properties in another or can perform adaptively in certain environmental contexts.

Conclusion

The polysemic meaning-making model is both complex and inclusive, allowing psychoanalysts to converse and share ideas with scientific colleagues without changing their vocabulary, as well as offering a useful theory to guide them in their clinical work. One of the advantages to the foundational principle of growth in complexity is that the analyst is alerted to the smallest new events—an insight or the expression of an affect previously avoided. A more traditional and linear psychoanalytic theory might acknowledge this new feature as positive in an impressionistic sense, but this model allows the analyst to recognize the event as one small part of an evolving process that might—at some future point—gain the energy needed to jump into a higher level of organization as a new, more adaptive meaning. Gregory Rochlin used to describe the analytic technique of offering an interpretation to the patient without knowing whether or not it makes sense to him—a "lob," as in tennis; neither analyst nor patient knows exactly where or when it will come down, but at some future, unpredictable time, if the treatment is moving along, the context may be right to embrace the new meaning, as—we might say—an emergent property of the system.

20. Infant Research-Rooted US Therapies	
Main, general underlying assumptions	1 Human beings are living systems that grow and change in a manner consistent with the general principles of non-linear dynamic systems theory; these principles require the individual to grow in complexity and coherence, gaining resources through this process. 2 Human development occurs through making meanings in an evolving process of exchange that occurs in multiple simultaneous domains—including the conscious, dynamic unconscious, and nonconscious, as well as bodily domains such as in the neurosensory, motor, and endocrine systems—constituting "polysemic bundles" of meaning. 3 This exchange of meanings takes place in a match, mismatch, and repair process which is typically more effective when two individuals exchange meanings than when an individual makes meaning alone; the new meanings resulting from this exchange can then be incorporated into the private inner world of each individual.
Specific theoretical assumptions	
psychic structure	Psychic structure is an emergent property of the constantly and messily evolving laminated flow of meanings. The organization that results from this flow creates a sense of continuity in the individual's perceptions of and reactions to the world, and his sense of himself as a unique individual.
energy	Sources of energy are comprised of a multiplicity of information about how an individual feels, what he perceives, what he desires, what he intends to do, and what he thinks. It is through the exchange of these meanings within and between individuals that new meanings are created and energy resources are gained. More energy is available from the exchange of information between two individuals than one individual can generate alone or in the exchange of information with the inanimate world.
relationships	Development—growth—depends on the exchange of meanings in a relationship.

(Continued)

developmental stages	Development is at once empirically predictable and individually variable and unpredictable; there is no blueprint for human development. Each individual arrives at these developmental accomplishments through intentional engagements with their environment.
body	The body plays an active role in the meaning-making that creates the individual's sense of herself. The nervous, motor, endocrine, and sensory systems are in constant meaning-making activity, within each system and with the others, creating patterns of perception and reaction that give meaning to the individual's experience.
anxieties/instincts and defenses	A hierarchically organized response to threat and the associated meanings.
Assumptions concerning etiology	Retrospective formulations about etiology are misleading in that they ignore the multiplicity of factors influencing an individual's development.
Implications for technique	The messy process of growth, including multiple simultaneous meanings, indicates that there is not "one answer," nor "one best way of doing something" and suggests that the analyst support the patient's agency, while creating a rhythm of exchange using words and silence.
Subsequent developments of the core concept	N/A

Note

1 Originally comprised of Louis Sander, Daniel Stern, Ed Tronick, Karlen Lyons-Ruth, Alexandra Harrison, Jeremy Nahum, and Alexander Morgan.

References

Bowlby, J. (1950). *Maternal care and mental health. Bulletin of the World Health Organization. The master work series.* (2nd ed., pp. 355–533). Jason Aronson.

Burlingham, D., & Freud, A. (1942). *Foster parents plan for war children.* Hampstead Nursery Annual Report.

Erikson, E. (1950). *Childhood and society.* Norton.

Harrison, A. (2014). The sandwich model: The "music and dance" of therapeutic action. *International Journal of Psychoanalysis, 95*(2), 313–340.

Harrison, A., & Beebe, B. (2018). Rhythms of dialogue in infant research and child analysis: Implicit/explicit therapeutic action. *Psychoanalytic Psychology*, *35*(4), 367–381.
Harrison, A. M., & Tronick, E. Z. (2007). Now we have a playground: Emerging new ideas of therapeutic action. *Journal of the American Psychoanalytic Association*, *55*(3), 853–874.
Harrison, A., & Tronick, E. Z. (2011). "The noise monitor": A developmental perspective of verbal and non-verbal meaning-making in psychoanalysis. *Journal of the American Psychoanalytic Association*, *59*(5), 961–983.
Harrison, A., & Tronick, E. (In publication). Intersubjectivity: Conceptual considerations in meaning-making with a clinical illustration. *Frontiers in Psychology*.
Klein, M. (1952). The origins of transference. *International Journal of Psychoanalysis*, *33*, 433–438.
Kris, E. (1950). Notes on the development and on some current problems of psychoanalytic child psychology. *Psychoanalytic Study of the Child*, *5*, 24–46.
Porges, S. (2003). The polyvagal theory: Phylogenetic contributions to social behavior. *Physiology & Behavior*, *79*, 503–513.
Sander, L. (2008). *Living systems, evolving consciousness, and the emerging person*. The Analytic Press.
Spitz, R. (1959). *A genetic field theory of ego formation*. International Universities Press.
Stern, D. N., Sander, L. W., Nahum, J. P., Harrison, A. M., Lyons-Ruth, K., Morgan, A. C., Bruschweiler-Stern, N., & Tronick, E. Z. (1998). Non-interpretive mechanisms in psychoanalytic therapy: The "something more" than interpretation. *International Journal of Psychoanalysis*, *79*, 903–921.
Tronick, E. (2007). *The neurobehavioral and social-emotional development of infants and children*. Norton.
Tronick, E., & Cohn, J. (1989). Infant-mother face-to-face interaction: Age and gender differences in coordination and the occurrence of miscoordination. *Child Development*, *60*, 85–92.
Waddell, M. (2006). Infant observation in Britain: The Tavistock approach. *International Journal of Psychoanalysis*, *87*(4), 1103–1120.

Chapter 21

Neuropsychoanalysis: A Widening Scope for Psychoanalysis

Iréne Matthis

In this chapter, I will present some basic assumptions and grounding concepts for neuropsychoanalysis. This means presenting the philosophical ideas, in particular ontological assumptions, occurring in neuropsychoanalysis and their relation to central psychoanalytic concepts. The clinical situation and its psychology, with the close relationship between therapist and patient, will not be dealt with in this context. However, I will add some thoughts related to the special field of somatic illness, still mostly unexplored, that are closely related to the development of neuropsychoanalysis and thus to the widening scope of psychoanalysis. But let me start with a short exposition of the history from which neuropsychoanalysis grew. As the name indicates it deals with at least three fields: neurology, psychology, and especially, psychoanalysis.

The Historical Background

Neurology is an old branch of medical science dating back to the Egyptians and the Greeks. Psychology, which also dates back a long time, is the study of mind and behavior. It was considered a branch of philosophy and thus belonged to the humanities. During the 19th century, both neurology and psychology were more clearly defined. At the same time, psychiatry as a special field was born, considered as a middle ground between neurology and psychology. Psychiatry literally means "medical treatment of the soul." It studied disturbances like schizophrenia, hysterical paralysis, obsessive diseases, etc., for which there were no good medical explanations.

It is perhaps not well known that Sigmund Freud, the creator of psychoanalysis, was one of the foremost brain specialists in Europe at the end of the 19th century. He wrote a long, detailed article on the development, anatomy, and physiology of the brain in the German encyclopedia (Freud, 1888/1990). At this time localizationist ideas about the brain were prevalent, i.e., it was thought that each function, for example, speech, had a specific localization in the brain. This was an easily accepted idea—it was simple and nice, and matched well with the cause-effect theorizing that gained much

DOI: 10.4324/9781003027768-22

acclaim within medicine at the time. This line of thought was part of what has been called the German school (Helmholtz) where it was thought that all manifest phenomena could be fully explained by tracing them back to some primary causes: physical, chemical, mechanical; today we would add genetical. Broca's finding in 1861 that a lesion of the base of the third frontal gyrus of the left hemisphere gave a loss of expressive speech, and Wernicke's discovery, in 1874, that a damage to the superior left temporal gyrus likewise gave a loss of ability to understand speech were hard evidence for this idea. From Freud's encyclopedia article it is, however, clear that he did not fully agree with such a simple reductionist viewpoint. He writes:

> If a specific change in the material state of a specific brain element connects with a change in the state of our consciousness, then the latter is entirely specific as well; however, it is not dependent on the change in the material state alone *whether* or not this connection occurs. If the same brain element undergoes the same change in state at different times, then the corresponding mental process can be linked with it on one occasion (it can cross the threshold of consciousness), [at] another time not.
>
> (1888/1990, p. 62)

This view is closely related to the French school at the end of the 19th century (Charcot). It stated that *regardless* of physiological cause, every clinical syndrome had to be investigated and described in as much detail as possible. This represents a more dynamic and complex view of human behavior. What Freud did was to introduce this perspective in the analysis of the structure and functioning, not only of somatic processes in general in his work with patients with bodily disorders but of the brain itself. Based on clinical studies he argued that psychological considerations must be taken into account in anatomical and physiological theorizing. But he added: "For the present we are unable to formulate the ruling over the laws governing this [any] closer" (1888/1990, p. 62). He spent the rest of his life elucidating these relationships, clinically and theoretically, mainly from a psychological perspective. Such a complexity is described under the heading of "the unconscious" in psychoanalytic theory and practice.

The Question of Dualism

But before entering into the subject of the unconscious, we need to say something about the question of dualism. Let us for a moment look more closely at the quote from Freud where he writes that "if a specific change in the material state of a specific brain element connects with a change in the state of our consciousness, then the latter is entirely specific as well" (1888/1990, p. 62). This is a statement claiming for mental phenomena, such as feelings and ideas, an equal but different status in relation to material brain elements. They are "entirely specific as well." And it is, of course, a proposition directed against the reductionistic claim that mental phenomena are only the epiphenomena of material states; in somewhat the same way as steam, apparently different from water, easily can be reduced to water again, by cooling.

If the above sentence is isolated from the rest of the quote, it could however be interpreted as a statement supporting a special aspect of dualism, one in which physical reality is the *only* reality. But this reality would have two equally important *aspects*. In such an interpretation it could be understood as a reductive materialism in disguise. But the next phrase: "However, it is not dependent on the change in the material state alone *whether* or not this connection occurs" (1888/1990, p. 62) warns us against such a conclusion, and brings into the equation psychological, i.e., immaterial elements that have to be brought into the equation if it is to have a solution. Mental events matter and they do have a case for themselves. Or as the neuroscientist Antonio Damasio writes:

> The conscious mind and its constituent properties are real entities, not illusions, and they must be investigated as the personal, private, subjective experiences that they are .... The idea that subjective experiences are not scientifically accessible is nonsense .... The idea that the nature of subjective experiences can be grasped effectively by the study of their behavioral correlates is wrong. Although both mind and behavior are biological phenomena, mind is mind and behavior is behavior. Mind and behavior can be correlated, and the correlation will become closer as science progresses, but in their respective specifications, mind and behavior are different.
>
> (1999, pp. 308–309)

This proposition is not, in my opinion, a step backward into a Cartesian substance dualistic tradition, where brain circuits and mental ideas would both have an ontology of their own. Instead, we could try to understand the physical and the psychical as two manifestations of something more fundamental, a reality matrix, which is neither physical nor psychical in the same way as we perceive ordinary physical and psychical phenomena through our consciousness.[1] This position is usually called neutral monism.

But if the physical and the psychical both are expressions of a basic phenomenon, whatever we choose to call it, we should expect some kind of correlation between the two. What we find in this enigmatic field of body-mind interaction is complexity, not to say uncertainty. No one clinical fact, whether dealing with sociological, psychological, or physiological findings, can be fully explained by only taking one perspective into account, be it the physical or the psychological. In clinical practice this is an everyday experience for a physician. This also seems to go for the functioning of the brain. In cases of a right hemisphere lesion, which causes paralysis of the left side of the body, some of the patients seem unaware of their predicament (*anosognosia*). Some of these patients, reported by Ramachandran, will for example insist that they are fine and able to walk, although they are sitting in a wheelchair.[2] Ramachandran (1998) summarizes his presentations with the declaration that "Denial stems not merely from a sensory motor deficit … [but] … whole system of beliefs about himself … [are involved]" (p. 140), and he continues: "The experiments … suggest that a denial patient is not just trying to save face; the denial is anchored deep in the psyche" (p. 143). This is now the field for neuropsychoanalytical research.[3]

Clinical Practice and Psychological Schools

Now, how do we relate this to the clinical practice of psychoanalysis, to its many different schools, and to the psychological concepts involved in the work, such as defenses, identification, projection, transference, etc.? The simplest answer is that neuropsychoanalysis is, as Mark Solms and Oliver Turnbull (two of the founders of neuropsychoanalysis) write:

> Neuropsychoanalysis is not … a "school" of psychoanalysis, in the way that we currently speak of Freudian, Kleinian, Intersubjective, and Self Psychology schools. Neuropsychoanalysis, … is far better conceptualized as a link between *all* of psychoanalysis and the neurosciences. Alternatively, it might be described as an attempt to insert psychoanalysis into the neurosciences, as a member of the family of neurosciences—the one that studies the mental apparatus from the *subjective* point of view. (2011, p. 141)

The same thing can be claimed regarding the medical study and treatment of disorders of bodily organs, such as the heart, liver, lungs, etc. Psychoanalysis brings into the field of medical science "the subjective point of view." Working with these patients Freud made his first revolutionary discoveries, which led to psychoanalysis, and it could well have earned a chapter of its own. My own doctoral dissertation was dedicated to this subject (Matthis, 1997). I will also mention the work of my two mentors in the field: Joyce McDougall (1985) and Luis Chiozza (1998, 1999). I would not hesitate to call their works, with their many differences, a kind of *SomaPsychoanalysis*.

One assumption behind the subjective perspective is, of course, that what people believe, wish or fear, usually unconsciously, is important in relation to how they act and what will happen. Let me give an example. Jesper Hoffmeyer, a Danish professor of biochemistry and semiotics, reports on a study of male sperm production carried out in Manchester. It was demonstrated that the production of sperm cells rose when the man thought that his woman was unfaithful. In traditional biological science this would be explained merely by reference to competitive behavior: the competition with other men for children stimulates sperm production. Even if this is true, it is not an adequate explanation of the phenomenon. We must also ask ourselves "how can a man's testicles know that the woman is unfaithful, or rather, that the man believes this?" (Hoffmeyer, 1997, pp. 99–100)

In the Cartesian tradition we have learned that doubt, not belief, is at the center of epistemology, but a contemporary of Freud, the philosopher Charles Sander Peirce, maintained that belief, rather than doubt, was the primary asset, and that man always tries to rid himself of the unpleasure attached to doubt in order to reach a state of belief or conviction. Believing strongly in something gives a positive feeling, which in biological self-generating systems is part and parcel of establishing homeostasis (Freud's pleasure principle). If this is true, it means that everything, including observations accepted as objective facts, depends to some extent on a human value-system. Convictions are to some extent based on human judgments that are made in contexts where the interactive relationships with the world and to other living beings are of fundamental importance. The question of how the testicles react to what the man believes cannot at the present moment be fully answered unless we take into account the extent to which the body is influenced by mental phenomena, such as fantasies, feelings, wishes, and hopes. This is a strong reason to take the subjective perspective seriously.

In this special field, Freud's concepts of displacement and condensation are important. They are the fruits of his work with hysterical and psychosomatic patients from the 1880s and onwards. The concepts have become indispensable tools in all psychoanalytic work and are, of course, a result of the symbolic capacity anchored not only in our ideational world, created by upper and frontal brain areas, but also having a deep bodily anchorage: in motor behavior (movements and rhythms) and finally, of course, in the affective processes of the nervous and humorous systems of the body. This, however, does not reduce thought processes, nor conscious human feelings, to impulses and energies of nervous and muscular tissues. In this field the old problem of cause-effect will reach new complexities.

New Trends in Brain-Mind Research

As to research in this in-between-field of brain-mind interaction, there is one new way of approach that has proven to be exceptionally important. This new model for brain functioning takes the necessity of "guessing" seriously and introduces computational prediction-error modeling to create a theoretical method to deal with complexity and uncertainty. This can give a better understanding of the mentalizing process, which eventually leads to cognitive consciousness. As regards the role of memory we can for example claim that the purpose of learning and memorizing is not really to create a "memory box of facts" with which to impress the world or remember one's history. It is basically a means for generating predictions based on which we act. This might be the most important part of memory processing. All or most of this goes on unconsciously. When the prediction (the guessing) fails we become conscious by necessity because it generates feelings that we have to deal with. This leads to a need for more learning. These affective processes[4] are driven by a Free Energy Principle and for homeostatic reasons, but for a fuller presentation of this field I have to refer to other writers. (Fotopoulou & Tsakiris, 2017; Friston, 2010, 2012; Solms & Friston, 2018).[5]

We could however ask, more generally, what need there is for probability calculations when dealing with subjective problems of decision-making in real life or in psychoanalysis. If a theory does not help the clinician to sort out the issues raised in the treatment situation, then, of course, that theory is of no value to him clinically. However, that is not an argument against the consistency of the theory, just a statement of the use a person can make, or not make, of it. We do not need the theories of light (wave and particle) to turn on the light in the room. We just need to believe that pressing the button will make the light come on. For many of us, it is, however, interesting to find out what the structures and functions are behind the actual phenomena of the light turning on. How does it work? This knowledge might improve the usage we make of the function. That is what metapsychology, so important to Freud's psychoanalysis, is all about. This brings us to the question of the unconscious.

The Question of the Unconscious and Its Relation to the Brain and Body

The fact of unconscious mental processes being the most important part of human psychic life and the role of consciousness being overvalued in traditional psychology is of course fundamental to psychoanalysis. This line of thought stems from Freud's *Project for a Scientific Psychology* (1895/1950) and is reworked in psychological terms in *The Interpretation of Dreams*, where he writes:

> It is essential to abandon the overvaluation of the property of being conscious before it becomes possible to form any correct view of the origin of what is mental .... the unconscious must be assumed to be the general basis of psychical life .... Everything conscious has an unconscious preliminary stage; whereas what is unconscious may remain at that stage and nevertheless claim to be regarded as having the full value of a psychical process. The unconscious is the true psychical reality; *in its innermost nature it is as much unknown to us as the external world, and it is as incompletely presented by the data of consciousness as is the external world by the communications of our sense organs.*
>
> (1900/1964, pp. 612–613)

From these basic assumptions of psychoanalysis Freud never wavered. They are important for psychoanalysis both in its clinical work (working with the dynamic unconscious) and in a metatheoretical context especially in regard to its scientific standing. Concerning the last claim, Freud returns to it very clearly in his last article, *An Outline of Psychoanalysis*, written the year before he died, as a testament to the psychoanalytic movement.

> Whereas the psychology of consciousness never went beyond the broken sequences which were obviously dependent on something else, the other view, which held that the psychical is unconscious in itself, enabled psychology to take its place as a natural science like any other. The processes with which it is concerned are in themselves just as unknowable as those dealt with by other sciences, by chemistry and physics, for example; but it is possible to establish the laws which they obey and to follow their mutual relations and interdependencies unbroken over long stretches—in short, to arrive at what is described as an "understanding" of the field of natural phenomena in question.
>
> (Freud, 1938/1940, p. 158).

This is what a neuropsychoanalytic approach represents for me. And it takes us back to the question of dualism that we raised in the beginning, claiming for mental phenomena, such as feelings and ideas, an equal but different status in relation to the material brain and other bodily elements. This perspective gives to psychoanalysis a widening scope for the future. In relation to clinical practice psychoanalytic treatment will not be relevant only for strictly psychic illnesses or ordinary human discontent, but it can also be used to deal with unconscious processes related to diseases of the body and brain. And in the realm of scientific investigation of nature, it will, as Freud wished, stand on an equal footing with all of science "in understanding … the field of natural phenomena." (Freud, 1938/1940, p. 158).

21. Neuropsychoanalysis	
Main, general underlying assumptions	1 The physical and the psychical are two different expressions (dual aspects) of a basic phenomenon (neutral monism). There are correlations between the two marked by complexity and uncertainty. 2 "Objectivity and subjectivity are observational perspectives, not causes and effects. Neurophysiological events can no more produce psychological events than lightning can produce thunder. They are parallel manifestations of a single underlying process." (Solms, 2021, p. 301)

(Continued)

	3 Neuropsychoanalysis is a link between psychoanalysis and the neurosciences. 4 "The unconscious is the true psychical reality; *in its innermost nature it is as much unknown to us as the external world, and it is as incompletely presented by the data of consciousness as is the external world by the communications of our sense organs.*" (Freud, 1900/1964, pp. 612–613)

Notes

1 For a more thorough presentation of this theme see Matthis, 2000.
2 For a full description of these delusional states of denial see Ramachandran & Blakeslee, 1998; Kaplan-Solms & Solms, 2000; and Solms & Turnbull, 2002.
3 For further information on this kind of research follow *The International Journal of Neuropsychoanalysis*. Or visit the website: www.neuro-psa.org
4 A good presentation of these primal emotional systems you will find in Jaak Panksepp's (1998) *Affective Neuroscience. The Foundations of Human and Animal Emotions*.
5 When I was finishing this chapter a new book on these issues was just launched, which carry these ideas much further: Mark Solms (2021): *The Hidden Spring. A Journey to the Source of Consciousness*.

References

Chiozza, L. (1998). *Affects in somatic disorders*. Psychosocial Press.

Chiozza, L. (1999). *Why do we fall ill?* Psychosocial Press.

Damasio, A. (1999). *The feeling of what happens: Body and emotion in the making of consciousness*. Harcourt Brace.

Fotopoulou, A., & Tsakiris, M. (2017). Mentalizing homeostasis: The social origins of interoceptive inference. *Neuropsychoanalysis, 19*(1), 3–28.

Freud, S. (1940). An outline of psychoanalysis. In J. Strachey (Ed. and Trans.), *The standard edition of the complete psychological works of Sigmund Freud* (Vol. 23, pp. 140–207). Hogarth Press. (Original work published 1938).

Freud, S. (1950). Project for a scientific psychology. In J. Strachey (Ed. and Trans.), *The standard edition of the complete psychological works of Sigmund Freud* (Vol. 1, pp. 283–387). Hogarth Press. (Original work written 1895).

Freud, S. (1964). The interpretation of dreams. In J. Strachey (Ed. and Trans.), *The standard edition of the complete psychological works of Sigmund Freud* (Vol. 5, pp. 339–686). Hogarth Press. (Original work published 1900).

Freud, S. (1990). *A moment of transition. Two neuroscientific articles by Sigmund Freud*. Institute of Psychoanalysis & Karnac. (Original work published 1888).

Friston, K. (2010). The free-energy principle: A unified brain theory. *Nature Reviews Neuroscience, 11*, 127–138.

Friston, K. (2012). A free energy principle for biological systems. *Entropy, 14*, 2100–2121.

Hoffmeyer, J. (1997). *Signs of meaning in the universe*. Indiana University Press.

Kaplan-Solms, K., & Solms, M. (2000). *Clinical studies in neuro-psychoanalysis*. Karnac Books.
Matthis, I. (1997). *Den tänkande kroppen. Studier i det hysteriska symptomet.* [*The Thinking Body. Studies on the Hysterical Symptom*]. Natur och Kultur.
Matthis, I. (2000). Sketch for a metapsychology of affects. *International Journal of Psychoanalysis*, *81*(2), 215–227.
McDougall, J. (1985). *Theaters of the mind*. Basic Books.
Panksepp, J. (1998). *Affective neuroscience. The foundations of human and animal emotions*. Oxford University Press.
Ramachandran, V. S., & Blakeslee, S. (1998). *Phantoms in the brain*. Morrow.
Solms, M. (2021). *The hidden spring. A journey to the source of consciousness*. Profile Books.
Solms, M., & Friston, K. (2018). How and why consciousness arises: Some considerations from physics and physiology. *Journal of Consciousness Studies*, *15*(5–6), 202–238.
Solms, M., & Turnbull, O. (2002). *The brain and the inner world. An introduction to the neuroscience of subjective experience*. Routledge.
Solms, M., & Turnbull, O. (2011). What is neuropsychoanalysis. *NeuroPsychoanalysis*, *13*(2), 133–145.

Chapter 22

Italian Psychoanalytic Thought

Massimo Vigna-Taglianti

Main Theoretical Assumptions

The "Italian school," which stemmed from a fecund interplay among several "classic" matrices of the psychoanalytic tradition, is characterized by multiple approaches that create a variegated theoretical panorama. While, on the one hand, it is firmly anchored in the Freudian tradition from which it started (thanks to the impulse of founding fathers like Weiss, Perrotti, Servadio, Musatti); on the other, it was able to progressively integrate—in the wake of "our" secular cultural habit accustomed to a fertile compromise of different perspectives—the great caesura of the European and non-European psychoanalytic thinking. This ability to resolve theoretical disagreements through a dialectic discussion is not the mark of an accommodating eclecticism but is rather the product of a tendency to creative synthesis that in some respects is comparable to the intellectual tradition of the British independent group, in which ideas are respected for their actual value independently of their origin (Rayner, 1991).

Over the years, a peculiarly Italian tension has developed, aimed at integrating, without easy shortcuts, a metapsychological vertical paradigm and a hermeneutic-constructivist horizontal paradigm.

The vertical paradigm—following Di Chiara (2003, p. 18)—is based on temporality and unconscious, and refers to the theory of drives, sexuality, and dream, as well as the theory of representation, memory, repression, and splitting. Deconstruction and reconstruction, transference analysis, and interpretation are the cornerstones of the analytic process. This paradigm is still linked to a scientific-reductionist explanation that requires some persistence of theories, operational rules, and criteria for an objective approach (Riolo, 1999, p. 17). The horizontal paradigm rejects the idea of a foundation (historical, biological, instinct-driven) in favor of a continuous production of the subject and meaning-making through the analytic relationship, conceived as a "hermeneutic circuit" (Riolo, 1999, p. 17). In its folds, though, lie the risks—at a theoretical level—of abandoning metapsychology, and—at a clinical level—of relinquishing the patient-analyst asymmetry.

DOI: 10.4324/9781003027768-23

Generations of Italian psychoanalysts devoted their efforts to integrate these two seemingly irreconcilable paradigms, in order to continue to use analytic tools inspired by a firm theory and a rigorous methodology, preserving them from an excessive hermeneutic drift.

From this patient and arduous work of "cultivating," an Italian psychoanalytic landscape has come about, whereof the analytic relationship, the analytic narrative, and the analytic field are the hallmarks (Chianese, 1997/2007). This landscape is characterized by multiple theoretical frameworks which inevitably cross-fertilized and produced innovative theoretical contributions. They range from the Freudian one—based on a classic drive model or a model revisited in light of the contributions of the French school—to the Kleinian/post-Kleinian model, with its theoretical assumptions standing on a crucial duality and conflict of love and hate drives in relation to the object, to contributions that are more clearly related to the object relations theories informed by the British independent approach, or associated with the North-American relational model, and lastly to the post-Bionian developments that range from the enrichment of the late Bion's thinking to the most recent conceptualization of the post-Bion's/post-field model.

In this chapter, besides mentioning the theoretical assumptions related to this range of perspectives, I will try to highlight some developmental lines (let me paraphrase Anna Freud here) typical of the Italian psychoanalytic thinking. They bear witness, in my view, to a trajectory that from the idea of an unconscious functioning mainly aimed at removing drives, affects, and desires incompatible with consciousness got to the conception of an unconscious that is more physiologically symbol-poietic, that can be thought of as a psychic organ capable of performing an osmotic-representative functioning in relation to the internal and the external realities.

In this short and partial examination, I will only mention the authors who stand along the "developmental lines" that I highlight, as it is impossible—for reasons of space—to mention all the rich contributions that concurred not only to give the Italian psychoanalytic thinking its specific identity but also to state its unquestioned credibility internationally (for an extensive study of topics of Italian psychoanalytic thought, see Ferruta (2016) in *Reading Italian Psychoanalysis* [Borgogno et al., 2016]).

From the Intrapsychic to the Analytic Relationship

The first developmental line that can be detected in the Italian psychoanalytic thinking is related to an increasing importance of the presence of the object (and/or its absence) and some indispensable qualities of such presence as crucial elements for both the construction of the basic mental structures and their implications in the analytic relationship. These structures create the possibility of attuning with the mind of the Other and define the characteristic approach of each subject—during their entire life—in relation to the affective modulation implied in the relation with oneself and others.

A turning point in Italian psychoanalysis—which started in the 1970s—was characterized by an original revision of the intuition that the individual's development occurs through interpersonal rather than internal maturational processes: the growth and the formation of psychic functions depend on the kind and the qualities of the intersubjective encounter. This becomes the informing principle of a "treatment" of which the crucial factor is the observation of the "doing" and "undoing" of the analytic relationship.

In the ensuing years, once the road to the internal world and the primitive levels of the affective and mental experience in the analytic relationship was paved, research was addressed to several aspects of it: the metapsychological apparatus (Conrotto, 1995; Traversa, 1981; Vergine, 1980); the object relation and its re-actualization in the transference/counter-transference dynamic (Amati Mehler, 1985; Borgogno & Vigna-Taglianti, 2008/2009; Nicolò, 2007; Turillazzi Manfredi, 1994); the different facets of the analyst's interpretative and transformative work (Canestri, 1994; Carloni, 1984/2016, Riolo, 2007; Speziale-Bagliacca, 1991); and a progressive recognition of the analyst's participation not only as an observer but also as co-author and co-actor in the analytic process (Bezoari & Ferro, 1991; Bonaminio, 2008; Ferro, 1992/1999b; Gaburri, 1992/2016; Nissim Momigliano & Robutti, 1992).

Relation and Introjection

So, in the Italian psychoanalytic thinking, we have seen a progressive rise of an object relations model. In terms of theoretical assumptions, this model particularly emphasizes the early life acquisitions and the structuring of mental functions, starting with the representational working-through of whatever comes from the context of primary sensory-motor experiences that occur within the mother-child matrix. These representations evolve to increasingly symbolic, differentiated, and coherent levels of the Self in relation to the object, but the general assumption of the current object relations theories is that the previous levels of the representations of the interactions are stored in the mind and continue to exert a determinant weight in the psychic life of the person, as since the beginning of life all the internalizations of the Self-Other relations have different features, depending on whether the interactions occur in intense affective states or in conditions of low affective activation (Fonagy, 2005; Kernberg, 2005).

An increasing interest of Italian psychoanalysts in these phenomena generated another "line of thought" that gives similar importance to the phenomena of internalization of early relational experiences and their strong emotional connotations as key elements for the constitution of mental structures. In this regard, a large group of Italian analysts has inherited from Ferenczi a deep interest in the importance of the mother and the emotions in the affective development of the child. The Hungarian analyst anticipated the concept of internalization of the object relations as "active" elements in the foundation of the individual's unconscious mental functioning. Many of his writings emphasize that the infant, just like the analysand, not only has an attitude for projection, but she is much inclined to incorporate and introject whatever comes from the adult in terms of relational atmosphere, hypnotic suggestions, and unconscious mandates (Ferenczi, 1916, 1955).

Such inborn imitative-introjective predisposition (Gaddini, 1969), were it not adequately supported and modulated by the object that provides primary care in the interpsychic relationship, will produce unconscious identifications with strong alienating power, interfering with the rise and development of the Self (Ammaniti & Gallese, 2014; Bolognini, 2008/2010). This is another field of study, proper to the Italian school that has always paid attention to the trauma and the transgenerational transmission of pathological identifications. (Badoni, 2002; Borgogno, 1999/2007; Meotti, 1996/2016; Neri, 1993/2016; Vallino & Macciò, 2004; Vigna-Taglianti, 2015a).

From Vis a Tergo to Learning from Experience and Beyond …

During his life and work, Freud progressively formulated, starting with his study on sexuality and the psychosexual development, an energy-drive theory of the mind based on the operating of a *vis a tergo*, that he identified in the *Trieb* (Freud, 1915). To this end, he hypothesized the cathexis of reality and formulated the notions of conflict, repression, and psychic reality informed by the drive economy.

Many Italian analysts are deeply in debt to this classic tradition, characterized by an economic-topographical vertex in which the concepts of libido, drive, psychic energy, discharge, repression, and representation are the keystones of a metapsychological construction (Petrella, 1988). From this there also stems, consistently, a specific theory of technique mainly based on interpretation and recollection (Semi, 2006/2007).

However, the concept of drive, as *vis a tergo* that is shaped by the clash with reality, appears—at least to another part of the Italian psychoanalytic community—partially superseded and not in line with the findings about the importance of the primary experience at play in the constitution of the basic mental structures, nor with the activity that these structures explicate from the very beginning in relation to the external reality, through a selection, understanding, and working-through of every piece of sensory information. To several Italian psychoanalysts, in fact, the classic formulations of dynamic unconscious and repression do not seem sufficient to explain either the early operations of the human psyche or the complex yet apparently chaotic operations of a mind that became disorganized following an early trauma that deeply interfered, during early development, with the creation of these basic structures.

Following Bion (1962)—the first analyst who spoke about the importance of *learning from experience*—and the post-Bionian school that has emphasized learning and subjective working-through of the experience as an engine for the structuring of the mind, currently several Italian authors tend to think in terms of innate predispositions to attribute a given meaning to specific experiential configurations which are being learned (Bion Talamo et al., 1999; Imbasciati, 2006). Thus, a model of the unconscious was theorized—emphasizing the working through of the subjective emotional experience rather than a development coming from endogenous forces—that proposes that the mind is gradually formed within an interpersonal context and configured as a system of understanding and transformation of the stimuli from the external and internal realities: an ever-evolving structure generating meanings from raw proto-sensory elements into meaningful affective elements (Ferro, 2007/2011; Vigna-Taglianti, 2021).

In this direction, a specific hallmark of the Italian school was the shifting of the conceptual frontier from a bi-personal epistemic vertex to the assimilation of the field theory (Baranger & Baranger, 2008) and the original revisitation of the narratological model (Corrao, 1991/1998). The psychoanalytic narrative, along with interpretation and construction, is one of the *royal roads* to access the derivatives of the human unconscious, allowing the indirect manifestation of its irrepresentable reality.

In particular, Ferro, in his conception of the analytic field, has emphasized the narrative as a matrix of potential stories. By narrative he means

> a specific way of the analyst being in the session in which he participates with the patient in a "construction of meaning" in a strongly dialogical way, without specific interpretive caesura: as if analyst and patient were building a play together in which the plots arise, intertwine, develop, at times even unpredictably and unimaginably to the two co-narrators, without either being a strong holder of a pre-established truth. In this way of progressing, the co-narrative transformation replaces the interpretation.
>
> (1999a, p. 747)

The theorization of the analytic field—to which Italian psychoanalysis has crucially contributed (Corrao, 1986/1997; Ferro & Civitarese, 2015/2019; Gaburri, 1997)—has allowed the full recognition of the value of co-construction and co-determination of what comes to life in analysis. In short, for the authors who refer to the concept of the field, the text is also a function of the actual interaction between the analyst and the patient and of the emotional field they generate in an analytic setting characterized by two peculiar elements. First, the shift of the analyst's primary function from interpretation, mostly understood as a decoding of a latent meaning, to his availability to take in the emotions that develop in the field from the patient's utterances. Second, the importance of the analyst's negative capability, understood as a non-intrusive, non-decodifying and not-colonizing quality of the interpretation of the text of the patient (Ferro, 1996/2002).

In this model—which can be called the oneiric field (Ferro, 2009)—the focus of analysis is the preliminary development of the capacities to dream one's own subjective psychic experience rather than working on repression or splitting. This is an aspect that several Italian authors have highlighted: by following Bion's concept of *becoming* (Grotstein, 2007), they maintain that the analyst, committed to making a contact with the unconscious of the analysand, needs to let the field get ill of the analysand's illness so as to lend parts of the analyst's own thinking apparatus, indispensable in repairing or conveying the tools for thinking (Borgogno, 2011/2013; Civitarese, 2008/2010; Vigna-Taglianti, 2014/2015b).

Implicit Memories and Unrepressed Unconscious

In continuity with the discourse that I have articulated thus far, there unfolds another "developmental line" detectable in the Italian psychoanalytic thinking: it concerns the progressive importance given to a pre-verbal, pre-representative unconscious procedural system and to its correlated mental automatisms.

An interest in this dimension of the unconscious has produced a thriving line of research focused on how early subjective experiences are acquired, settled, and transformed; in short, on the formation and inscription of mnestic traces, since it is the affective content and not the semantic content that crucially affects the "stocking" mechanism of the implicit memories of the subject. These memories are not objective memories stored in some sort of psychic hard drive, but inscriptions of a functional acquisition: they have a very nuanced character and are influenced by the apparatus in charge of their codifying interpretation; essentially, in their layering, they undergo a continuous meaning-making (Imbasciati, 2017; Mancia, 2004/2007).

This is one reason why today it is easier to understand why the infant's unconscious functioning persists in the older child and in the adult, and manifests—at times in elusive forms, at times in blatant forms—in the transference/counter-transference dynamic: the non-verbal expressive current, which ties the child to the parent throughout life, continues to be a primary means for exchanging affective-relational communications that people perceive at intuitive and pre-symbolic levels (Schore, 2003). Transference re-actualization of implicit memories, during an analytic treatment, is therefore more frequently considered by many Italian authors as a condition that is not only ineludible but also indispensable to allow the patient to have a transformative interpersonal experience that will allow for the construction of a mind that is finally capable of experiencing psychically what had not been possible up to that point (Boccara et al., 2018; Borgogno & Vigna-Taglianti, 2013).

If what cannot be remembered is acted out—like Freud (1905, 1912, 1914) intuited since he wrote the case of Dora by introducing the concept of *agieren*—only apparently *where there is action there is not representation*; or better: where there cannot be representation we will find enactment sequences that preempt the symbolic and represent the only possible way to give voice to an intrapsychic dimension that has not been repressed but is mute and still wordless. Listening to what is acted out can just swing between personification, dramatization, and narrative of some disavowed and dissociated aspects of the infantile experience. This is a point shared also by Bolognini (2002/2004) who claims that a deep knowledge of the patient depends on the analyst's capacity to activate a continuous and dynamic play of identification and disidentification with the patient herself; a kind of empathic immersion and emersion that allow such an emotional proximity that is cure and knowledge at the same time.

In conclusion, the following theoretical-technical cornerstones of the so-called Italian school date back in time and their roots come from the most noble tradition of psychoanalytic thinking: 1) the hypothesis of an unconscious not only based on an energy-drive theory of the mind, but also structured according to sediments of internalized interpsychic relations that take on a structuring character that is determinant in the psychic life of the individuals; 2) relinquishing the idea of a treatment that occurs through the recovery of repressed or split verbal memories only, but rather through the construction and/or reconstruction of those mind's symbolic capacities necessary to become able to deal with a psychic suffering that previously was not bearable nor figurable; 3) the intuition that what was not understood by the ego's verbal logic will show up again on the analytic scene only through *agieren*—that is, through enactment (Jacobs, 1986)—by choosing the analyst as the object by which to represent a specific relational script, whose title and conclusion are still unknown.

22. Italian Psychoanalytic Thought	
Main, general underlying assumptions	1 Integration between a metapsychological vertical paradigm and a hermeneutic-constructivist horizontal paradigm. 2 The conception of an unconscious functioning mainly aimed at removing drives, affects, and desires incompatible with consciousness. 3 The conception of an unconscious that is more physiologically symbol-poietic: a psychic organ capable of performing an osmotic-representative functioning in relation to the internal and the external realities. 4 Hallmarks of Italian psychoanalytic landscape: analytic relationship, analytic narrative, analytic field

(*Continued*)

Specific theoretical assumptions	
psychic structure	The structuring of mental functions starts with the representational working-through of whatever comes from the context of primary sensory-motor experiences that occur within the mother-child matrix.
energy	An energy-drive theory of the mind in which the drive is seen as *vis a tergo* shaped by the clash with reality and by the cathexis of reality.
relationships	Importance of phenomena of internalization of early relational experiences and their strong emotional connotation as key elements for the constitution of mental structures.
developmental stages	The development of psychic functions depends on the kind and the qualities of the intersubjective encounter, and occurs through interpersonal rather than internal maturational processes.
body	N/A
anxieties/instincts and defenses	N/A
Assumptions concerning etiology	Internalized interpsychic pathogenic relations are determinant in the psychic life of the individuals: previous levels of the representations of the interactions are stored in the mind and continue to exert a determinant weight in the person's psychic life.
Implications for technique	The analyst's primary function shifts from interpretation, mostly understood as a decoding of a latent meaning, to his availability to make contact with the unconscious of the analysand, in order to let the field get ill of the analysand's illness and to lend parts of the analyst's own thinking apparatus, indispensable in repairing or conveying the tools for thinking.
Subsequent developments of the core concept	The focus of analysis is the preliminary development of the capacities to dream one's own subjective psychic experience rather than working on repression or splitting; transference re-actualization of implicit memories allows the construction of a mind that is finally capable of experiencing psychically what had not been possible up to that point.

References

Amati Mehler, J. (1985). Transitional objects, transitional phenomena and transitional area. *Rivista di Psicoanalisi, 31*(3), 4–46.

Ammaniti, M., & Gallese, V. (2014). *The birth of intersubjectivity: Psychodynamics, neurobiology and the self.* W. W. Norton & Company.

Badoni, M. (2002). Parents and their child—and the analyst in the middle: Working with a transgenerational mandate. *International Journal of Psycho-Analysis, 83*, 1111–1131.

Baranger, M., & Baranger, W. (2008). The analytic situation as a dynamic field. *International Journal of Psycho-Analysis, 89*, 795–826.

Bezoari, M., & Ferro, A. (1991). A journey through the bipersonal field of analysis. In Roleplaying to transformations in the couple. *Rivista di Psicoanalisi, 37*(1), 4–46.

Bion, W. R. (1962). *Learning from experience.* Tavistock Publications.

Bion Talamo, P., Borgogno, F., & Merciai, S. (Eds.). (1999). *W. R. Bion: Between past and future.* Karnac Books.

Boccara, P., Meterangelis, G., & Riefolo, G. (2018). *Enactment.* FrancoAngeli.

Bolognini, S. (2004). *The psychoanalytic empathy.* Free Association. (Original work published 2002).

Bolognini, S. (2010). *Secret passages: The theory and technique of interpsychic relations.* Routledge. (Original work published 2008).

Bonaminio, V. (2008).The person of the analyst: Interpreting, not interpreting, and countertransference. *Psychoanalytic Quarterly, 77*, 1105–1146.

Borgogno, F. (2007). *Psychoanalysis as a journey.* Open Gate Press. (Original work published 1999).

Borgogno, F. (2013). *The girl who committed hara-kiri and other clinical and historical essays.* Karnac Books. (Original work published 2011).

Borgogno, F., Luchetti, A., & Marino Coe, L. (Eds.). (2016). *Reading Italian psychoanalysis.* Routledge.

Borgogno, F., & Vigna-Taglianti, M. (2009). Role-reversal: A somewhat neglected mirror of heritages of the past. *Italian Psychoanalytic Annual, 3*, 93–102. (Original work published 2008).

Borgogno, F., & Vigna-Taglianti, M. (2013). Role-reversal and dissociation of the self. Actions signalling memories to be recovered: An exploration of a somewhat neglected transference-countertransference process. In R. Oelsner (Ed.), *Transference and countertransference today* (pp. 289–313). Routledge.

Canestri, J. (1994). Transformations. *International Journal of Psycho-Analysis, 75*, 1079–1092.

Carloni, G. (2016). Tact, contact, and tacticts. In F. Borgogno, A. Luchetti, & L. Marino Coe (Eds.), *Reading Italian psychoanalysis* (pp. 198–208). Routledge. (Original work published 1984).

Chianese, D. (2007). *Constructions and the analytic field: History, scenes and destiny.* Routledge. (Original work published 1997).

Civitarese, G. (2010). *The intimate room: Theory and technique of the analytic field.* Routledge. (Original work published 2008).

Conrotto, F. (1995). Pulsione o relazione: Una opposizione irriducibile? [Drive or relationship: An irreducible opposition?] *Rivista di Psicoanalisi, 41*, 583–610.

Corrao, F. (1997). Il concetto di campo come modello teorico [The field's concept as a theoretical model]. In E. Gaburri (Ed.), *Emozione e interpretazione* [*Emotion and interpretation*] (pp. 33–38). Bollati Boringhieri. (Original work published 1986).

Corrao, F. (1998). *Orme, vol. 1 : Contributi alla psicoanalisi* [*Footsteps. Contributions to psychoanalysis*] (Vol. 1). R. Cortina. (Original work published 1991).

Di Chiara, G. (2003). *Curare con la psicoanalisi* [*Curing with psychoanalysis*]. R. Cortina.

Ferenczi, S. (1916). Introjection and transference. In E. Jones (Trans.), *Contributions to psychoanalysis* (pp. 30–80). Richard G. Badger. (Original work published 1909).

Ferenczi, S. (1955). Confusion of tongues between adults and the child. In *Final contributions to the problems and methods of psychoanalysis* (pp. 156–167). Hogarth Press. (Original work published 1932).

Ferro, A. (1999a). Interpretazioni, decostruzioni, narrazioni. Ovvero: le ragioni di Jacques [Interpretations, deconstructions, narrations. That is: Jacques' reasons]. *Rivista di Psicoanalisi*, *45*, 743–758.

Ferro, A. (1999b). *The bi-personal field: Experiences in child analysis*. Routledge. (Original work published 1992).

Ferro, A. (2002). *In the analyst's consulting room*. Brunner-Routledge. (Original work published 1996).

Ferro, A. (2009). Transformations in dreaming and characters in the psychoanalytic field. *International Journal of Psycho-Analysis*, *90*, 209–230.

Ferro, A. (2011). *Avoiding emotions, living emotions*. Routledge. (Original work published 2007).

Ferro, A., & Civitarese G. (2019). *The analytic field and its transformations*. Karnac. (Original work published 2015).

Ferruta, A. (2016). Themes and developments of psychoanalytic thought in Italy. In F. Borgogno, A. Luchetti, & L. Marino Coe (Eds.), *Reading Italian psychoanalysis* (pp. 18–35). Routledge.

Fonagy, P. (2005). The psychoanalytic evolutive theory. In S. E. Person, A. M. Cooper, & G. O. Gabbard (Eds.), *The American psychiatric publishing* textbook of psychoanalysis (pp. 131–146). Psychiatric Publishing.

Freud, S. (1905). Fragment of an analysis of a case of hysteria. In J. Strachey (Ed. and Trans.), *The standard edition of the complete works of Sigmund Freud* (Vol. 7, pp. 7–122). Hogarth Press.

Freud, S. (1912). The dynamics of transference. In J. Strachey (Ed. and Trans.), *The standard edition of the complete works of Sigmund Freud* (Vol. 12, pp. 97–108). Hogarth Press.

Freud, S. (1914). Remembering, repeating and working-through. In J. Strachey (Ed. and Trans.), *The standard edition of the complete works of Sigmund Freud* (Vol. 12, pp. 145–156). Hogarth Press.

Freud, S. (1915). Instincts and their vicissitudes. In J. Strachey (Ed. and Trans.), *The standard edition of the complete works of Sigmund Freud* (Vol. 14, pp. 117–140). Hogarth Press.

Gaburri, E. (Ed.). (1997). *Emozione e interpretazione* [*Emotion and interpretation*]. Bollati Boringhieri.

Gaburri, E. (2016). Personification. In F. Borgogno, A. Luchetti, & L. Marino Coe (Eds.), *Reading Italian psychoanalysis* (pp. 614–621). Routledge. (Original work published 1992).

Gaddini, E. (1969). On imitation. *International Journal of Psycho-Analysis, 50*, 475–484.

Grotstein, J. S. (2007). *A beam of intense darkness. Wilfred's Bion legacy to psychoanalysis*. Karnac.

Imbasciati, A. (2006). *Constructing a mind: A new base for psychoanalytic theory*. Routledge.

Imbasciati, A. (2017). *Mindbrain, psychoanalytic institutions, and psychoanalysts: A new metapsychology consistent with neuroscience*. Routledge.

Jacobs, T. (1986). On countertransference enactments. *Journal of the American Psychoanalytic Association, 34*, 289–307.

Kernberg, O. F. (2005). Object relations theories and psychoanalytic technique. In S. E. Person, A. M. Cooper, & G. O. Gabbard (Eds.), *The American psychiatric publishing* textbook of psychoanalysis (pp. 57–76). Psychiatric Publishing.

Mancia, M. (2007). *Feeling the words. Neuropsychoanalytic understanding of memory and the unconscious*. Routledge. (Original work published 2004).

Meotti, F. (2016). Some thoughts on inauthenticity. In F. Borgogno, A. Luchetti, & L. Marino Coe (Eds.), *Reading Italian Psychoanalysis* (pp. 502–506). Routledge. (Original work published 1996).

Neri, C. (2016). Field theory and trans-generational phantasies. In F. Borgogno, A. Luchetti, & L. Marino Coe (Eds.), *Reading Italian psychoanalysis* (pp. 406–416). Routledge. (Original work published 1993).

Nicolò, A. M. (2007) (Ed.). *Attualità del transfert* [*On the current relevance of transference*]. FrancoAngeli.

Nissim Momigliano, L., & Robutti, A. (Eds.). (1992). *Shared experience: The psychoanalytic dialogue*. Karnac Books.

Petrella, F. (1988). Il modello freudiano [The Freudian model]. In A. A. Semi (Ed.), *Trattato di psicoanalisi* [*Treatise on psychoanalysis*] (Vol. 1, pp. 41–146). R. Cortina.

Rayner, E. (1991). *The independent mind in British psychoanalysis*. Free Association Books.

Riolo, F. (1999). Il paradigma della "cura" [The Paradigm of the Cure]. *Rivista di Psicoanalisi, 45*, 7–26.

Riolo, F. (2007). Psychoanalytic transformations. *International Journal of Psycho-Analysis, 88*, 1375–1389.

Schore, A. N. (2003). *Affect regulation and the repair of the self*. W. W. Norton & Company.

Semi, A. A. (2007). Transference and unconscious communication: Countertransference, theories and the analyst's narcissism. *Italian Psychoanalytic Annual, 1*, 29–47 (Original work published 2006).

Speziale-Bagliacca, R. (1991). The capacity to contain: Notes on its function in psychic change. *International Journal of Psycho-Analysis, 72*(1), 27–33.

Traversa, C. (Ed.). (1981). *La relazione analitica* [*The analytic relationship*]. Borla.

Turillazzi Manfredi, S. (1994). *Le certezze perdute della psicoanalisi clinica* [*The lost certainties of clinical psychoanalysis*]. R. Cortina.

Vallino, D., & Macciò, M. (2004). The child's sense of existence and the fatal attraction of identification. *International Forum of Psychoanalysis, 13*, 71–77.

Vergine, A. (1980). La relazione analitica come struttura: Una ipotesi metapsicologica del funzionamento psichico come "relazione" [The analytic relationship as a

structure: A metapsychological hypothesis of psychic functioning as a "relationship"]. *Rivista di Psicoanalisi*, *41*, 611–631.
Vigna-Taglianti, M. (2015a). Death instinct, death passion and unconscious pathological identifications: Too much and not enough. *Psychoanalysis in Europe*. Bullettin EPF, 69.
Vigna-Taglianti, M. (2015b). Ruptures and reconnections: Play as a thread for sewing up? In G. Saragnano, & C. Seulin (Eds.), *Playing and reality revisited* (pp. 175–200). Karnac Books. (Original work published 2014).
Vigna-Taglianti, M. (2021). Il pezzo mancante. Sulle tracce di una metapsicologia al passo con i tempi [The missing piece. On the trail of a metapsychology in step with the times]. *Rivista di Psicoanalisi*, *67*(2), 327–346.

Chapter 23

Argentine Psychoanalysis and the Psycho-Social Perspective[1]

Samuel Arbiser

Since 1942, the year in which the Argentine Psychoanalytic Association was founded, in Argentine society there has been a clinical practice under theoretical, technical, and ethical precepts in line with those of other world centers of psychoanalysis. From that time on, scientific activity has resulted in a remarkable expansion outward in different directions, one which sprung from the fertile ground that gave rise to the most influential currents of psychoanalytic thinking as they interacted with the most representative local authors and ideas. Amongst the influential currents, the most resonant were those which proposed early object relations—especially Melanie Klein, Harry Guntrip, and Ronald Fairbairn—as opposed to those inclined towards ego psychology. Later, in 1970, these influences multiplied and became more diversified with Heinz Kohut, Otto Kernberg, Donald Winnicott and post-Kleinians such as Wilfred Bion, Donald Meltzer and the thriving French current with Jaques Lacan and post-Lacanians such as André Green and Piera Aulagnier. One of the many offshoots that this initial intense intellectual atmosphere flowed into went on to shape what I call "psychosocial perspective." This perspective has its roots in the original impact left by the innovative thinking of Enrique Pichon Rivière and his most creative disciples amongst whom I should mention (while being unjustly limited in an effort to be brief) José Bleger, David Liberman, Madeleine, and Willy Baranger. Even if it is impossible to quiet my own bias, in this chapter I will attempt to set out a general and concise panorama of the thinking of these authors.

This perspective—and here I attribute the aforementioned originality—is based on a conception of a "human being" different from the traditional, predominantly anthropocentric one. To be precise, it differs from that conception in understanding man as immersed in and inseparable from his historic and socio-cultural context: "the man in situation," a designation borrowed by Pichon Rivière from J. P. Sartre. The French philosopher placed emphasis on the "existence" of man over and above and rummaging into his "essence." Given the inherent imperfection of this sociocultural context—in contrast to the stance taken by classical psychoanalysis which traces the shortcoming to the conflict between drives and defenses from this perspective,

DOI: 10.4324/9781003027768-24

both in the collective and the individual dimension, the shortcoming is inextinguishable as it is inherent to the aforementioned imperfection. As a consequence, therefore, the adaptive equilibrium achieved (health) is essentially precarious, as David Liberman (1976) explained when he stated that:

> Mental equilibrium can be considered an **unstable equilibrium** that may be disturbed as an effect of variations which occur **inside of the communicative networks in which a given individual interacts** and also the place of origin of the disturbance may consist in **an intrasystemic disturbance** (p. 53).

This understood, in this formulation, both the imperfection of the psychosocial context (the communicative networks in which they interact) on the one hand and the personal "dispositional series" (intrasystemic disturbance) on the other are connoted.

I would now like to choose some selected excerpts from contributions made by the aforementioned authors in the hope that they will help illustrate the differing positions that they held within the heterogeneous and nuanced field of the psychoanalytic theory of those days.

The Design of the Psyche: The Internal Group

Enrique Pichon Rivière and Samuel Arbiser

The visualization of man and his reality sustained by this sector of Argentine psychosocial psychoanalytic thought involves the need to design a model of the psychic apparatus in accordance with this (socio-cultural-historic) collective conception. This is the concept of the "internal group" to which Pichon Rivière made just scant mention in his written work. Given the lack of systematic and detailed development of this psychic model on the part of its creator himself, in a number of works (especially Arbiser, 2001, 2013) I have attempted to do just that. Considering these premises, I can now suggest my own definition as a conclusion:

> The internal group is a way of visualising and conceptualising in an operational sense the human psyche in terms of a repertoire of organising link structures into a unit which (ideally) makes them coherent. These link structures are in a permanent state of feedback interchange with the link structures of the current surrounding external world. They were incorporated during evolutionary development and reproduce, in a refracted manner, in the internal world each subject's own social and cultural world. The infinite variety of personal histories determines their singularity and, moreover, which psychic resources are used to decode and process the social universes and cultural inheritance (2001, p. 113).

It should also be mentioned that this proposal of a model of the psyche does not exclude, but rather includes the previous models which came about progressively starting with the initial proposals made by Freud of his "first topology." With the phrase "operational sense," I am attempting to highlight the fact that the model of the internal group is ubiquitous and is equally suitable for both individual and collective analytic frames (i.e., small therapeutic or operative groups, couples, families).

A Vision of Psychopathology

Enrique Pichon Rivière

Enrique Pichon Rivière holds that health and illness are not static categories, but rather dynamic modalities in which the subject reads [judgement of attribution (Freud, 1925)] and adapts to reality. The "active adaptation to reality" is defined by Pichon Rivière when he states that "… [the subject] *transforms* things from things-in-themselves into things-for-themselves. By way of a continuous praxis, to the extent that he modifies himself he modifies the world, in a *continuously spiral* movement" (1971, p. 340). The term "transformation" is the key term in this statement with regards to the importance it allows to *change*. Meanwhile, the term "spiral" points to overcoming on the circularity which is part of "repetition compulsion." On the other hand, the author places "passive adaptation to reality" in neuroses in the general sense and would add in this category, even as its paradigm, the "overadapted personalities" described by David Liberman (1982) (see below Arbiser, 2014), personalities which, according to this author, adapt to reality in an uncritical way. The passive maladjustment to reality includes—and here I speak in general terms once again—psychotic patients, that is to say, those cases where helplessness marginalizes them from contact with reality, and condemns them to the need of some sort of assistance by agents that will allow them to survive in that reality. Finally, active maladjustment to reality refers to the psychopath and those people of action who, instead of adapting themselves, have the ability to use reality, detecting the specific weaknesses of the human context.

David Liberman and the Systemization of Clinical Psychoanalysis

Firstly, it would seem appropriate to differentiate between psychopathology and clinical psychoanalysis. The former is theoretical, and a guiding discipline that addresses the latter, which is empirical. For Liberman, the session and the process (the progressive succession of sessions), that is to say, clinical psychoanalysis, was the starting point of all investigation. Thus, he suggested that the discipline should have a method of its own based on the study of its own empirical core: the "psychoanalytic dialogue." To study this dialogue, it would be necessary to have indicators that are testable, and—in this search—he in succession turns to the theory of communication, semiotics, and finally linguistics. In *La Comunicación en Terapéutica Psicoanalítica* (Liberman, 1962), he uses the theory of communication, and especially contributions by Ruesch (1957), to classify different types of "person" by the way they communicate with the interlocutor, correlating them in the process with phases of the development of the libido (Abraham, 1924; Freud 1905, 1932/1933). Later, Liberman turns to semiotics (Morris, 1946) in order to group and systematize analysands, from the objective distortions of the semiotic areas: syntactic, semantic, and pragmatic. Finally, the factors and the functions of the communication model of Román Jakobson (1960) allows him to formulate his doctrine of "the styles." Here, he differentiates six styles according to each factor and function: 1) the reflexive style, which corresponds to schizoid personalities; 2) the lyrical style, with depressions and depressive personalities; 3) the epic style, with its action personalities; 4) the narrative style, with an obsessive character and neurosis; 5) the dramatic style which searches out the unknown and creates suspense; 6) the dramatic style which has an aesthetic impact in hysterical personalities and in successful advertising messages. This doctrine of the styles incorporates the development of notions of "stylistic complementarity," "functions of the Ego," and the "ideally plastic Ego." [For a better understanding of the topic, see, in English, Arbiser, 2014 and, in Spanish, the author himself in Liberman, 1970].

The Body and Psychosomatic Impact

David Liberman

For Liberman (1982), what was conspicuous, what stood out with regards to the characterization of those patients referred to as psychosomatic, was not a result of the event of the organic disorder, but rather of an overadaptation to the unquestioned environment and to the dominant cultural values. As mentioned above, these patients could be said to constitute the paradigmatic example of passive adaptation to reality. The consequence of this environmental overadaptation—and this is the essential part—is the postponement and the rejection of the corporal and emotional self; in this way the signals coming from the emotional and corporal sphere are ignored because of a deficit in the construction of symbols, a construction normally carried out by a supposed symbolic apparatus. From the point of view of early development, research locates the responsibility for these results in a flaw in the normal evolutionary symbiosis. These cases of overadaptation are to be found in mothers who abridge or avoid this step of compulsory mutual rapport (symbiosis), favoring and celebrating the adaptive achievements of the breastfed child. This favors and stimulates the premature development of the distal sensory receptors (sight and hearing) to the detriment and delays in the development of the proximal receptors (taste, smell, touch) and the enteroceptive (kinesthesia, coenesthesia, thermal, pain, and equilibrium). The hypertrophy of the distal receptors, therefore, allows for rapid adaptation, which is however mimetic in the environmental reality. Therefore, concepts of time and space are registered in a Euclidean geometry and are not integrated in the meanings of organic and affective inner rhythms.

José Bleger: His Psychopathology Based on His Personal Vision of Early Evolutionary Development

In psychopathology, José Bleger (1967) undertook the study of symbiosis, ambiguity, and also accessional episodes such as epilepsy or syncope and sudden fainting. The ambiguity would express itself in fictitious, factual, and Manichaean personalities, and in psychopathy. Theorizing on these cases led him to reformulate the Kleinian theory of early psychological development postulating a primitive phase of indifferentiation prior to the paranoid-schizoid position that this author suggests. He refers to this as the "glischrocaric position" (from *glischros* meaning "viscous" and *karion* meaning "nucleus") as it contains a "viscous nucleus." In this position, there is a predominance of fusion and confusional anxieties which don't reach the stage of discrimination until the next paranoid-schizoid stage through the establishment of polarities (divalency). This is especially the case with the "I"-"you" and "inside"-"outside" and can be seen as a necessary condition for the restitution of the process of projection and introjection. What is left behind in this phase of differentiation will go on to become the "psychotic part of the personality." All Bleger's psychopathology rests on the greater or lesser persistence of this viscous nucleus in shaping this psychotic part of the personality and in the vicissitudes and necessity to use the diverse forms of its neutralization through control, cleavage, fragmentation, evacuation, or immobilization in a depository.

The psychoanalysis of the psychoanalytic frame was another of Bleger's insightful theoretical contributions. Referred to in a straightforward way, he distinguishes two parts in the analytic situation: a) the frame as the constant of the method and b) the process where he identifies the variables. When, by some accident or other, a change occurs in the frame, it becomes variable and we discover that relevant aspects of the psychotic part of the personality were deposited and immobilized there.

Madeleine and Willy Baranger and the Analytic Situation as a "Dynamic Field"

With a solid French academic training under their belts, Madeleine and Willy arrived and lived on both sides of the River Plate: first Buenos Aires, then Montevideo and, finally, settling back in Buenos Aires. Considered as continuing the work of Pichon Rivière, they contributed (while applying the Field Theory [Lewin, 1958]) to the psychosocial perspective of psychoanalysis which could be seen clearly in the proposal of the analytic situation as a dynamic field in Chapter 7 of *Problemas del campo psicoanalítico* (Problems in the Psychoanalytic Field, 1969). There, they established:

> The analytic situation must therefore formulate itself not as a situation of one person facing himself, but rather of two people inevitably linked in a complementary manner for the duration of the situation and involved in the same dynamic process [emphasis added].
>
> (Baranger & Baranger, 1969, p. 129)

The patient and the analyst—the analytic couple—shape a field inside of which all the phenomena emerging from that same field depend on the interaction between those two participants who are "inevitably linked in a complementary manner."

Conceptual, Referential, and Operative Schema (CROS)

Enrique Pichon Rivière

This creative thinker came from the world of culture and psychiatric practice. His background led him to test, and practice as a psychoanalyst, positions which came from a wide range of sources, not only from psychoanalysis but from diverse humanistic disciplines, from art and even from popular culture. It could be said that he practiced the broadest pluralism and the multidisciplinary in his theorizing and in his clinical practice itself. From the already mentioned Marxist and Sartrean philosophical background, he borrowed from the symbolic interactionism of George Mead (1972), Kurt Lewin's field theory (1958), and *Communication* by Gregory Bateson and Jurgen Ruesch (1951/1984).

Considering this, therefore, the question arises: how do we reconcile such diversity? Answering this led Pichon Rivière to propose CROS, an acronym for the Conceptual, Referential, and Operative Schema. This name refers to the baggage of knowledge that an operator uses to approach the object to be investigated, with the emphasis on a receptive and permeable attitude that tends more toward the expectation of discovery and change rather than the confirmation of an expectation. This baggage we can understand as a metaphorical toolbox that gathers together constantly renewed paradigms that have been created by formative events and experiences and crises of life which have been processed through personal and didactic analysis. From this large and versatile toolbox, the operator chooses what is most suitable for each particular situation.

Breaking down the acronym, we see that he uses **C**onceptual to indicate the fact that the knowledge is expressed in the form of statements with a certain degree of abstraction and generalization typical to science; **R**eferential traces the territorial limits of the object of study; **O**perative for its part attempts not to limit itself only to the traditional epistemological criteria of the "truth" of our efforts, but rather also implies the production of changes—hence the idea of praxis; and finally, **S**chema refers to a joined set of knowledge.

Underlying Assumptions

Principles

After Pichon Rivière and the most significant of those who continued in his wake, the thinking of man, inseparable from his social, cultural, and historic context, took root in the most innovative philosophy and ideology of its times (K. Marx and J. P. Sartre). Without straying too far from his fundamental principles, I have to admit that in my own version I attempt to sidestep the philosophy and the ideology in order to base myself on grounds that are more centered on biology and anthropology. In other words, this current of psychoanalytic thought rejects the classical notion of isolated man who becomes part of society gradually, driven by the desexualized libido (Freud, 1921), upholding instead the social essence of man and, therefore, discarding the concept of a primary narcissism. It could be that for many of the followers of this current, these assumptions were implicit but, in fact, at least for Enrique Pichon Rivière, they were explicit, and indeed very assertive for José Bleger (1958). Yet another main assumption was based on broad pluralism and an unbiased multidisciplinary attitude.

Specific Theoretical Assumptions

Following the dominant influence of the Kleinian English school, the hypotheses were kept concerning early psychic development: the positions on the topic of partial and then total object relations, and persecutory, depressive, and confusional anxieties. As I have mentioned above, Bleger suggested a position of indifferentiation previous to the Kleinian paranoid-schizoid position.

Psychic Structure

With respect to the nature of the psychic structure, these authors implicitly follow the classical Freudian and Kleinian lines, but with more emphasis on the terms of the "unconscious phantasy" of Susan Isaacs (1950). Enrique Pichon Rivière alone suggests the concept of the internal group, even if he doesn't develop it conceptually. It is for that reason that I took on its theoretical development, as can be seen in my works, especially Arbiser, 2001 and 2013.

Energy

Concerning the nature of the sources and nature of energy, this current in general steered away from classical instinct theory. In other words, they tended more towards phantasy (dramatic: scenes with arguments) than to theorization in vectorial language.

Relationship

I have already stated that object relations are considered immediate, disregarding primary narcissism, however, this does not prevent them from having to transit an evolutionary and regressive path.

Development Stages

The assumptions on the classical evolutionary development of Abraham-Freud coexist with the Kleinian position theory while questioning the linear path inherited from the neurological model of the time. It should better be understood in a way that is more simultaneous, structuralist, or dialectical.

Body

I have already mentioned this topic with the concept of the somatic impact in overadapted patients (David Liberman).

Anxieties/Instinct Defenses

Pichon Rivière limits the dynamic of life and that which appears in treatments to two basic anxieties: the fear of the new and the fear of loss. Even if these can overlap with Kleinian persecutory and depressive anxieties, this author places most emphasis on the general dynamic of man—which is "change"—and defines the development of human life and even that of humanity in a struggle between the "tendency to change" and what he calls the "resistance to change."

Etiological Assumptions

An answer is alluded to in the first pages of the present text in the quotation by David Liberman. From my point of view, the topic of etiology in psychoanalysis could be expressed thus: the varied contexts present in the lives of the patients jeopardize the strengths and plasticity of the dispositional repertoire of the patient to deal with the contingencies of life. In summary, much more relevance is given to the current context while the psychological resources (dispositional series) to confront this are tested. The psychoanalytical treatment should deal with and give an opportunity to a new, corrected, and augmented edition of this dispositional series which is updated in the transference-countertransference.

Implications for Technique

The transference and the countertransference are subsumed and mutually interdependent in the idea of psychoanalytic dialogue at the level of greatest inclusion, the same as the concept of field as mentioned in the section dedicated to Willy and Madeleine Baranger. Without dismissing the theme of pathology because of a deficiency and its differentiation from the pathology of the conflicts of life, I would add in contemporary psychopathology the inconsistency—due to a loss of density and solidity—in the identificatory systems. It would appear that, in the cultural climate of the velocity and volatility of the stimuli and the prevalence of image above thought, liquid modernity (Bauman, 2000/2002) takes precedence in personality.

Finally, it is appropriate to state that the psychoanalytic perspective which I put forward in this work constitutes neither a compact nor monolithic set of analysts. Each author develops their own version derived from their own conceptual interests in accordance with their multiple and changing formative experiences and the particular vicissitudes of the life and sciences of each. However, it could be of interest to differentiate this perspective from another which is currently widespread in Argentina and which also addresses the collective. Considering the purposes of this text, I would only conclude: Berenstein and Puget (1997) developed a considerable theoretical and technical body of work to address couple and family frames using an instrumental and conceptual psychoanalytic approach—I personally would qualify these developments as link psychoanalysis. On the other hand, the thinkers who were inspired by the work of Pichon Rivière point to what I would term a link perspective of psychoanalysis. Furthermore, it would be inconceivable for Puget and Berenstein's followers to understand the configuration of the psyche in terms of links as they insist on defining the link exclusively in its concrete manifestation of factual reality. Moreover, they strive to differentiate the intrasubjective object relation from the intersubjective link.

23. Argentine Psychoanalysis	
Main, general underlying assumptions	1 Man is inseparable from his social, cultural, and historic context. 2 Unrestricted and multidisciplinary pluralism.
Specific theoretical assumptions	
psychic structure	The structure adopts a configuration in terms of object links. Pichon Rivière and Arbiser develop the concept of the "internal group."
energy	Pichon Rivière and Bleger discuss and reject the classical instinctive theory. Primary narcissism is rejected.
relationships	In terms of "links" where the subject and the object are mutually conditioned and terms such as "roles" and "belonging" from Social Psychology are used.
developmental stages	Freud's and Abraham's classic contributions are used for the later development stages and those of Melanie Klein for early development.
body	For Bleger and Pichon Rivière, the body constitutes an area of expression of behavior and Liberman suggests a theory of psychosomatic pathology.
anxieties/instincts and defenses	For his part, Pichon Rivière focuses on the dialectic concept of "change," redefining anxieties as "resistance to change," fear of the loss of the known and fear of the unknown.
Assumptions concerning etiology	The imperfections of the environment in which we live and the resources provided during upbringing (complementary series) are sufficient in explaining human shortcomings.
Implications for technique	Attention is paid to the coherence and support of the frame even if this can be flexible and adapted to the times.
Subsequent developments of the core concept	The concept of man as inseparable from his contexts and that of the internal group allows for approaches through individual and group therapies, the latter having therapeutic or pedagogical objectives.

Note

1 A longer consideration of the topic can be found in English in the American Psychoanalytic Association (Arbiser, 2003). In this paper, I limit myself to what I have termed "the psychosocial perspective of psychoanalysis."

References

Abraham, K. (Ed.). (1924). Un breve estudio de la evolución de la libido, considerada a la luz de los trastornos mentales. [A brief study of the evolution of libido, considered in the light of mental disorders]. In *Psicoanálisis Clínico*. Hormé.
Arbiser, S. (2001). El grupo interno. [The internal group]. *Revista de la Sociedad Argentina de Psicoanálisis*, (4), 97–114.
Arbiser, S. (2003). A brief history of psychoanalysis in Argentina. *Journal of the American Psychoanalytic Association*, 51S(Supplement), 323–335.
Arbiser, S. (2013). *El grupo interno: Psiquis y cultura*. [The internal group: Psyche and culture]. Ediciones Biebel.
Arbiser, S. (2014). David Liberman's legacy. *International Journal of Psychoanalysis*, *95*(4), 719–738.
Baranger, W., & Baranger, M. (1969). *Problemas del campo psicoanalítico*. [Problems in the psychoanalytic field]. Kargieman.
Bateson, G., & Ruesh, J. (1984). *Comunicación: La matriz social de la psiquiatría*. [Communication: The social matrix of psychiatry]. Paidós. (Original work published 1951).
Bauman, Z. (2002). *Modernidad liquida*. [Liquid modernity]. Fondo de Cultura Económica de Argentina. (Original work published 2000).
Berenstein, I., & Puget, J. (1997). *Lo vincular: Clínica y técnica psicoanalítica*. [Link it: Clinical and psychoanalytic technique]. Paidós.
Bleger, J. (1958). *Psicoanálisis y dialéctica materialista*. [Psychoanalysis and materialistic dialectics]. Paidós.
Bleger, J. (1967). *Simbiosis y ambigüedad: Estudio psicoanalítico*. [Symbiosis and ambiguity: Psychoanalytic study]. Paidós.
Freud, S. (1905). Tres ensayos sobre una teoría sexual. [Three essays on a sexual theory]. In J. L. Etcheverry (Trans.), *Obras Completas*, (Vol. 7). Amorrortu.
Freud, S. (1921). Psicología de las masas y análisis del yo. [Psychology of the masses and analysis of the self]. In J. L. Etcheverry (Trans.), *Obras Completas*, (Vol. 18). Amorrortu.
Freud, S. (1925). La Negación. [The negation]. In J. L. Etcheverry (Trans.), *Obras Completas*, (Vol. 19). Amorrortu.
Freud, S. (1932/1933). Nuevas conferencias de introducción al psicoanálisis. [New introductory lectures on psychoanalysis]. In J. L. Etcheverry (Trans.), *Obras Completas* (Vol. 22). Amorrortu.
Isaacs, S. (1950). Naturaleza y función de la fantasía. [Nature and function of fantasy]. *Revista de Pscicoanálisis*, *7*(4), 555–609.
Jakobson, R. (1960). *Lingüistique et poétique: Essais de lingüistique general*. [Linguistic and poetic: General linguistic tests]. Minuit.
Lewin, K. (1958). *Teoría del campo y experimentación en psicología social*. [Field theory and experimentation in social psychology]. Notebook 10. Universidad de Buenos Aires.
Liberman, D. (1962). *La comunicación en terapéutica psicoanalítica*. [Communication in psychoanalytic therapy]. Eudeba.
Liberman, D. (1970). *Lingüística, interacción comunicativa y proceso psicoanalítico*. [Linguistics, communicative interaction and psychoanalytic process]. Nueva Visión.

Liberman, D. (1976). *Comunicación y psicoanálisis.* [Communication and psychoanalysis]. Alex Editor.
Liberman, D. (1982). *Del cuerpo al símbolo.* [From the body to the symbol]. Kargieman Editores.
Mead, G. (1972). *Espíritu, persona y sociedad.* (1927–1930). [Spirit, person and society]. Paidós.
Morris, C. (1946). *Signs, language and behavior*. Prentice Hall.
Pichon Rivière, E. (1971). *Del psicoanálisis a la psicología social.* [From psychoanalysis to social psychology]. Editorial Galerna.
Ruesch, J. (1957). *Disturbed communication.* W. W. Norton.

Chapter 24

Psychoanalyses in Asia

Koichi Togashi

My assignment in this chapter is to describe psychoanalysis in Asia, but this is not so easy to accomplish, because Asia is comprised of many nations or regions, all with unique histories, languages, and political backgrounds. The history of psychoanalysis in Asia is diverse, and raises the question of what, precisely, we mean when we speak of "Asia."

If we limit our focus to the East and South Asian countries in which psychoanalysis has become relatively more popular, we find that one of the most salient differences in the history of psychoanalysis in these nations is the development of training and practice. In this regard, India and Japan have particularly long histories. The Indian Psychoanalytic Society was founded in 1922, by Girindrasekhar Bose (Dhar, 2018), with the assistance of Ernest Jones. The Japanese psychiatrist Kiyoyasu Marui visited Freud in 1933 and obtained a certification in psychoanalysis. Returning to Japan, Marui founded the precursor of the Japan Psychoanalytic Society in 1934.

In Taiwan, China, and Korea, it was not until the end of the Second World War that internationally standardized societies were established to provide psychoanalytic training. These countries needed time to heal the wounds of the war—in some cases, to deal with subsequent civil wars—while negotiating internal political conflicts, and economic turmoil. But in each of these nations, academic psychoanalysis had been imported before the Second World War, and people had learned of psychoanalysis through books and journals (Huang & Kirsner, 2020; Jeong & Sachs, 2009).

Despite significant differences between Asian nations, only one chapter in this ambitious and groundbreaking book project *Underlying Assumptions in Psychoanalysis* is devoted to Asian psychoanalyses. Elsewhere, a chapter is devoted to each psychoanalytic school in the English-speaking world, and each non-English speaking Western country. With no disrespect to the superb editing of Doctor Bernd Huppertz, I ask, why?

First, it may be because the countries of eastern and southern Asia are generally seen as a loosely defined region that shares similar thoughts and values. Of course, the same is true of schools in the English world and non-English speaking Western countries, each of which contains multiple

DOI: 10.4324/9781003027768-25

thoughts and theories but is addressed as a single entity, so it's not surprising that Asian psychoanalyses are also grouped into one discussion.

But it may also be the case that Asian psychoanalyses are lumped together because the psychoanalytic world assumes that its prevailing thoughts and practices live in the West, not in Asia, and Asian psychoanalyses are marginalized as "non-Western psychoanalysis." They are nothing less than a "foreign psychoanalysis" in the psychoanalytic community. Notwithstanding the global nature of this project, it exposes a Euro-centricity in the culture of psychoanalysis that all of us in the field are embedded in, not only Western analysts but also Eastern.

In this chapter, I will discuss some of the problems of psychoanalytic culture which are manifested in this tendency to see Asian psychoanalyses as a unitary group. First, however, I will briefly review the histories of psychoanalyses in several East and South Asian nations, and summarize several themes frequently discussed by Asian psychoanalysts. I would like to note that I was trained in the US, but was born and raised in Japan, where I currently practice psychoanalysis and psychoanalytic psychotherapy. Thus, my descriptions in this chapter are necessarily the product of my own cultural, social, and historical context.

Historical Reviews in Asian Psychoanalyses

Psychoanalysis in China

The history of psychoanalysis in China has been strongly influenced by political situations before and after the Second World War. It was in the 1910s that Freud's ideas were imported to China (Li, 2021, personal communication), and "Freudian theories were familiar to many Chinese intellectuals and, in reductive forms, to a surprisingly broad sector of the Chinese population" (Zhang, 1992, p. 34) until the Japanese invasion changed the environment in 1930. Even so, from 1935 through 1939, Bringham Dai, a psychiatrist trained in psychoanalysis in New York and Chicago, taught classes at Peking Medical College (Varvin & Gerlach, 2011). After the Second World War, psychoanalytic ideas and practices gradually became known to Chinese intellectuals, but this development was abruptly ended by the Chinese revolution.

In the 1980s, an era of reform, psychoanalysis in China entered into a new age. According to Huang and Kirsner (2020), Wen-Shing Tseng, a psychiatrist, who was trained in Taiwan and taught mental health in the US, came to the mainland and introduced a Western style of psychotherapy, and Chinese psychiatrist Zhong Youbin began practicing his original form of psychotherapy using the psychoanalytic framework.

With rapid economic growth in 2000s, China entered the age of the "Psycho-Boom," during which many psychoanalytic institutes or training groups were established in major cities. The psychoanalytic section of the

Sino-German Program currently educates analysts in Shanghai and a training program of the Sino-Norwegian Course was founded in Beijing in 2006. The China American Psychoanalytic Alliance, which began its activity in 2008, was established in Beijing and offers a nationwide program using digital technology. Recent developments include a training program for couples therapy, begun by David & Jill Scharff; an academy of Winnicottian psychoanalysis, founded in Beijing; and a training institute of psychoanalytic psychotherapy, taught in Mandarin and established in Chengdu. In light of this great success, the International Psychoanalytic Association (IPA) organized a China committee in 2008, and hosted the 2010 IPA conference in Beijing, its first international conference in Asia.

Despite these developments, Huang and Kirsner (2020) maintain that psychoanalysis and psychoanalytic psychotherapy in China are still on an upward learning curve. Original academic writings, for them, suggest that Chinese psychoanalysis is still at the stage of assimilating itself in Western thinking, rather than developing its own original ideas.

Cai (2009) explores a famous Chinese allegory, a story of Liang Shanbo and Zhu Yingtai, to illustrate Chinese patients' conflict between the pressure to conform to the family tradition and a wish to fulfill an individual sexual desire. She states that this story symbolically describes a conflict between Confucian tradition and modern values. Gu (2009) also extracts a variation of Oedipus conflicts which are often seen in psychoanalytic practice in China. Yang (2013) draws attention to the ideas of Wei Pan, a Chinese researcher who sees the family as the basic unit of society in Chinese culture. Yang maintains that one of the most important themes in psychoanalytic practice in China is patients' anguish over sacrificing their individual autonomy in order to fulfill their obligation to remain a "dependent being." Zhong (2013) addresses conflicts between psychoanalytic practice and Chinese culture on three levels: philosophical, social, and psychological. The philosophical conflict has to do with a traditional value, *He-Yi* (oneness), which places a high priority on social and familial harmony and peace and regards individual needs and autonomy as secondary. The social conflict is organized between the traditional "authoritarian system," based on Confucianism, and modern Chinese culture; the psychological conflict shows an individual's "agreeable attitude on the surface" and "disagreeable thoughts inside" about the authoritarian system.

Psychoanalysis in South Korea

According to Jeong and Sachs (2009), it was in the late 1960s that psychoanalysis and psychoanalytic psychotherapy in South Korea began taking shape. It was through the 1970s that psychodynamic psychotherapy training programs became more widely known. The development of psychoanalysis in South Korea runs alongside the economic growth known as the *Miracle on the Han River*. Since the 1980s, many psychoanalysts have been invited to

South Korea from abroad—including the United States, United Kingdom, and Japan—and South Korean clinicians gained significant insights into psychoanalysis through discussions with international clinicians. The Seoul Psychoanalytic Study Group was established by Doo-Young Cho in 1980 and began providing psychoanalytic study and training (Jeong & Sachs, 2009). The Group changed its name to the Korean Psychoanalytic Society in 1989, and published the first psychoanalytic journal in Korea, to which many international and domestic psychoanalysts have contributed. The society was approved as an affiliate of the IPA in 2008.

Korean and Korean-origin American psychoanalysts often discuss cultural features of Korean families and human relationships, and a unique expression of aggression. Lee (2013), for example, argues that in Korean culture, which values the family system over individual autonomy, the social community is often treated as a family, and an individual is expected to assume a role in the community. An individual who is seen as a part of a family or intimate group system is often expected to recognize and fulfill the needs of other people before they are verbally requested. Lee believes that this value affects a self-other boundary in many Korean people.

Choi-Kain (2009) and Lee (2013) both suggest that one of the important themes for Korean patients is aggression. Choi-Kain (2009) links this aggression with *haan*, an indigenous cultural value that can be described in "the Korean phrase, 'I will show you who will eventually win'" (Kim et al., 2006, p. 152). According to Choi-Kain (2009), *haan* should be understood with reference to Korea's historical context, which was one of repeated invasions and occupation over centuries by many powerful countries such as China, Russia, and Japan. As a positive value, *haan* is a feeling associated with an individual bearing up under adversity and being motivated toward his or her goal. The negative pole of the same value is often expressed in self-destructive emotional outbursts.

Haan should not be seen as simply anger or envy. Kim (2015) states that the term originally means one or coherence—oneness, as well as wholeness. She states that it is a sophisticated cultural value in which an individual strives to find essential rightness, superlativeness, and peace. She also says that it is an expression of emotional crisis or sorrow when a person witnesses the destruction of oneness or wholeness.

Psychoanalysis in Taiwan

As in China and Korea, the history of psychoanalysis in Taiwan began with the importation and study of psychoanalytic literature. According to Liu (2011), many psychoanalytic writings were translated into Mandarin from the late 1960s through the 1980s.

In the 1990s, systemized psychoanalytic trainings and practices were introduced in Taiwan, and clinicians were able to attend training programs and seminars in various psychoanalytical schools of thought. It was in 2001 that the Taiwan Association of Psychotherapy and Taiwan Institute of Psychotherapy were founded, followed in 2004 by an organization dedicated specifically to psychoanalysis, The Taiwan Center for the Development of Psychoanalysis (TCDP). TCDP became an affiliate of the IPA in 2006. It has since changed its name to the Taiwan Psychoanalytic Association, and currently is active in encouraging psychoanalytic training and education. In 2010, the Taiwan Study Group was formed, and at the IPA Congress in Boston in 2015, five members were qualified as IPA psychoanalysts (Lin, 2021, personal communication).

The "Formosa Model" (Liu, 2011) of psychoanalytic training is worthy of special mention. Formosa is the symbolic appellative of Taiwan, derived from the Portuguese, "*Ilha Formosa*" (beautiful island). Liu (2011) proudly uses this word to symbolize the history and culture of Taiwan, which includes diverse languages, values, races, ethnicities, cultures, and thoughts. Training in the Formosa Model asks analysts to be open to various schools of thought, values, and techniques. Liu calls this approach "an emerging tradition," which is, interestingly, also the subtitle of Mitchell and Aron's "Relational Psychoanalysis: The Emergence of a Tradition" (Mitchell & Aron, 1999). The two schools of thought, Taiwanese and American relational, share a basic philosophy, in which democratic dialogues create a new culture.

Like other Asian analysts, most Taiwanese researchers tend to discuss Asian or Chinese culture through comparison to Western culture. For example, Huang and Yang (2013) discuss a particular form of shame among Taiwanese people that is different from a Western sense of shame. They posit that shame should not be considered as a single emotional experience, but seen as having different faces, related to different cultural values, and often mixed with guilt.

Psychoanalysis in Japan

The history of psychoanalysis in Japan begins with the first Japanese-certified psychoanalyst, Yaekichi Yabe. He went to Europe and met Freud personally in 1930 and returned to establish the Japanese branch of the International Psychoanalytic Association in Tokyo. Around the same time, Kiyoyasu Marui founded the Sendai Branch of the IPA, which ultimately came to be the Japan Psychoanalytic Society. Heisaku Kosawa, who studied psychiatry in Marui's office, went to Vienna in 1932; underwent analysis with Sterba and was supervised by Federn (Nishi, 2019).

Kosawa proposed his original idea of the *Ajase Complex*, a unique form of guilt embedded in Japanese culture. Ajase Complex is a theory of an Eastern sense of guilt and human development, based on Kosawa's exploration of the allegory of Ajatashatru in ancient India. According to Okonogi (2009), it assumes three developmental stages in the relationship between a mother who is afraid of a baby's birth and a baby who holds a grudge. This begins with the baby united with an ideal mother, develops through abandonment from the mother, then finally reaches a mother and child connectedness beyond grudge.

The most famous psychoanalytic theory provided by a Japanese analyst is "*Amae* Theory" advocated by Takeo Doi (1962, 1973, 1989). *Amae* is the term the Japanese use to refer to a person's presumption of a right to another's favors. Doi describes it as "an emotion that takes the other person's love for granted" (1973, p. 168). Doi traced the genesis of this idea to his own analysis with an American analyst. Doi felt that he was not able to experience the analyst's sensitivity and receptivity of Doi's *amae* feelings. He states that "passive object love or primary love as defined by Michael Balint can be equated with *amae* in its pure form and as such his concept becomes something quite tangible" (Doi, 1989, p. 350).

Passive love is not a person's longing for an object, but a longing for being loved. As Doi states,

> If the prototype of *amae* is the infant's desire to be close to its mother, who, it has come vaguely to realize, is a separate existence from itself, then one may perhaps describe *amae* as, ultimately, an attempt psychologically to deny the fact of separation from the mother.
>
> (Doi, 1973, p. 75)

A person finally recognizes that the longing is not always fulfilled. In a healthy form, a person recognizes how much they have *amae*-ed others and failed to experience their being. In this sense, *amae* would often function to sublate a tension between mother-child union and separation.

The term *amae* is deeply connected to the Japanese language and culture. But the feeling is experienced in Western cultures as well. Doi (1962) states that *amae* is a theory that is broadly applicable to any patient, regardless of their cultural background. In this sense, *amae* is an original psychoanalytic theory with original models of ego, development, object relation, and self-experience. Like Bose's *Opposite Wish* model discussed in the next section, it is not a psychoanalytic interpretation of a specific culture or people, but a broadly applicable theory for our psychoanalytic practice, regardless of cultural background.

Psychoanalysis in India

Indian psychoanalysis has two histories. One history is domestic, the psychoanalysis built by Girindrasekhar Bose and others who established the Indian Psychoanalytic Society (Dhar, 2018; Mukherjee, 2017). The other history of Indian psychoanalysis is international, the work of Indian-origin psychoanalysts who were trained and achieved fame in the Western psychoanalytic world, such as Masud Khan, and more recently, Akhtar and Kakar.

Bose developed an original psychoanalytic concept that he called "Opposite Wish," and sent his book, *Concept of Repression* (1922), to Freud, beginning a correspondence between them about this theory (Jones, 1922). The concept is interesting from a modern psychoanalytic perspective. It assumes two ego states and proposes an Oedipus conflict that is different from Freud's idea. Bose maintains that the Oedipus complex is not always organized around a wish to be a man with a penis and a fear of castration; rather, as he states in a letter to Freud, it is organized "between the desire to be a male and its opposite, the desire to be a female" (Bose, 1929; as cited in Sinha, 1966, p. 430). Sinha (1966) expounds on the theory as follows.

> He [Bose] showed that when A wishes to strike B, he has also the wish to be struck by B, but such a wish is usually repressed. When A wishes to strike B it may be that A feels hurt by B in some way and then retaliates. Anyway A has the experience of being hurt and by that identification feels that B will suffer pain which A desires to inflict on B; or, in other words, A as an active person hits B and by his partial ego-identification with B feels hurt too.
>
> (Sinha, 1966, p. 432)

The uniqueness of Bose's work lies in his intention to propose an original psychoanalytic theory, with original models of psychic structure, development, and therapeutic approach, that looked beyond an analysis of Indian culture. He theorized aspects of the general human experience that Freud had overlooked.

Common Themes Discussed by Asian Psychoanalysts

Themes that appear across the spectrum of Asian analyses include (1) self-experience, (2) object and interpersonal relationships, (3) psychological structure, and (4) transference and countertransference. These themes are usually examined through a discussion of traditions or customs in each region, or through the exploration of unique linguistic expressions in local communities. An example of the former is the conflict between the individual's needs and traditionally required familial roles in China, as described by Yang (2013). Examples of the latter are, *haan*, the Korean expression Choi-Kain (2009) discusses, and '*chi*' a culturally unique form of shame that Huang and Yang (2013) illustrate. In most cases, these discussions are based on the theorists' recognition of their own cultural, historical, and linguistic backgrounds in relation to Western culture.

The Self Experience

If, for a moment, we leave aside the issues of diversity among Asian nations, the self-experience that Asian analysts address most frequently can be called "self-in-relationship," which is a sense of self-organized around a psychological union with significant others, families, or communities. It is often contrasted to the Western individual self, which is described as ideally *disconnected* from others, family, or community. The self-in-relationship is often manifested in a custom, common to many regions in Asia, of, for example, calling a member of a community by a name that signifies a family role, such as "uncle," "aunt," "mother," or "father." Roland (1996) calls it the "we-self" as opposed to the Western "I-Self." Nevertheless, I believe the distinction between we-self and I-self is an artificial one.

Some relational theories (Kohut, 1977; Mitchell, 1997; Stolorow & Atwood, 1994; Togashi, 2020) criticize self-theories in traditional psychoanalysis as being embedded in Western values and propose some models of self-in-relationship. Sobel (2000), an anthropologist, notes that the so-called "we-self" was manifested in Western societies in the Middle Ages. From this historical perspective, we can say that there is no substantial difference between self-experience in Asian and Western people. Rather, I would suggest that the differences between Western and Asian self-experience theories are reflecting aspects of the theorists' own values or beliefs.

The Object and Interpersonal Relationship

The object and interpersonal relationship frequently discussed by Asian analysts can be described as the duty to sacrifice oneself for others—family or community—and accompanying guilt, shame, or rage when one fails to fulfill that duty. Zhong (2013) illustrates how Chinese people do not divulge family scandals to outsiders, in order to uphold the traditional value of *He-Yi* (oneness), and how they may be overwhelmed by a deep sense of guilt if anything they do reflects poorly on the family. Kitayama (1998) explores a Japanese allegory, "A Crane's Repayment of Her Debt" and illustrates the object relationship manifested in a Japanese expression, *On*, a unique emotion experienced when people are given something by another. *On* is often translated as obligation, debt, or guilt, and people often experience shame and guilt when they fail to fulfill a duty of requital or repayment.

While these theories mainly focus on the cultural pressure for a person to recognize others' expectations, there are other theories that focus on a person's yearning for his or her expectations to be recognized and fulfilled by others. In Doi's (1962, 1973, 1989) *amae* theory, children long to be loved and accepted by their caregivers in a special way. Choi-Kain's (2009) idea of *haan* is also a person's need for others to keep the oneness in an interpersonal relationship. In my own attempt to explore the twinship experience (Togashi, 2009), I illustrate how a Japanese patient often longs for his therapist to find herself in him, before he can find himself in her. Without confirmation of the therapist's willingness, the patient cannot allow himself to experience his therapist as essentially akin to him.

As with the self-experience, we should not consider that these theories reveal the substance of object and interpersonal relationships that are exclusive to Asian people. Rather, they illustrate a form of human relationship which is often found in Western culture as well but goes unrecognized. Indeed, Doi's *amae* is broadly accepted in the psychoanalytic community.

Psychological Structure

Asian analysts are frequently critical of a theoretical dichotomy between conscious and unconscious. The Freudian topographical model defines the unconscious as a psychological space in which previously experienced feelings or memories are repressed. The repressed materials cannot be approved as part of an individual self, in light of the person's cultural values and ego ideals. In this model, "approved" experience and "not approved" are constructed as an antithesis: love and hate, good and bad. Giving love full play means hate would be killed; giving good full play, bad would be repressed.

Asian analysts, instead, are more accepting of dissociated or multiple states of mind. For example, Bose (1922) argues the existence of two ego modes that manifest themselves as a "wish to love and wish to be loved" and a "wish to attack and wish to be attacked." Love and hate, however, are seen as related forms that cannot be considered to constitute an antithesis. As Sinha (1966) explains, in this model, giving the "wish to love or strike" full play means that what is repressed is a "wish to *be* loved or struck." Kitayama (2013) also illustrates two modes of 'I,' manifested as a social I and a private I, and best described in the Japanese phrase "*Omote* and *Ura* (face and tail)." They are not considered to be an antithesis; giving either one full play does not, and cannot, repress the other.

Again, the psychological structures that Asian analysts propose should not be considered to be unique to Asian people, and the discussion of multiple modes of psychological structure are not limited to Asian psychoanalysis in Asia. Western theorists have also illustrated multiple states of self or psychological structure (Bromberg, 1993; Mitchell, 1997; Stern, 2002).

Transference and Countertransference

Asian analysts often suggest that, in the transference, Asian patients expect them to behave or guide them more actively, beyond the traditional analytic attitude. Zhong (2013) states that Chinese patients often seek for their therapists to be directive, and a non-directive therapeutic approach often leads to resistance. A Japanese psychiatrist, Taketomo (1989), proposes the idea of "teacher transference," in which patients need their therapists to guide them and to take responsibility for their lives. Needless to say, this type of transference is not limited to Asian patients. Some Western analysts such as Kohut (1977) and Bacal (1998) emphasize the importance of analysts not disrupting the development of optimal idealization in the transference.

In terms of countertransference, some important suggestions are given by Asian analysts. Cai (2009) maintains that clinicians trained in psychoanalysis tend to value a Western form of autonomy, and can be ambivalent about traditional Chinese values and thoughts. Zhong (2013) posits that analysts are deeply embedded in psychoanalytic theory and values through their training, and thus cannot be free from Western values and beliefs.

Psychoanalysis itself is a culture, and analysts are not only embedded in their indigenous culture but also in the psychoanalytic one (Togashi, 2020). We need to recognize that the type of countertransference Zhong and Cai warn of may make our patients more conflicted about the regional, social, and cultural values they live in. As Brandchaft (2007) says, analysts often develop loyalty toward and an identification with psychoanalytic culture through their training. Thus, analysts may see their patients' needs and wishes which do not fit with "psychoanalytic culture" as pathological or "something to be fixed." Even analysts who value and respect indigenous cultures face the same risks, for they can experience their own "open" attitude as a betrayal of psychoanalytic culture, and may attempt to assimilate their patients to it in order to avoid and deny their own sense of guilt or shame.

Some Problems of Psychoanalytic Culture

Our review of the psychoanalytic literature by Asian analysts indicates two trends: first, Asian analysts frequently filter their experience in the light of Western psychoanalysis when developing theory, and second, they are always and already embedded in the psychoanalytic culture. What do these two ideas suggest about Asian or Western analysts? How are they related to the problem of seeing Asian psychoanalyses as a single unified group?

In his book, "*Orientalism*," Edward Said (1978) argues that classifying people and regions by groups necessitates objectifying and abstracting people from a position of superiority. He maintains that the "Orient" referred to by European Orientalists is an imagined area that is intended to imply the Middle East, and "Orientals" are a romanticized imagined people. Neither Orient nor Orientals exist anywhere; the construct is used by Western Orientalists to mean "non-Europe."

As Said (1978) posits, "the Orient is the stage on which the whole East is confined. On this stage will appear figures whose role it is to represent the larger whole from which they emanate" (p. 63). He argues that this "representation" comes from European Orientalists' mixed feelings about the Middle East—envy as well as a feeling of superiority—and that it is consciously and unconsciously used to support the West's political strategies of invasion and colonization. Representing a variety of peoples and cultures with one name serves not only to categorize them but also to define them in contrast to "normal culture" and "superior people." Paradoxically, Orientalists' efforts to define Orientals do not aid them in understanding non-Western people but do serve to define themselves in a position of rightfulness and meliority.

Said's reasoning suggests that we are always on the precipice of "re-presenting" or objectifying Asian psychoanalyses and analysts. We must be aware that any categorization contains the risk of denying the diversity of Asian psychoanalyses in order to uphold the traditions of Western psychoanalysis. We are always deeply embedded in psychoanalytic culture through our psychoanalytic training and develop a loyalty toward it. No analysts or theorists can consider their experiences without referring to the traditional Western psychoanalytic perspective. We must constantly check ourselves to ensure that we are not confined by the culture of psychoanalysis—as well as our local and native cultures—when we see our patients.

We need to ask ourselves how free we are from colonial thoughts in the psychoanalytic culture, in which Western psychoanalysis is valid and superior and Asian is foreign. In a recent book, I discussed the history of Japanese psychoanalysis and how Japanese pioneers such as Yabe or Marui, who visited Freud and were trained in Europe, have been relegated to the role of "foreign student" (Togashi, 2021). I also argued that Japanese analysts themselves tend to value the writings of Western analysts more than those of Asian analysts, with notable exceptions such as Doi's (1962) work, which crosses swords with Western analysis as an equal in the international literature.

Löwith, a philosopher who studied under Heidegger and taught philosophy at Tohoku University in Japan before the Second World War, criticizes the Japanese attitude toward Western thoughts as self-divisive, and states:

> [Japanese] seem like they live in a two-story house; in the first floor they think and feel in a Japanese form, while they store European literature in orderly rows on the second floor. Then, a European teacher wonders where the ladder is to move up and down.
>
> (1974, p. 188, my translation)

What Löwith sees here is a relational and cultural context often faced by Japanese scholars, one that is likely faced by other Asian academics as well. In other words, it is a form of transference-countertransference among the international psychoanalytic community. For Asian analysts, Western analysts are the teachers for all time, authorities who are identified with and who are expected to act as guides. In the West, Asian analysts will always be students. The relationship can be described as "valid and superior psychoanalysis" over "inferior and foreign psychoanalysis." But Asian psychoanalysts have been and continue to produce original and valuable perspectives, and today is a good time to re-evaluate relationships among the international psychoanalytic community.

24. Psychoanalysis in Asia		
1 Regional, social, and cultural differences in specific theoretical assumptions of Asian psychoanalytical schools 2 Common themes in Asian psychanalysis discussed through conceptual, but the artificial distinction between Eastern and Western minds, developments, and cultural peculiarities		
	Eastern	**Western**
1. The Self Experience	self-in-relationship	self isolated
2. The Object and Interpersonal Relation	Sacrificing for other and yearning for one's expectation to be recognized	Organized around self and object distinguished
3. Psychological Structure	multiple modes and states of psychological structures	conscious and unconscious
4. Transference	Seeking for guidance	Seeking for free-expression
5. Cultural program of Countertransference	Idealization with Western psychoanalytic culture	Loyalty toward psychoanalytic culture
6. Problem of psychoanalytic culture	Unfree from colonial thoughts in psychoanalytic culture	

Acknowledgment

I am grateful to dear friends and colleagues, Liling Lin, MSW., Kotagal Shyamsundar, MBA, PsyD., and Mr. Xin Li for their thoughtful comments about this article.

References

Bacal, H. A. (1998). Optimal responsiveness and the specificity of selfobject experience. In H. A. Bacal (Ed.), *Optimal responsiveness: How therapists heal their patients* (pp. 141–170). Jason Aronson.

Bose, G. (1922). *Concept of repression*. Sri Gauranga Press and Kegan Paul, Trench, Troubner.

Brandchaft, B. (2007). Systems of pathological accommodation and change in analysis. *Psychoanalytic Psychology*, *24*(4), 667–687.

Bromberg, P. M. (1993). Shadow and substance: A relational perspective on clinical process. *Psychoanalytic Psychology*, *10*(2), 147–168.

Cai, J. (2009). The butterfly lovers: Psychodynamic reflections on the ancient Chinese love story "Liang-Zhu." In S. Akhter (Ed.), *Freud and Far East: Psychoanalytic perspectives on the people and culture of China, Japan, and Korea* (pp. 105–113). Jason Aronson.

Choi-Kain, L. (2009). Second generation Korean Americans. In S. Akhter (Ed.), *Freud and Far East: Psychoanalytic perspectives on the people and culture of China, Japan, and Korea* (pp. 215–233). Jason Aronson.

Dhar, A. (2018). Girindrasekhar Bose and the history of psychoanalysis in India. *Indian Journal of History of Science*, 53 (4), T198–T204.

Doi, T. (1962). Amae: A key concept for understanding Japanese personality structure. In R. J. Smith & R. K. Beardsley (Eds.), *Japanese culture: Its development and characteristics* (pp. 132–139). Aldine.

Doi, T. (1973). *The anatomy of dependence (Revised paperback ed.)*. Kodansha International.

Doi, T. (1989). The concept of amae and its psychoanalytic implications. *International Review of Psycho-Analysis, 16*, 349–354.

Gu, M. D. (2009). The filial piety complex: Variations on the Oedipus theme in Chinese literature and culture. In S. Akhter (Ed.), *Freud and Far East: Psychoanalytic perspectives on the people and culture of China, Japan, and Korea* (pp. 115–136). Jason Aronson.

Huang H-Y & Kirsner, D. (2020). The history of psychoanalysis in China. *Psychoanalytic Inquiry*, *40*(1), 3–15.

Huang H-Y. & Yang, M-M. (2013). Shame and losing face in Taiwanese culture: A clinical and cultural perspective. In A. Gerlach, M. T. S. Hook, & S. Varvin (Eds.), *Psychoanalysis in Asia: China, India, Japan, South Korea, Taiwan* (pp. 237–246). Routledge.

Jeong, D-U & Sachs, D. (2009). Psychoanalysis in Korea. In S. Akhter (Ed.), *Freud and Far East: Psychoanalytic perspectives on the people and culture of China, Japan, and Korea* (pp. 27–41). Jason Aronson.

Jones, E. (1922). Letter from Ernest Jones to Sigmund Freud, February 13, 1922. *The complete correspondence of Sigmund Freud and Ernest Jones 1908–1939*, 460.

Kim, I. J., Kim, L. I. C., & Kelly, J. G. (2006). Developing cultural competence in working with Korean immigrant families. *Journal of Community Psychology, 34*(2), 149–165.

Kim, K. (2015). *Haan no kuni Kankou* [*Korea as the country of Haan*]. Shodensha.

Kitayama, O. (1998). Transience: Its beauty and danger. *International Journal of Psycho-Analysis, 79*(5), 937–942.

Kitayama, O. (2013). Psychoanalysis in a "shame culture": A drama-based viewpoint. In A. Gerlach, M. T. S. Hook, & S. Varvin (Eds.), *Psychoanalysis in Asia: China, India, Japan, South Korea, Taiwan* (pp. 151–168). Routledge.

Kohut, H. (1977). *The restoration of the self.* International University Press.

Lee, M-S. (2013). Korean culture and psychoanalysis. In A. Gerlach, M. T. S. Hook, & S. Varvin (Eds.), *Psychoanalysis in Asia: China, India, Japan, South Korea, Taiwan* (pp. 197–208). Routledge.

Liu, C-C. (2011). The Formosa model: An emerging tradition of developing psychoanalysis in Taiwan. In P. Loewenberg & N. L. Thompson (Eds.), *100 years of the IPA: The centenary history of the International Psychoanalytic Association 1910–2010. Evolution and change* (pp. 412–418). Routledge.

Löwith, K. (1974). *European Nihilism* [in Japanese]. Chikuma Shobo.

Mitchell, S. A. (1997). Psychoanalysis and the degradation of romance. *Psychoanalytic Dialogues*, *7*(1), 23–41.

Mitchell, S. & Aron, L. (1999). *Relational psychoanalysis: The emergence of a tradition*. The Analytic Press.
Mukherjee, D. G. (2017). Girindrasekhar Bose. In B. Bhaushan (Ed.), *Eminent Indian psychologists: 100 years of psychology in India* (pp. 30–38). Sage Publications.
Nishi, M. (2019). *Ikanishite Nihon no Seishinbunseki wa Hajimattaka* [*How psychoanalysis in Japan began*?]. Misuzu Shobo.
Okonogi, K. (2009). Psychoanalysis in Japan. In S. Akhter (Ed.), *Freud and Far East: Psychoanalytic perspectives on the people and culture of China, Japan, and Korea* (pp. 9–25). Jason Aronson.
Roland, A. (1996). *Cultural pluralism and psychoanalysis: An Asian and North American experience*. Routledge.
Said, E. W. (1978). *Orientalism*. Pantheon.
Sinha, T. C. (1966). Development of psycho-analysis in India. *International Journal of Psycho-Analysis*, *47*, 427–439.
Sobel, M. (2000). *Teach me dreams: The search for self in the Revolutionary Era*. Princeton University Press.
Stern, S. (2002). The self as a relational structure: A dialogue with multiple-self theory. *Psychoanalytic Dialogues*, *12*(5), 693–714.
Stolorow, R. D. & Atwood, G. E. (1994). The myth of the isolated mind. *Progress in Self Psychology*, *10*, 233–250.
Taketomo, Y. (1989). An American-Japanese transcultural psychoanalysis and the issue of teacher transference. *Journal of the American Academy of Psychoanalysis*, *17*, 427–450.
Togashi, K. (2009). A new dimension of twinship selfobject experience and transference. *International Journal of Psychoanalytic Self Psychology*, *4*(1), 21–39.
Togashi, K. (2020). *The psychoanalytic zero: A decolonizing study of therapeutic dialogues*. Routledge.
Togashi, K. (2021). *Tojisha tositeno Chiryosha: Sabetsu to Shihai eno Osore to Yokubo* [*The therapist as a player-witness: Fears and lusts for discrimination and domination*]. Iwasaki Gakujyutsu shuppan.
Varvin, S. & Gerlach, A. (2011). The development of psychodynamic psychotherapy and psychoanalysis in China. *International Journal of Applied Psychoanalytic Studies*, *8*(3), 261–267.
Yang, Y. (2013). Psychoanalytic psychotherapy in the Chinese context: Development and challenges. In A. Gerlach, M. T. S. Hook, & S. Varvin (Eds.), *Psychoanalysis in Asia: China, India, Japan, South Korea, Taiwan* (pp. 73–86). Routledge.
Zhang, J. (1992). *Psychoanalysis in China: Literary transformations, 1919–1949*. East Asia Program, Cornell University.
Zhong, J. (2013). Working with Chinese patients: Are there conflicts between Chinese culture and psychoanalysis? In A. Gerlach, M. T. S. Hook, & S. Varvin (Eds.), *Psychoanalysis in Asia: China, India, Japan, South Korea, Taiwan* (pp. 125–135). Routledge.

Chapter 25

Jung and the Jungians: The Jungian Perspective

Isabelle Meier

Main, General Underlying Assumptions of the Perspective of Jungian School

Jung's theory of the psyche is (like Freud's) based on the assumption that our conscious experience represents only a relatively small part of our total psychic world. Much of our affects, experiences, body feelings, and behavior exist outside our awareness, in areas of the psyche that are unconscious, only to become experienced through symbols (e.g., in dreams).

By psyche, Jung understood the totality of all psychic processes, conscious as well as unconscious (Jung, 1921/1967). Jung distinguished between a personal unconscious and a collective unconscious. Whereas the contents of the personal unconscious are acquired during the individual's life and include personal memories, the contents of the collective unconscious are invariable and present from the beginning of time in every culture (Jung, 1912/1967, 1954/1970). They are visible as symbolic images, and stories in all cultures, in art, myths, fairy tales, religion, and philosophy. The cultural themes and symbolic forms comprise the archetypes (prototype of image, pattern, etc.) of the collective unconscious.

Consciousness and the unconscious are in a compensatory, dynamic relationship to each other, i.e., the ego or persona (parts of the consciousness) are opposite of the self or the anima (archetypes in the unconscious). The goal of life is to transcend the opposites within one's psyche and to develop a personality in which the conscious and unconscious are balanced. Jung's conception of the psyche is grounded in opposites (Jung, 1948/1970).

Jung assumed an autonomous, dynamic potential in us acting without our consciousness, tending towards a wholeness of the personality (Jung, 1912/1967). Jung assumed furthermore a self-regulation drive as a result of the evolution process in the psyche that leads to the compensatory relationship between conscious and unconscious (Jung, 1935/1967).

The early Jung assumed that archetypes are genetically imprinted and transmitted from one generation to the next via biological pathways.

DOI: 10.4324/9781003027768-26

Specific Theoretical Assumptions

Assumptions about the Nature of Psychic Structure

The human psyche can metaphorically be seen as being built up in layers; with the ego at the top, embedded in the consciousness, followed by the personal unconscious, the collective unconscious and at the bottom, the never-conscious part of the unconscious.

According to Jung, the ego is the organizer of our thoughts, feelings, and not repressed memories. It is responsible for maintaining personality, its continuity, and identity. The personal unconscious contains repressed memories, and subliminally perceived emotions and thoughts, but contrary to Freud, also not yet developed human potential and possibilities. Jung outlined moreover the theory of the collective unconscious comprising latent archetypes and a creative quality containing developmental impulses. These are innate universal predispositions stemming from our evolutionary past (Jung, 1954/1970).

Archetypes are at the center of Jung's interest. He assumed there was an ordering power in them. The archetypes themselves are deeply unconscious and unknowable. They are only capable of being known in images, affects, symbols, stories, or events (as birth, marriage, death, separation, etc.).

One of the most important archetypes would be the self that reaches into the transcendental area. It is characterized as the whole personality, conscious and unconscious, as well as the process of becoming the whole personality. It urges the individual toward self-development. The relationship of the ego to the self is a lifelong process, neither an identification of the ego with the self (with the consequences of fantasies of grandeur, psychosis, etc.) nor a blockage between both is healthy. The goal is a related ego-self-axis. Individuation (self-realization or self-development) is seen as a final arduous process of dealing with one's own repressed sides (shadow), adapting to the outside (persona), and adapting to the inside (anima, self, other unconscious content).

Assumptions about the Sources and Nature of Energy

Jung assumed that the psychic nature has an energetic structure, he saw the wholeness of the organism as something that is in constant energetic movement.

In contrast to Freud's concept of libido, he believed the libido is not just sexual energy, but instead generalized psychic energy that can manifest itself as drives in sexuality, aggression, affects, creative impulses, and in the drive to individuation.

According to Jung, energy only flows if there is an opposite tension. Within the psychic system, the amount of energy is constant to a certain extent. If the natural polarity and the associated compensation is disturbed (e.g., by a defense mechanism), the energy passes into the unconscious, animates, and strengthens its contents, that—if not made conscious, differentiated, and integrated—can cause mental disorders and symptoms (Jung, 1948/1970).

In his association studies, Jung discovered that the free flow of psychic energy could be blocked. He called this phenomenon "complex." The unconscious complex has an energetic value that lacks consciousness and, if activated, can promote, or inhibit psychological contents (Jung, 1934/1967). In this respect, the energetic point of view is an important part of diagnostics and therapy in analytical psychology. The energetic point of view also reflects an important role in self-regulation, in the dialectical relationship between the conscious and the unconscious, and the ego and the self.

Assumptions about the Nature of Relationship

The relationship is perceived in Jungian psychology on three levels. On the one hand, on the intrapsychic level (relationship of consciousness and unconscious with integration of shadow, complex, and differentiation of unconscious archetypal material), on the interpersonal level (the relationship to the object with the withdrawal of the projections from the other), and on the transpersonal level (the relationship of the subject to the self, and to the infinite). The self is the goal of the process of individuation, which can be achieved with a balanced self-ego-axis. The individuation process depends on all three levels, it is an internal subjective integration process, but on the other hand, it is an equally objective relationship process (Jung, 1946/1966).

On the intrapsychic and interpersonal level, Jung assumed that unconscious complexes can only be experienced by projecting onto an object. Unconscious contents must dock at an external content or appear in dreams or in imaginations, only then does their reality arise (Jung, 1934/1967). The ego projects complexes or identifies with them. Only through the withdrawal of the unconscious parts (e.g., of the shadow, and of complexes), a real relationship with others becomes possible.

The transpersonal level is related to the other two levels because being in a relationship with the deeper parts of the psyche is necessary for an authentic relationship. "The relationship to the self is at once relationship to our fellow man, and no one can be related to the latter until he is related to himself" (Jung, 1946/1966, §445).

Assumptions about Developmental Stages

In general, maladaptive patterns of complexes from childhood can create disorders and problems later in life, but they are not fixed in developmental stages.

Particularly important for Jung was the separation from the mother, during puberty, to become an adult (Jung, 1912/1967). He called this process the hero journey, due to the fact, that numerous tales and myths were written about this process. The classic hero is a youthful hero who emancipates himself from his parental images to be able to grow up. It is necessary to overcome the desire for regression as a mental danger to sink back into the instinctual level of childhood. The incest taboo stands in the way of this, which is why symbolic forms must be found for the mother.

The hero fights on the objective level against the mother image and on the subjective level against the power of the unconscious. When the regression into the unconscious gets out of hand, the mother image acts like a paralyzing poison on the hero's energy and makes the person depressed. Only if the hero's journey is successful, the teenager can develop a relationship with a girlfriend or to his inner female part (anima) (Jung, 1912/1967).

Jung viewed the process of individuation as a lifelong, incomplete process, coming up especially in transition periods when questions of meaning are urgent (as in times of illness, midlife-crisis, retirement, etc.). Individuation means not following "what you should" or "what would be right," but rather listening to yourself to find out what the inner wholeness (the self) can be. Jung's view of the individuation process set him apart from Freud's etiological (causal) thinking in favor of a final, goal-oriented thinking.

Assumptions about the Body

Jung assumed the archetypes link body (instinct) with psyche (image) because the body and mind have the same psychoid root. The body (instincts, drives, impulses, and patterns of behaviors) is noticeable for the ego via archetypal and symbolic images (Jung, 1954/1970). Jung argued in some works for an instinctual source of the archetypes, they seem to be located in the old, so-called reptilian brain (hypothalamus and brain stem) (Samuels et al., 1986).

A long debate is to be observed amongst Jungians, some favor the opinion that archetypes are more biologically conditioned, while others are more culturally conditioned (Roesler, 2012). The goal of individuation is to accept the body, without being driven unconsciously by its drives and instincts.

Assumptions about Anxieties/Instincts and Defenses

Jung saw instincts and archaic mode meet in the "patterns of behavior" that mean an innate readiness to react. The relationship between archetype and instincts or patterns of behavior plays a major role in dealing with the archetype. Jung suspects that there is no such thing as a drive per se, but that drives are always tied to images, affects, situations, or behavior (Jung, 1935/1967, 1948/1970, 1954/1970).

If an archetype is at work, the human being experiences numerous strong affects such as lust, panic, rage, play, fear, etc. The archetypal fear can be seen in dreams and indicate that a new development is pending, and insofar anxieties may have a positive aspect. If a person flees from this challenge, his life becomes narrow and impoverished (Samuels et al., 1986).

Analytical psychology has largely adopted the defense mechanisms described by psychoanalysis. However, the defense mechanisms serve not only as a neurotic defense but also as constructive self-regulation.

Assumptions Concerning Etiology

Analytical psychology sees the causes of psychological and psychosomatic disorders by the fact that the ego develops in another direction as the unconscious, it becomes one-sided. The causes lie, on the one hand, in complexes such as the minority complex. Some of those complexes arise from our personal unconscious (personal complex of negative childhood experiences), yet some seem to come from the collective unconscious (collective complex; e.g. witch image, eternal child image). Jung assumed that complexes are autonomous parts of the psyche, consisting of unconscious representations grouped around a strong affect and an archetype. Further on, the complex representations concern emotions, body feelings, thoughts, memories of internalized interactions, symbolic images, and coping strategies (Jung, 1934/1967; Meier, 2019). When complexes arise, the ego-functioning is disrupted.

On the other hand, the causes lie in crises due to unused potential. These can appear at some point in life events such as separation, midlife-crisis, menopause, retirement, illness, or death, especially when a person is developing one-sided. The unconscious reacts complementarily e.g., in dreams, showing possible ways out of the situation. Jung saw crises of meaning as a division of consciousness from the intentions of the self (Jung, 1954/1970).

Implications for Technique

Work with the Unconscious

The goal of Jungian psychology is to explore the unconscious, both personal and collective, and integrate them into consciousness through a variety of methods. The aim of psychotherapy is to help the patient to reestablish a healthy relationship to the unconscious. That means neither to be overwhelmed by the unconscious (psychosis), nor to be blocked from it (depression, compulsiveness, etc.).

Symbol Work

According to Jung, problems and symptoms manifest themselves by symbols. Understanding the symbolic material takes place in a therapeutic process with dream work, drawing pictures, active imaginations, etc. Working with the transcendent function is a further method to bring the opposite of consciousness and unconscious together, by forming symbols that include both areas. Jung assumed working with the symbolic and complex material of the client is the royal road in the treatment, not working with the transference.

Transference Work

However, the transference process may also help in this process. Unconscious complexes, as the father complex, are rising up in analysis and may be projected to the analyst. The analyst himself experiences the complex constellation in the countertransference and can react as the father if he is not realizing what is happening. In some cases—when a complex is strong—the analyst realizes only afterward, what has happened.

Complex Work

Instead of automatically "falling" into a complex, the analyst's goal is to realize what is happening here and now, with the patient as the subject and the other as the object, and to learn to take the projection of the complex back.

Individuation Work

The aim of (Jungian) psychotherapy is to assist the individual to establish a relationship to the self so that the full potential of the individuum can be realized. That means, exploring the dark, inferior, and repressed aspects of the psyche (shadow); and the inner woman and man image (anima and animus), in general, all different parts of the own psyche.

Subsequent Development of the Concepts of the Jungian School

The successors Mario Jacoby (2001), Kathrin Asper (1993), Jean Knox (2003), and others incorporated the results of the infant research into Jungian psychology.

Christian Roesler is arguing that Jung's assumption of a biological/genetic transmission of archetypes can no longer be supported (Roesler, 2019). Roesler states, even if there are genetically preformed mental patterns, they are subject to strong influence from the environment via epigenetic processes (Roesler, 2012). Cultural influences and socialization strongly form unconscious symbolization as well as the way we organize our inner imagery. He proposes to restrict the use of the term "archetype" to a small set of motifs and patterns, which constitute a map of transformational processes of the individuation process.

Isabelle Meier redefines the complex definition assuming they are formed when basic needs are not met. These basic needs as attachment, play, autonomy, meaning, and others can be found universally as psychologists or neuroscientists are claiming (Panksepp, 1998). Basic needs include subcortical primordial affects, body reactions, and action-systems. With maturation, higher brain mechanisms as memories of internalized interactions, thoughts, and images come into view. These processes form feeling-toned complexes. The complex consists of unconscious representations grouped around a strong affect, and concern for emotions, body feelings, thoughts, memories of internalized interactions (of subject and object), a symbolic image (i.e., in dreams), and coping strategies (Meier, 2019).

25. Jung and the Jungians	
Main, general underlying assumptions	• Jung distinguished between a personal unconscious and a collective unconscious. • Some basic structures of the collective unconscious are invariable and present from the beginning of time in every culture (archetypes). • Consciousness and unconscious stand in a compensatory, dynamic relationship to each another. • An autonomous, dynamic potential in us acts without our consciousness, tending towards a wholeness of the personality
Specific theoretical assumptions	
psychic structure	• The human psyche can metaphorically be seen as being built up in layers; at the top the ego, embedded in the consciousness, followed by the personal unconscious, the collective unconscious, and the never conscious part of the unconscious. • The archetypes have an ordering power that can be experienced in symbolic stories, images, affects, symbols, behavior. • Individuation is seen as a process of integration of the different parts of the personality (persona, shadow, anima, animus, self, etc.).
energy	• The psychic nature has an energetic structure. • In contrast to Freud's concept of libido, the libido is not just sexual energy but generalized psychic energy. • Mental disturbances arise when the natural polarity and compensation is disturbed. The energy passes then into the unconscious, and strengthens its contents (complexes, archetypes). • If the free flow of psychic energy is blocked, complexes arise in the unconscious that withdraw energy from the consciousness.

(*Continued*)

relationships	• Relationship is perceived on three levels; on the intrapsychic level, on the interpersonal level, and on the transpersonal level. • Unconscious complexes can be experienced by projecting onto an object and by identifying with the complex content.
developmental stages	• Maladaptive patterns of complexes from childhood can create later in life disorders and problems. • The psychology of puberty was important for Jung, especially the separation from the mother (image) to become an adult (hero's journey). • The process of individuation is a lifelong process.
body	• Jung argued for an instinctual source of the archetypes, which he located in the old, "reptilian" brain. • The archetypes link body (instinct) with psyche (image) because they have the same psychoid root.
anxieties/instincts and defenses	• Drives and instincts are always tied to archetypal images, affects, situations, or behavior. • If an archetype is at work the human being experiences numerous, strong affects such as lust, panic, rage, play or fear etc. • Anxiety may be seen as avoidance to becoming conscious and has therefore not only a sexual base as in psychoanalysis. • The Jungian psychology has largely adopted the defense mechanisms described by psychoanalysis. However, the defense mechanisms are not only seen as neurotic defenses, but also help the person for self-regulation.
Assumptions concerning etiology	• The causes of psychological disturbances lay in complexes (similar to the term "schema" of schema therapy). Some of those complexes arise from our personal unconscious, some from the collective unconscious. • Complexes are autonomous parts of the psyche, consisting of unconscious representations grouped around a strong affect and an archetype. • The complex representations concern emotions, body feelings, thoughts, memories of internalized interactions, symbolic images, and coping strategies. • Crises arise due to unused potential. That can appear in times of transition. Jung saw crises of meaning as a division of consciousness from the intentions of the self.

(*Continued*)

Implications for technique	• The goal is to explore the unconscious, both personal and collective, and integrate them into consciousness through dream work, symbol work, complex work, transference/counter-transference work, and the work to find out what the symptoms mean.
Subsequent developments of the core concept	• Incorporation of child research results into Jungian Psychology. • Elaboration of the archetype definition. Originally, they are seen as genetically formed patterns. The new view is that cultural transmission and epigenetic processes play a much bigger role than usually admitted. The term "archetype" shall therefore be restricted to a small set of motifs and patterns in transformation processes (Roesler, 2019) • Elaboration of the complex definition: Feeling-toned complex arises when basic needs are not met. The complex consists of unconscious representations grouped around a strong affect, and concern emotions, body feelings, thoughts, memories of internalized interactions (of subject and object), symbolic images, and coping strategies. The feeling-toned complex can be triggered by a perception, leads to a disruption of ego-functioning, and pursues a goal via constellation, projection, or identification (Meier, 2019).

References

Asper, K. (1993). *The abandoned child within: On losing and regaining self-worth*. Fromm Intl.

Jacoby, M. (2001). *Jungian psychotherapy and contemporary infant research*. Routledge.

Jung, C. G. (1966). The psychology of transference. In G. Adler & R.F.C. Hull (Eds. and trans.), *The Collected Works of C. G. Jung, Vol. 16*, pp. 163–203. Princeton University Press. (Original work published 1946).

Jung, C. G. (1967). Symbols of transformation. In G. Adler & R.F.C. Hull (Eds. and trans.), *The Collected Works of C. G. Jung, Vol. 5*. Princeton University Press. (Original work published 1912).

Jung, C. G. (1967). Psychological types. In G. Adler & R.F.C. Hull (Eds. and trans.), *The Collected Works of C. G. Jung, Vol. 6*. Princeton University Press. (Original work published 1921).

Jung, C. G. (1967). A review of the complex theory. In G. Adler & R.F.C. Hull (Eds. and trans.), *The Collected Works of C. G. Jung, Vol. 8*, pp. 92–104. Princeton University Press. (Original work published 1934).

Jung, C. G. (1967). The relationship between the ego and the unconscious. In G. Adler & R.F.C. Hull (Eds. and trans.), *The Collected Works of C. G. Jung, Vol. 7*, pp. 123–305. Princeton University Press. (Original work published 1935).

Jung, C. G. (1970). On psychic energy. In G. Adler & R.F.C. Hull (Eds. and trans.), *The Collected Works of C. G. Jung, Vol. 8*, pp. 3–66. Princeton University Press. (Original work published 1948).

Jung, C. G. (1970). On the nature of Psyche. In G. Adler & R.F.C. Hull (Eds. and trans.), *The Collected Works of C. G. Jung, Vol. 8*, pp. 159–236. Princeton University Press. (Original work published 1954).

Knox, J. (2003). *Archetype, attachment, analysis: Jungian psychology and the emergent mind*. Brunner-Routledge.

Meier, I. (2019). Basis needs and complexes: Similarities between feeling-toned complexes, emotional schema and affective states. *Journal of Analytical Psychology*, *64*(5), 761–779.

Panksepp, J. (1998). *Affective neuroscience: The foundations of human and animal emotions*. Oxford University Press.

Roesler, C. (2012). Are archetypes transmitted more by culture than biology? Questions arising from conceptualizations of the archetype. *Journal of Analytical Psychology*, *57*(2), 224–247.

Roesler, C. (2019). Theoretical foundations of analytical psychology: Recent developments and controversies. *Journal of Analytical Psychology*, *64*(5), 658–681.

Samuels, A., Shorter, B., & Plaut, F. (1986). *A critical dictionary of Jungian analysis*. Routledge.

Chapter 26

The Post-Jungians

Ann Addison

Introduction

Since the publication of Jung's Red Book in 2009, analytical psychology has entered a new phase in the appreciation of Jung's work, and contemporary post-Jungians have gained a greater understanding of his conceptual shift from a scientific to a hermeneutic approach and a deeper engagement with the meaning of some of his original concepts. The present chapter is written primarily from this vertex, in view of the wealth of recent scholarship and in the face of the difficulty in so confined a space of satisfactorily tracing a complete timeline from Jung's previous work.

Underlying Assumptions in Analytical Psychology

When talking about basic underlying assumptions in analytical psychology, it is common to lift out certain key concepts in Jung's thinking, such as complexes, archetypes, and the collective unconscious, and then to be left with an impression of a model of the psyche that is somewhat static. So, before focussing on these central assumptions, I want to highlight that Jung's theory is essentially process-oriented and concerns the ebb and flow of energy in the tension that arises between conscious and unconscious. Jung sought to harness that energy symbolically in the service of the patient's healing and in the life-long work of individuation.

Jung's model of the psyche was developed through years of scientific work (his Word Association Tests—WATs—conducted at the Burghölzli Clinic), self-reflection and hermeneutic study (his Red Book work, and his subsequent theoretical conceptualizations), comparative study in other disciplines, and empirical observation of his clinic patients' hallucinations and his analytic patients' dreams and imaginal material. This model embraces all the elements that feed into the analytic process. For the early post-Jungians, not all of his work was available but contemporary post-Jungians have access to his personal self-experimentation, with the publication of his Red Book in 2009 and the publication of his Black Books in 2019, and considerable research (e.g.,

DOI: 10.4324/9781003027768-27

Kirsch & Hogenson, 2014; Stein, 2011; Stein & Arzt, 2017, 2018, 2019) has gone into this new material. Thus, we now have far greater insight into Jung's hermeneutic approach and its implications for analytical psychology, clinically, theoretically, and culturally. We also have Jung's own example of his individuation process through his repeated working and re-working of the material from his unconscious as displayed in the Red Book.

Certain of Jung's ideas that are not prominent in his previously published work have come to the fore, most notably his psychoid concept and his notion of synchronicity. There is not space here to address all the developments, so I propose simply to draw out certain main strands of post-Jungian thought from their historical base in Jung's work while weaving in contemporary changes in emphasis and picking up on just some of the aspects of post-Jungian thinking that have an important place in clinical practice.

Main, General Underlying Assumptions

Structure of the Psyche (Personal and Collective Unconscious); Complexes; Archetypes; Individuation

From his early WATs, Jung conceived the idea of a *personal unconscious* including accumulations of ideas clustered around emotionally charged events in our lived experience. He termed these clusters *complexes*. Jung described a complex as:

> The *image* of a certain psychic situation which is strongly accentuated emotionally and is, moreover, incompatible with the habitual attitude of consciousness. This image has a … high degree of autonomy, so that it is subject to the control of the conscious mind to only a limited extent.
>
> (Jung, 1934/1969, para. 201)

His experiments demonstrated scientifically that complexes exert a strong energic influence in which emotion and physical reaction are seen to be intimately combined. This was the beginning of his understanding of a monistic relation between mind and body.

From his subsequent hermeneutic study in the multi-layer work of imagination that gave rise to his Red Book, and from his empirical observation of his patients, he discovered the existence of universal ideas and patterns of behavior common to all mankind, and he conceived the notion of *a collective unconscious* that is inhabited by primordial images.

The flood of unconscious fantasy, unleashed in the autumn of 1913 following two dreams of a terrible sea of blood, prompted him to begin his "most difficult experiment" of actively engaging with the unconscious, by plunging himself into his fantasies and entering into dialogue with them. Such dialogue involved encouraging his visions, reflecting on the primordial images that arose, and engaging in a multi-layer process of imaginal elaboration, which he continued over many years. He termed this process *active imagination*, seeing it as a means for fostering the symbolic expression of an unconscious determinant and harnessing the associated energy in the service of transformation and individuation.

His self-experimentation showed that primordial images have a numinous quality, echoing mythological motifs, and possess a vitality and fascination that activates the psyche:

> [I]n dreams, fantasies, and other exceptional states of mind the most far-fetched mythological motifs and symbols can appear autochthonously at any time .... These "primordial images" ... make up that psychic stratum which I have called the collective unconscious.
>
> (Jung, 1929/1969, para. 229)

After developing a view of the collective unconscious as a locus of deeply unconscious sources of potential, the *archetypes*, serving as generators of psychic form, he gave these images the name *archetypal images*. "[T]he archetype is ... a dynamism which makes itself felt in the ... fascinating power of the archetypal image." (Jung, 1947/1954/1969, para. 414). He saw this dynamism as potentially transformative.

Specific Theoretical Assumptions

Psychoid Unconscious; Archetype as Such; Unus Mundus; Body and Mind; Transcendent Function

At the deepest level of the psyche, Jung conceived a *psychoid unconscious* that was so deep as to be unknowable:

> The archetypal representations (images and ideas) mediated to us by the unconscious should not be confused with the archetype as such. They are very varied structures which all point back to one essentially "irrepresentable" form. The latter is characterised by certain formal elements ... although these can be grasped only approximately. The archetype as such is a *psychoid* factor .... It does not appear to be capable of reaching consciousness.
>
> (Jung, 1936/1969, para. 417)

His psychoid concept has some very far-reaching implications since he saw this aspect of the unconscious as possessing particular qualities of organization taking effect through the archetypes, and as being associated with an *unus mundus* or unitary world in which body and mind, later even mind and matter (cf. his synchronicity concept), and self and other are undifferentiated.

Describing the archetype as having a "gripping" quality, Jung writes:

> This remarkable effect points to the "psychoid" and essentially transcendental nature of the archetype as an "arranger" of psychic forms inside and outside the psyche.
>
> (Adler, 1976, p. 22)

He thought of this as a vital force or life-energy. Addison (2019) argues that the archetype as such can be seen as a potential in the psychoid unconscious for organizing and shaping elements of an instinctual or imaginal character to engender new and more complex emergent positions depicted as the instinctual image or the archetypal image, respectively. As a result of the psychoid nature of the archetype, these images may emerge in embodied form anywhere along the psyche-soma continuum between instinct and spirit, and thence become conscious. This is important in the analytic process.

Jung himself saw the archetypes as "formal factors responsible for the organization of unconscious psychic processes" and "at the same time they have a 'specific charge' and develop numinous effects which express themselves as *affects*." (Jung, 1952/1969, para. 841). Such affects withdraw energy from the contents of consciousness and allow unconscious contents, generally of an archetypal nature, to break through, or emerge, and find expression as images. These instinctual and archetypal images enrich and clarify the affect and are symbolic in that they portray the meaning of the affect in terms of the best possible expression for a complex fact not yet clearly consciously apprehended. Such transformation of energy is an emergent process having a vitalizing effect on the personality for enabling the conscious ego to come to terms with the unconscious in a symbolic way to achieve a resolution of internal conflict through a new position. Jung described this effect as the transcendent function, a mediator and transformer of psychic energy.

Assumptions Concerning Etiology

Reductive Method; Synthetic Method; Emergence

As can be seen from the above, Jung's model is dynamic and emergent. Although he does write about the psychology of childhood development, his work is directed more toward the nature of the unconscious and the dynamics of the psyche in the adult. Furthermore, he eschews causal interpretations of psychic material, which look to childhood for an explanation, in favor of understandings based on prospective meaning, which contemplate potential future unfolding.

> No psychological fact can ever be explained in terms of causality alone; as a living phenomenon, it is always indissolubly bound up with the continuity of the vital process, so that it is not only something evolved but also continually evolving and creative.
>
> (Jung, 1921/1971, para. 717)

In this, Jung makes plain that he is distinguishing himself from Freud, describing Freud's method as reductive in its attempts to depict unconscious material in terms of infantile, instinctual motivations and past deficits, and as limiting to the ongoing development of the personality. He describes his own method as constructive or synthetic because it attends to the full meaning and potential for growth represented by unconscious contents, thereby seeking to integrate these unconscious contents into the personality as a whole. More especially, he acknowledges that, whilst it may be necessary at the outset of analysis to employ Freud's method to uncover and deal with childhood issues, thereafter the reductive viewpoint tends to lead to a limited, mechanistic effect whereas the synthetic viewpoint leads to an emergent life-enhancing result.

In Jung's view, it is important to reach the vital meaning of unconscious symbolism. Such unconscious material, he believed, has a prospective function compensating for the conscious attitude and anticipating lines of future development. A symbol is the best current formulation of an unknown fact, a numinous structural element in the collective unconscious attracting conscious content to itself to generate an archetypal image representing the unknown fact, an intimation of a meaning beyond our present comprehension. Thus, the synthetic approach, based on the question, what is the purpose of this material, offers a more complete understanding better suited to the future adaptation of the personality.

Amongst the post-Jungians, Colman (2007) describes the symbol as representing living, emergent meaning. He refers to the idea of the third to describe the emergence of a new level of mental functioning, linking this with Jung's concept of the transcendent function. The transcendent function arises through an active confrontation between the conscious and unconscious leading to the emergence of new symbolic forms. The new symbolic forms transcend internal conflicts and lead to a greater psychic wholeness. Such third (area or position) may thus be described as a representational space for the occurrence of emergent meaning (p. 566).

Urban (2008) contemplates a symbol as a vital process. She takes issue with the use of the terms "image" and "representation" for symbolic expression, on the grounds that they imply something static. She suggests instead that consciousness and unconsciousness are in ceaseless movement, constantly blending into and clashing against one another to create "symbolic expressions [that] are ephemeral and elusive, rising up, emerging into consciousness seemingly from nowhere and disappearing again" (p. 346).

Implications for Technique

Transference; Countertransference; Active Imagination; Relationship

The synthetic approach has considerable implications for analytic technique. The analyst, seeking to mediate the relations of unconscious and conscious, and hence the transcendent function, with and for the patient in order to help the patient arrive at a new position, is all the time monitoring and evaluating the purpose of the *transference*. Unconscious manifestations, slips, spontaneous fantasies, and dreams, are noted for emotional intensity and energic value and the analyst engages with the patient in what Jung described as a form of active imagination to assist the patient in giving symbolic shape to this charged material. In view of Jung's psychoid concept, the shape may emerge anywhere along the psyche-soma continuum and anywhere along the relational continuum between patient and analyst, depending upon numerous factors including the ego strength of the patient, the stage of the analysis, and the current transference-countertransference relationship.

A description of this emergent process in the transference, from confidential interview material, is given below:

> For me, the important [thing] is not the phenomena itself, it is how the phenomena is going to shape our thoughts. And to allow us to think what we would be unable to think without that. It is an emergent process. [… T] hese phenomena are linked to the complex system, which is the encounter. [F]rom this system emerges something which would not have emerged in another system. I would say that, in this moment, the important thing for the analysis is that you have been able to accept to lose your boundaries, so that's this complex system, which is the transference, will then take the place of your ego, inside your psyche, inside your body first, and then your psyche. And will create inside you some shape or representation, using your consciousness for that. And then you recovered your boundaries, and you have been able to think something, to be conscious of a thinking, which has emerged from this experience inside you. [… There is also] the necessity of time for the analyst to lose his boundaries and the necessity of time for the patient to be able to hear something about an important insight. And what is very mysterious for me is that this necessity of time is coming from the encounter, and no one decides, it emerges. And usually, when it emerges like this, if the analyst is able to say something, usually the analysand is able to hear.
>
> (Addison, 2019, pp. 138–139)

In post-Jungian thinking, there is a significant body of work (e.g., Cambray, 2002; Hogenson, 2004) attending to questions of emergence relating to this synthetic understanding.

Subsequent Developments

In the above, I have woven contemporary post-Jungian thinking into observations on certain of Jung's key concepts. I have embraced some of the current ideas concerning his model of the psyche, and its deeply unknowable strata designated the psychoid unconscious and the emergent dynamic associated with that. I have not covered his views on synchronicity, seen as a locus of meaningful coincidence or an acausal connecting principle, nor have I highlighted the considerable amount of research addressing this concept (see, by way of example only, Atmanspacher, 2014; Aziz, 2007; Cambray, 2009; Hogenson, 2009; Main, 2004).

Many other aspects of Jung's thinking have also been critiqued and expanded by the post-Jungians, and space permits me to select a few key areas only. There exist important critiques on the validity of his central notion of the archetype, its nature, its function, and its basis in the psyche. Significant among these discussions are Pietikainen, 1998; Knox, 2003; Stevens, 2015; and Hogenson, 2019. There is, in addition, an evolving area of post-Jungian study devoted to gender and queer theory (e.g., McKenzie, 2006; Samuels, 1984), critiquing Jung's ideas concerning the two specific contra-sexual archetypes, anima, and animus.

Specific applications of Jung's theory have also received attention, including studies of development (e.g., Fordham, 1957, 1986; Jacoby, 1999; Neumann, 1973), studies of trauma (e.g., Kalsched, 1996), studies on therapeutic care for refugees (e.g., Papadopoulos, 2002), and studies of politics and diversity (e.g., Samuels, 1993).

Finally, recent work by various post-Jungians has identified and elaborated an additional important aspect of Jung's model of the psyche, designated the cultural complex (Singer, 2000, 2018; Singer & Kimbles, 2004), which relates to the influences of cultural background on individuals and on the unconscious behaviors of social groups.

26. The Post-Jungians	
Main, general underlying assumptions	A dynamic model of the psyche having a personal and a collective unconscious, in which individuation is a key function.
Specific theoretical assumptions	
psychic structure	A personal unconscious characterized by complexes, a collective unconscious characterized by archetypes and archetypal images, and a deeply unknowable stratum, the psychoid unconscious.
energy	A purposive vital principle or life-force governs an emergent dynamism in the psyche.

(Continued)

relationships	Relationship is seen in terms of transference, wherein analyst and patient together strive to give symbolic form to emerging material.
developmental stages	N/A
body	A body-mind monism applies so that unconscious material may manifest anywhere along a continuum from physiologic to psychic.
anxieties/instincts and defenses	N/A
Assumptions concerning etiology	Jung's synthetic method focuses on the purpose of the transference, in contrast to Freud's reductive method which focuses on the cause.
Implications for technique	The analyst mediates the relation of conscious and unconscious, hence the transcendent function, through a form of active imagination by monitoring the purpose of the transference.
Subsequent developments of the core concept	• Critiques of Jung's depiction of the archetype, elaborations of his psychoid concept and his notion of synchronicity, the conceptualisation of cultural complexes. • Applications of Jung's ideas address areas of development, gender, trauma, refugee care, politics, and diversity.

References

Addison, A. (2019). *Jung's psychoid concept contextualised.* Routledge.

Adler, G. (Ed.). (1976). *C. G. Jung Letters: 1951–1961* (Vol. 2). Routledge & Kegan Paul.

Atmanspacher, H. (2014). Psychophysical correlations, synchronicity and meaning. *Journal of Analytical Psychology*, *59*, 181–188.

Aziz, R. (2007). *The syndetic paradigm: The untrodden path beyond Freud and Jung.* State University of New York Press.

Cambray, J. (2002). Synchronicity and emergence. *American Imago*, *59*, 409–434.

Cambray, J. (2009). *Synchronicity: Nature and psyche in an interconnected universe.* Texas A&M University Press.

Colman, W. (2007). Symbolic conceptions: The idea of the third. *Journal of Analytical Psychology*, *52*, 565–583.

Fordham, M. (1957). *New developments in analytical psychology.* Routledge & Kegan Paul.

Fordham, M. (1986). *Explorations into the Self.* Academic Press.

Hogenson, G. B. (2004). Archetypes, emergence and the psyche's deep structure. In J. Cambray, & L. Carter (Eds.), *Analytical psychology: Contemporary perspectives in Jungian analysis* (pp. 32–55). Brunner-Routledge.

Hogenson, G. B. (2009). Synchronicity and moments of meeting. *Journal of Analytical Psychology, 54*, 183–197.

Hogenson, G. B. (2019). The controversy around the concept of archetypes. *Journal of Analytical Psychology, 64*, 682–700.

Jacoby, M. (1999). *Jungian psychotherapy and contemporary infant research: Basic patterns of emotional exchange*. Routledge.

Jung, C. G. (1969). The significance of the constitution and heredity in psychology. In H. Read, M. Fordham, & G. Adler (Eds.), *Collected works: The structure and dynamics of the psyche* (2nd ed, Vol. 8, pp. 107–113). Routledge. (Original work published 1929).

Jung, C. G. (1969). A review of the complex theory. In H. Read, M. Fordham, & G. Adler (Eds.), *Collected works: The structure and dynamics of the psyche* (2nd ed, Vol. 8, pp. 92–104). Routledge. (Original work published 1934).

Jung, C. G. (1969). Psychological factors determining human behaviour. In H. Read, M. Fordham, & G. Adler (Eds.), *Collected works: The structure and dynamics of the psyche* (2nd ed, Vol. 8, pp. 114–125). Routledge. (Original work published 1936).

Jung, C. G. (1969). On the nature of the psyche. In H. Read, M. Fordham, & G. Adler (Eds.), *Collected works: The structure and dynamics of the psyche* (2nd ed, Vol. 8, pp. 159–234). Routledge. (Original work published 1947/1957).

Jung, C. G. (1969). Synchronicity: An acausal connecting principle. In H. Read, M. Fordham, & G. Adler (Eds.) *Collected works: The structure and dynamics of the psyche* (2nd ed, Vol. 8, pp. 417–531). Routledge. (Original work published 1952).

Jung, C. G. (1971). Definitions. In H. Read, M. Fordham, & G. Adler (Eds.), *Collected works*: Psychological *types* (2nd ed, Vol. 6, pp. 408–486). Routledge. (Original work published 1921).

Jung, C. G. (2009). *The red book, liber novus: A reader's edition*. (S. Shamdasani, Ed.). W. W. Norton.

Kalsched, D. E. (1996). *The inner world of trauma*. Routledge.

Kirsch, T., & Hogenson, G. (2014). *The red book: Reflections on C. G. Jung's liber novus*. Routledge.

Knox, J. (2003). *Archetype, attachment, analysis*. Brunner-Routledge.

Main, R. (2004). *The rupture of time: Synchronicity and Jung's critique of modern western culture*. Brunner-Routledge.

McKenzie, S. (2006). Queering gender: Anima/Animus and the paradigm of emergence. *Journal of Analytical Psychology, 51*, 401–421.

Neumann, E. (1973). *The child: Structure and dynamics of the nascent personality*. G. P. Putnam's Sons.

Papadopoulos, R. K. (2002). *Therapeutic care for refugees—No place like home*. Karnac.

Pietikainen, P. (1998). Archetypes as symbolic forms. *Journal of Analytical Psychology, 43*, 325–343.

Samuels, A. (1984). Gender and psyche: Developments in analytical psychology. *British Journal of Psychotherapy, 1*, 31–49.

Samuels, A. (1993). *The political psyche*. Routledge.

Singer, T. (2000). *The vision thing: Myth, politics and psyche in the world.* Routledge.
Singer, T. (2018). The cultural complex theory: Scientific and mythopoetic ways of knowing. In J. Cambray & L. Sawin (Eds.), *Research in analytical psychology: Applications from scientific, historical and cross-cultural research* (pp. 69–82). Routledge.
Singer, T., & Kimbles, S. L. (Eds.). (2004). *The cultural complex: Contemporary Jungian perspectives on psyche and society*. Routledge.
Stein, M. (2011). What is the red book for analytical psychology? *Journal of Analytical Psychology*, *56*, 590–606.
Stein, M., & Arzt, T. (Eds.). (2017, 2018, 2019). *Jung's red book for our time: Searching for soul in post-modern conditions* (Vols. 1, 2, 3). Chiron Publications.
Stevens, A. (2015). *Archetype revisited: An updated natural history of the Self.* Routledge.
Urban, E. (2008). The "Self" in analytical psychology: The function of the "central archetype" within Fordham's model. *Journal of Analytical Psychology*, *53*, 329–350.

Chapter 27

Summary and Overview

Bernd Huppertz

In my early professional life, I was confused by the contrast between the agreed evidence-based medical thinking and the at times controversial and differing perspectives in the many psychoanalytic schools or societies around the world. I began a study of these latter approaches. This led to the idea of this book where authors were invited to declare their reasons for holding their particular views, beginning with their school's/society's/institute's underlying assumptions.

By observing the differences between these psychoanalytic schools of thought, we may see that these different schools exist because psychoanalysts have different views about certain essentials in addition to the issue of whether they use a "one-person" or a "two-person psychology." Mostly these models have tended to adapt to the changing social environment and have been made functional in their own way for the current periods of time. I recognized furthermore that between the so-called schools of thought are fluid transformations as in a rainbow. We shall discover many mutations and interpenetrations from one color to the next. The growth of the various schools of psychoanalysis and the evolution of psychoanalytical/psychodynamic theory and therapy resulted in tremendous developments.

I was able to differentiate four groups of schools of thought:

1 Groups of schools that were connected with a one-person psychology

The first group of schools was always strongly connected with a founder and tended to involve a one-person psychology. A one-person psychology tends to focus on intrapsychic (processes or interactions) and is also marked by observing and interpreting the unconscious experiences of individuals. After the names of the respective founders evolved into labels, their followers began to change their teachings and opinions. Nowadays, the same labels are used by various people in different ways and yet there is an overlap with other psychodynamic schools.

DOI: 10.4324/9781003027768-28

These are the Freudians, the contemporary UK-Freudians, the Kleinians and post-Kleinians, the Bionians and post-Bionians, the Lacanians, the New York Freudian group, US-Freudians and the contemporary US-Freudians, the American ego psychologists, and the American objects relations analysts.

However, there are some groups in a middle category (between Freud and Klein and between a one- and a two-person psychology): Fairbairn, Winnicott, and other British independents and the interpersonal analysts in the United States.

2 Groups of schools that were connected with a two-person psychology

After the advent of constructivism and social psychology, pragmatic and empiricist America developed various and different perspectives and schools of two-person psychology and broke away from the scientifically oriented, positivist, and objectivist-oriented one-person psychology (Wallerstein, 1988, 2002; Walsh et al., 2014). It must be recognized that the development of the psychoanalytic movement became very much influenced in the USA both by the development of social psychology and by the increase in interest of psychologists in psychoanalysis. At the same time, the classical psychoanalysis represented mostly by MDs remained and developed further. However, there became a split between classical psychoanalysis named by the founders and the newer schools of the two-person psychology (Aron, 1990; Ghent, 1989). These last are Sandor Ferenczi, the Budapest school of psychoanalysis, and the Ferenzci tradition, the interpersonalists, Bowlby and the attachment theorists, the neo-Freudians, the Kohutians, and the self psychologists, the post-Kohutian self psychologists, the relational psychoanalysts, and the intersubjectivists.

The Shift from a One-Person Psychology to a Two-Person Psychology

In Europe, the classical schools of one-person psychology continued to exist and spread successfully. In France, in the context of structuralism and linguistics, the school of Lacan and the Lacanians developed. However, in the United States, based on the Ferenzci tradition and Balint, at first, through Sullivan, a major shift took place in the change from a one-person psychology to a two-person psychology (Balint, 1950; Target, 2013). A two-person psychology was marked by a relationship-based treatment approach, focusing on the (interpsychic) interaction of real individuals with nevertheless considerable attention still paid to internal relations as well.

Nowadays, Europe seems to be characterized by a more classically based, (however, modified) one-person psychology, the United States more by the development of the two-person psychology.

3 Regional/Local/National Schools

Regional or country-specific psychoanalytic schools are often influenced by their respective local contexts. Cultural, national, temporal, social, historical, geographical, and/or political factors are likely to influence the development and design of the content of these regional schools, producing a different local weighting. Similarly, religious, ethnic, social and/or linguistic factors may influence, prevent, promote, enable, or block ideas. The different languages alone seem to have a great influence. After all, there are often non-congruent translations for the content of general terms in other languages. The content of a term we are generally familiar with cannot always be reproduced accordingly and must be reproduced in a rewritten manner. National psychoanalytic schools can be influenced by national history and/or historical trauma (Aron, 1996; Birksted-Breen, 2021; Mitchell & Harris, 2004). Examples are the Italian psychoanalysts, the French psychoanalysts, the Argentine psychoanalysts, and the Asian Psychoanalysts.

4 Other Schools

The Jungians and the post-Jungians.

The Jungian school approach, the analytical psychology, traditional and contemporary, is marked by its difference from the other more Freudian-oriented schools, in the distinction between a personal and a collective unconscious in Jung's complex theory. The ideas of Jung together with the post-Jungian approach vary depending on the influence of differing regional and cultural practices (Jung, 1995; Samuels, 1986).

Method of Differentiation

In order to differentiate the wide range of terms, conceptualizations, and models, sometimes with a variety of different meanings, I asked contributors to focus on the following main topics:

1. **Underlying Assumptions**
   These are defined as involving a willingness to accept something as true without question or proof. Basic assumptions usually involve a set of rules a person may hold involving themselves, others, and the world. These rules are seen as unquestionably right. They may be used to identify the essential nature of a phenomenon as well as its causes and effects. For example, all criminals have faulty genes and are dangerous. Some basic assumptions are held consciously and others unconsciously (Tuckett et al., 2008).

When looking at the questions, I listed the most common main assumptions and then started to examine the development of the respective terms and concepts. Subsequently, I have given brief hints on the further development of these terms. In detail, however, reference should be made to the review of the schematic overviews. Overall, it should be noted that the change from the one-person (Europe) to the two-person psychology (US) can reveal major changes in the respective perspectives of the different schools of mind. It is worth noting that, whereas in America the two-person psychologies tend to refer to relations between self and figures in the external world, in Europe, where some two-person emphasis does exist, it tends to describe relations within an inner world consisting of self and internal figures.

1.1 The Main, General Underlying Assumptions of the Perspective

(Contributors were asked to choose one or as many as two, three, or four basic assumptions.)

I will list only the most frequently claimed assumptions:

1.1.1 The Unconscious

Perhaps the most important assumption is that of the unconscious. First in psychoanalysis, the term and concept was coined and developed by Freud in "The Interpretation of Dreams." All other psychoanalytic perspectives, influenced by analysts such as Klein, Fromm, Lacan, Arlow, Stern, Langs, Stolorow and Atwood, and Lyons-Ruth have integrated the unconscious into their concepts in different ways. Depending on the school, it sometimes took on very different meanings and was used differently, such as with C. G. Jung, who differs from Freud by adding to the concept of a personal unconscious a collective one.

1.1.2 The Self

At first, Freud used the term and the concept of the self in psychoanalysis, to have a similar meaning to that of the ego. This term and concept can be found in different ways in the most diverse schools of thought (especially Klein, Fairbairn, Winnicott, Sullivan, Hartmann, Kohut, Wolf, Anna and Paul Ornstein, Kernberg, Stern, and Lichtenberg) with different meanings and emphases. The self usually means the whole that makes up the human being, always connected with subjective experience and in contrast to the other. In Britain, the mind is mostly seen as containing an inner world consisting of both self and internal objects.

1.1.3 The Mother-Child Relationship

The early mother-child relationship and infant research (also called early dyad or early object relationships, early infant-parent communication (verbal and non-verbal)) have become increasingly important for various psychoanalytic concepts. Early mother-child interaction was increasingly seen as crucial for psychological development and the shaping of relationships. These findings were integrated yet used differently by most schools of mind. It began with Freud and Ferenczi, later with Anna Freud, Klein, Bowlby, Bick, Piaget, Balint, Winnicott, Bion, Spitz, Mahler, Ainsworth, Stern, Beebe, Harrison, Lichtenberg, Fonagy, and Target. It started with regular clinical observation, infant observation, and research on interaction experiments and observation. Later, video microanalysis was developed, which could then show early bidirectional influence in the development of vocalization, emotional communication, and movements of the infant and caregiver. This field of research is now enormous.

1.2 **Specific Theoretical Assumptions** (Contributors were asked to choose one or as many as two, three, or four assumptions for each category.) They were asked to feel free to elaborate on the assumptions of their school so that the reader could become familiar with the ways in which the assumptions influenced conceptualizations and practice.

1.2.1 **Assumptions about the Nature of Psychic Structure**
Psychic structure was first described by Freud in his topographic model (the unconscious, the preconscious, and the conscious) and later in his structural model (id, ego, and superego). Using his theory of infantile sexual development, Freud developed an explanation of the development of personality types as well as psychological diseases. These were thought to be based on disturbances of respective developmental steps (s. etiology). After Freud, many other new concepts and extensions were developed by A. Freud, Hartmann, Arlow, Brenner, Jacobson, Loewald, Mahler, Rapaport and Gill, Sandler, Kernberg, Schafer, Kohut, Stern and other object relationists, interpersonal, and relational theorists.

1.2.2 **Assumptions about Sources and Nature of Energy**
The power of the drives (often translated as instincts that were equipped with a drive source, a drive aim, and a drive object) was seen as energy or a force by Freud. He saw psychic energy in his metapsychology in analogy to physical energy. Because of other newer concepts, Freud made various changes in the meaning of this term during his life. Later the concept was further developed by Hartmann and, more recently, by analysts influenced by neuroscience. However, often this idea has been rejected. Many British schools after Klein chose to abandon biological drives/instincts, and substitute

object-seeking (such as Fairbairn). These British schools now have influence around the globe, and use the idea of "unconscious phantasy," not "drive," "instinct," or "energy."

1.2.3 **Assumptions about the Nature of Relationships**

The ideas and assumptions about what is called relationship in psychotherapy and psychoanalysis on the one hand can refer to the meaning of a relationship to a real object, that is, an interpersonal object (external object) or, on the other hand, to the representation of an object in the mind, the object representation or so-called intrapsychic object (internal object). Starting with Freud, the schools of mind developed various definitions and variations about internal or external objects. Analysts such as Klein, Fairbairn, Winnicott, Sullivan, Bowlby, Hartmann, Spitz, Jacobson, Mahler, Kohut, Kernberg, Sandler, Stern, Greenberg and Mitchell, Blatt, Lichtenberg, and Fonagy developed these terms further.

Fairbairn coined the term object relationship theory (referring both to internal and external object relations), whereas the Americans followed with a view of object relations that tended to lay the emphasis on actual external interpersonal relationships.

1.2.4 **Assumptions about Developmental Stages**

Freud was the first who developed—with his sexual theory and the developmental steps of the so-called infantile sexuality—a concept of development stages. He had assumed that psychosexual development consisted of three phases each with its own dominant partial drives (an oral, anal (urogenital), and phallic-Oedipal phase), which ran along prevailing erogenous zones (oral mucosa, intestinal and genitourinary mucosa, genitals) and that the child would be still polymorphically perverse at that time. The mother-child relationship would lead to the Oedipus complex. After the biological changes during puberty, psychological restructuring would occur. Partial drives, part objects, and autoeroticism are replaced by attraction to sexual objects with the partial drives uniting under the primacy of the genital zone. This would be accompanied by psychosexual differentiation. The basic concept of developmental mental stages in psychic development is often found in subsequent schools and perspectives of thought such as A. Freud, Klein, Winnicott, Bowlby, Mahler, Erikson, Spitz, Kohut, or in other configurations in the interpersonal and intersubjective schools. Klein and now many non-Kleinians use the idea of "positions" instead of developmental steps. This can provide a much more flexible description of changes in mental state. Some child analysts are concerned that there may be some costs to the loss of the concept of development (Anne Alvarez, 2012).

1.2.5 **Assumptions about the Body**

Freud was very interested in the relation between body and mind for various reasons and the body was a very important concept in Freud's thinking. The soma would be the biological ground and the body the mental representation of the soma. Soma and body would provide the sources of the drives. In the development of the ego, the body as a body-ego, the representation of the earliest experiences of a baby would be the first manifestation of the developing ego. The theme of the body plays a great role in different psychoanalytical schools and perspectives and colleagues such as Abraham, Fliess, Kubie, Hoffer, Katz, Laufer, Lichtenberg, Balsam, Grotstein, Lemma, Schachter, Aron and Birksted-Breen. This is especially in the context of psychosomatic disorders for Fenichel, Alexander, Dunbar, Schur, and McDougall.

1.2.6 **Assumptions about Anxieties and Defenses**

Freud saw the anxieties as caused by inner-psychic conflicts connected with anxiety-generating thoughts, and/or external stress. By so-called defense mechanisms, the individual would be unconsciously protected from these. Freud described around ten defenses, which would distort the stimuli coming from the id or else block them unconsciously or consciously. Later his list was extended by Anna Freud and Hartmann. Sigmund Freud's concept was changed—and added to—by different schools and perspectives of thought, for example by Klein, Reich, Fenichel, Bibring, Kohut, Sullivan, Stern, Modell, Levenson, Brenner, Gray, Kernberg, Stolorow and Lachman.

1.3 **Assumptions Concerning Etiology**

For Freud it was the conflict between consciousness and the unconscious that was the cause of symptoms. These would show at the level of consciousness and leave traumatic reminiscences at the level of the unconscious. Trauma would be held back by repression in the unconscious. Symptoms would be seen as a kind of compromise between a trauma from puberty and/or childhood striving for consciousness or at least displacement. Freud's view was changed or seen differently by the newer schools and colleagues, such as Klein, Hartmann, Rangell, Kris, Arlow, Brenner, and the Tysons. Later the focus shifted to include deficits alongside conflicts as with Kohut. Finally, the relationists and the interpersonalists saw the cause in the relationship to the other.

1.4 **Implications for Technique**

Here for example, we have studied different assumptions about the level of attention to transference, countertransference, developmental thinking, defense, relationships, field, self, internal objects, and deficits.

Freud saw the task of his work to explore the unconscious processes that led to symptoms and to bring them into consciousness through his therapeutic method of free association and interpretation. Free association, transference, and later, countertransference were among the most important tools for the technique of psychoanalysis. The later schools and perspectives of thought changed and added to these terms or focused on particular aspects. However, the substantial content, analytical relationship, and associations remained mostly still relevant with Ferenzci, Klein, Heimann, Racker, Bion, Alexander, Mahler, Jacobson, Loewald, Winnicott, Kohut, Stolorow, Greenberg and Mitchell, Levenson, Stern, Bromberg, Fonagy and Target, Gabbard, Lichtenberg, Kernberg, and Wallerstein.

2 **Subsequent Development of the Core Concepts of the Respective Schools**

The core concepts of all of the respective schools have undergone major changes over more than 120 years through further developments, changes, and deviations in the respective schools. These have led to the creation of some exciting new basic concepts and perspectives.

Conclusion

My questions and topics raised in the book led back to Freud's early theories. At that time, almost all those interested who would later become important for psychoanalysis met at Berggasse 19 in Vienna, as did later Freudians, but also later founders or followers of other, new schools. Freud's thinking, however, influenced them all. This book was intended to present the development of these topics during the course of the history of psychoanalysis over the decades.

In schematic overviews, which are attached to the individual chapters, the development of the respective topics over the decades can be tracked.

Are these schools and perspectives now comparable? Can they be put together into one picture or not? Is there a unity or a non-unity in the psychoanalytic view? Can all these terms be compared? Can one respective term be compared with another?

Seeing these theories as points of view over the decades, I have had to conclude that all these schools and perspectives cannot be brought together theoretically. For the schools of the early period, this seems at least partially possible. However, the schools in their current form have their focus on different aspects or themes, which are not always comparable or compatible.

In addition, psychoanalysis worldwide developed regional manifestations with, for a foreigner, often unknown meanings and tints due to and interwoven with different contexts.

Looking at the clinic and the treatment of patients, theories were not so important to me in my life, only marginally helpful. Theories of the mind always seemed a bit suspect and daring to me due to the complexity of the content. For me, the theory is something that should emerge from practice. Superstructure, meta-practice, as it were, is by no means unimportant, but not the most important element for this work. In the course of my professional activity, I have seen many theories come and go, including the theories of Freud, then of Anna Freud, etc., and etc.

I was aware of the impossibility of summarizing these schools and perspectives from the very beginning. That's why my goal was simply to draw a picture of this diverse landscape of assumptions, a picture that consists of little mosaic pieces. Only in the case of the first early psychoanalytic schools, which still spoke the same language in a certain way, temporally and historically, can certain terms be compared and/or summarized with each other.

The common ground of these schools or perspectives is the framework, the respective framework. By frame, I mean the time frame, the location frame, the framework of interaction, the framework of whatever it is called that is equivalent to what is called transference and countertransference, and the framework of building that which—together with the analysand—is called the creation of meaning.

If this summary is experienced as boring, I can tell you that the phenomenological approach is often experienced in this way. It offers a summary of the opinions and findings of others and often, unfortunately, or thank God, nothing new of its own.

I believe that this approach reflects reality in the most appropriate way. The question of which school or perspective is right or the most appropriate cannot or can never be clarified on the basis of currently limited knowledge. The main thing with all of these approaches is that many patients can be successfully treated.

I would like to end this chapter with a quote from Wallerstein:

> That our overall and overarching general theoretical diversity and pluralism can be fully consonant with the shared clinical theory, basic clinical method, and common observational data that I trust I can demonstrate to be our psychoanalytic common ground, that unites the diversity represented in this hall today.
>
> (Wallerstein, 1990, p. 12)

References

Alvarez, A. (2012). *The thinking heart: Three levels of psychoanalytic therapy with disturbed children*. Routledge.

Aron, L. (1990). One person and two person psychologies and the method of psychoanalysis. *Psychoanalytic Psychology*, *7*(4), 475–485.

Aron, L. (1996). *A meeting of minds: Mutuality in psychoanalysis*. Analytic Press.

Balint, M. (1950). Changing therapeutical aims and techniques in psycho-analysis. *International Journal of Psychoanalysis*, *31*, 117–124.

Birksted-Breen, D. (Ed.). (2021). *Translation/Transformation: 100 years of the international journal of psychoanalysis*. Routledge.

Ghent, E. (1989). Credo—The dialectics of one-person and two-person psychologies. *Contemporary Psychoanalysis*, *25*, 169–211.

Jung, C. G. (1995). *Memories, dreams, reflections*. Flamingo.

Mitchell, S. A., & Harris, A. (2004). What's American about American psychoanalysis? *Psychoanalytic Dialogues*, *14*(2), 165–191.

Samuels, A. (1986). *Jung and the post-Jungians*. Routledge.

Target, M. (2013). Foreword. In B. Huppertz (Ed.), *Psychotherapy in the wake of war: Discovering multiple psychoanalytic traditions*. Aronson.

Tuckett, D., Basile, R., Birksted-Breen, D., Böhm, T., Denis, P., Ferro, A., Hinz, H., Jemstedt, A., Mariotti, P., & Schubert, J. (Eds.). (2008). *Psychoanalysis comparable & incomparable: The evolution of a method to describe and compare psychoanalytic approaches*. Routledge.

Wallerstein, R. S. (1988). One psychoanalysis or many? *International Journal of Psychoanalysis*, *69*, 5–21.

Wallerstein, R. (1990). Psychoanalysis: The common ground. *International Journal of Psychoanalysis*, *71*, 3–20.

Wallerstein, R. S. (2002). The trajectory of psychoanalysis: A prognostication. *International Journal of Psychoanalysis*, *83*, 1247–1267.

Walsh, R. T. G., Teo, T., & Baydala, A. (2014). *A critical history and philosophy of psychology*. Cambridge University Press.

Chapter 28

Epilogue: Psychanalysis and the Journey from Natural to Social Science

Bernd Huppertz

At the end of my studies for this book, I would like to raise some questions. Can psychoanalysis be a science? Have I discovered the reasons for so many psychoanalytic approaches? Is there one or are there many correct views among them?

When I started traveling to London around the turn of this century, I understood psychoanalysis to be mainly concerned with the issue of "unconscious mental activity" (Freud, 1914, p. 36).

However, I also realized I had to find a way to track the many developments that went beyond this original concept. I continued to be puzzled by the fact that, in spite of their common interests in unconscious mental activity, there were marked differences in emphases between the various schools. (I have begun to wonder if the differences were influenced by the unconscious mental preoccupations of their founders, but there remains no space to develop this). Like Freud in his introduction to the many previous theories of dreams, I wanted to examine their assumptions (Freud, 1917, p. 222; 1925, p. 47), especially the underlying assumptions (Freud, 1900, p. 75; 1927, p. 30) of the schools of thought.

The question arising for me was what the differences were in the assumptions of the respective schools and the ways in which they had each developed, especially after "the blossoming of a variety of psychoanalytic theories such as those of Kohut, Lacan, and many others" (Chessick, 1997). This is how my own long journey from European to American psychoanalysis began. Since the 1970s, after the establishment of various new psychoanalytic schools and perspectives, discussions developed over the years concerning the concept of "perspectivism." They began with Edgar A. Levenson's 1972 book, *The Fallacy of Understanding* and Lawrence Friedman's book review of it entitled "Perspectivism in Psychotherapy" (1974).

This led to more than two decades of discussions regarding this term (Hoffman, I. Z.; Levenson E. A., 1989, 1990; Chessick, R. D.; Stern, D. B.; Iannuzzi, V. P.; and Hinshelwood, R., 2012). (Protter discussed pluralism or perspectivism. He thought that "the view that there are multiple interpretive standpoints from which to see phenomena, touches on yet another more

DOI: 10.4324/9781003027768-29

recent controversy relating to the practice/theory, clinical/metapsychology themes" (Protter, 1988), and later coined the term of pluralistic perspectivism (Protter, 1996)).

Gabbard then observed that:

> A burgeoning literature on social constructivism, mutuality, intersubjectivity, relativism, and perspectivism has stressed that absolute objectivity is a myth and that the analyst's subjectivity inevitably enters into perceptions of the analysand (Aron, 1996; Gill, 1994; Greenberg, 1991; Hoffman, 1992; Levine, 1994; Mitchell, 1993; Natterson, 1991; Ogden, 1994; Renik, 1993; Stolorow et al., 1987).
>
> (Gabbard, 1997, p. 15)

He also wrote:

> As Hanly (1995), argues, psychoanalysis should consider the possibility of an epistemology that integrates objectivity and subjectivity. As analysts most of us oscillate between a one-person relatively objective intrapsychic focus and a two-person intersubjective focus (Gabbard, 1996b; Sandler, 1996). Even modernity and post-modernism need not be as polarised as they often are (1997, p. 16).

The Various Views and Divisions in Psychoanalysis, What Did All This Mean?

As I mentioned in the Introduction, while studying these differences in psychoanalytic schools, I found myself walking through an exhibition called "Constable: The Great Landscapes" and studying paintings, perspective, and standpoint/point of view. I began to understand better what Bion meant by the terms vertices, transformations, and invariants (see Introduction). To understand the development of the variety of different schools of thought I had to go deeper in search of clarification.

Historical Background and Development of the Terms

Standpoint/Point of View and Perspective

Perspective can be the view of spatial conditions, as Jacobson said "Perspective, in art, is a system of representation of objects in spatial recession, on a particular observer, in relation to a fixed point of view" (Jacobson, 1973, p. 11).

However, perspective does not only mean the "representation in a drawing or painting of parallel lines as converging in order to give the illusion of depth and distance," (Merriam-Webster, Inc., n.d., perspective 4a) or a "method of graphically depicting three-dimensional objects and spatial relationships on a two-dimensional plane or on a plane that is shallower than the original" (Encyclopædia Britannica, 2020).

Among the different meanings of this term, I was particularly interested in the fact that perspective nowadays is furthermore connected with the meaning of standpoint, not only as the "physical place where you stand" but also as connected with "the way you 'see' things as a result of who you are and what you do" (Merriam-Webster, Inc., n.d., perspective). That is, a certain attitude with which one sees something and assesses it from a particular point of view.

Perspective and Perspectivism in Philosophy

When we look at philosophy, we find not only the term perspective but also a concept in the philosophy of perspectivism, which means that "the world forms a complex of interacting interpretative processes in which every entity views every other entity and event from an orientation peculiar to itself" (Merriam-Webster, n.d., perspectivism).

Perspectivism can be seen in a second way as a "consciousness of or the process of using different points of view (as in literary criticism or artistic representation)" (Merriam-Webster, n.d., perspectivism).

Gottfried Wilhelm Leibniz was the first to introduce, in The Principles of Philosophy, or *The Monadology* (1714), the terms of perspective and standpoint into philosophy.

> Just as the same city viewed from different directions appears entirely different and, as it were, multiplied perspectively, in just the same way it happens that, because of the infinite multitude of simple substances, there are, as it were, just as many different universes, which are, nevertheless, only perspectives on a single one, corresponding to the different points of view of each monad (sec 147).
>
> (Leibniz, 1989, p. 220)

Friedrich Nietzsche even saw in "the perspectival, the basic condition of all life" (Nietzsche, 2014a).

The Measurability of Objectivity and the Variety of Subjectivity

Nietzsche distinguishes between subjectivity and objectivity as follows:

> "Essence," "essentially" is something perspectival and already presupposes a multiplicity. What underlies here is always "what is that for me?" (for us, for everything that lives etc.)
>
> (Nietzsche, 2020)

and

> "Objectivity,"—the latter not understood as "disinterested contemplation," ... "but as the capacity to have control over one's pro and con and to deploy them: so that we know precisely how to make the diversity of perspectives and affective interpretations useful for knowledge.
>
> (Nietzsche, 2014b)

> But everything for which the word "knowledge" alone makes sense refers to the realm where counting, weighing and measuring can occur, to the quantitative—; while, on the other hand, all our sensations of value (i.e., precisely our sensations) adhere exactly to the qualities, that is, adhere to our perspectival "truths" belonging to us alone, which simply cannot be "known." It is obvious that each being differing from us senses other qualities and thus lives in another world as do we.
>
> (Nietzsche, in press)

The concepts of perspective and standpoint play an important role, not only for Leibnitz or Nietzsche, but also in the philosophies of, for example, Immanuel Kant, Ludwig Wittgenstein, and Edmund Husserl. They appear also in psychology, that of Wilhelm Wundt, Gustav Theodor Fechner, and Jean Piaget, and in the ethnology of Eduardo Viveiros de Castro, and George Herbert Mead (König, 1989).

The so-called perspectival objectivism is based on an objective reality that is interpreted differently due to the different viewpoints and characteristics of the persons looking at it (Leibniz), while the so-called perspectival subjectivism is based on a variety of realities (Nietzsche) (König, 1989).

Ronald Giere (2006) prefers another position, a position between so-called objectivism/realism and so-called constructivism. "The result will be an account of science that brings observation and theory, perception and conception, closer together than they have seemed in objectivist accounts."

To Return to the So-Called Dichotomy Between Objectivity and Subjectivity

Here the foundation of the dichotomy or division of terms in object versus subject, objectivity versus subjectivity, and natural sciences versus social sciences becomes clear. Nowadays objectivity can be conceptually attributable to positivism, subjectivity rather than constructivism, in which man creates his own perceptions.

Object and Subject, Objectivity and Subjectivity: What Is a Science and Can Psychoanalysis Be a Science?

If we want to clarify this issue, we should first clarify the basic terms, concepts, and contexts.

What Is Science?

The term science in the modern sense is relatively new (Hepburn & Andersen, 2021; Hoyningen-Huene, 2015; "Science," 2021; Walsh et al., 2014).

Science, in the sense of all human knowledge and experience, can be understood as a system of scientific knowledge. It provides information in theory and practice about the laws, properties, and causalities of the world. This is expressed in terms of categories, theories, hypotheses, laws and/or units of measurement. The basis of this science is research in the sense of an intersubjectively comprehensible methodical process of investigation in theoretical as well as applied areas.

The goal of science is an ordered, well-founded, and secured knowledge of the world with the associated values of clarity, transparency, objectivity, verifiability, reliability, openness, honesty, novelty, and neutrality.

Science can be divided into sub-areas with appropriate differentiation. These in turn can be divided into those which are purely concerned with the theory and those with practical applications, that is, into rational and empirical sciences. Thus there are both the formal sciences (which use deductive logic), and also the empirical sciences (which use inductive logic) and these include the natural and other applied sciences. For example, medicine can be seen as an applied science along with the subsciences of natural and social sciences, whereas computer science and/or research and statistics form the theoretical, formal side of medicine.

History of Science

The history of science attempts to describe the historical development of science ("History of Science," 2021). Both the theory and practice of natural and social sciences are included in its study.

Science started in Classical Antiquity with the collecting of observations and practices. First there was an oral tradition, later a written one. These investigations were called natural philosophy and natural philosophers became thus the first scientists. In his famous mathematical treatise "Elements," Euclid (around 300 BC) collected, developed, and coordinated his concepts and mathematical terms, such as deduction, theorem, and axioms, terms that remain relevant up to the present. In this way, scientific inquiry was developed and later, encyclopedias about nature were published.

In the Middle Ages, both the monasteries and the medieval universities (with their "seven liberal arts"), gradually developed more modern methods of science. The fall of Constantinople (and the migration of men of knowledge), together with the advance of printing, all marked a new step in the development of science. The following Scientific Revolution during the Renaissance with a beginning around AD 1543 produced many scientific advances. This made modern mathematics, physics, and astronomy possible. With the rise of new technology, modern science was established on a more secure base. During the 19th century, the sciences became increasingly professionalized. Scientific institutions were founded. Thus, out of natural philosophy, the natural sciences were born.

History of Ideas/Intellectual History

The history of ideas/intellectual history, (Horowitz, 2004; "Intellectual History," 2021) whose content is the exploration of ideas and approaches, is a sub-area of the history of science. It has most of its roots in European cultural and intellectual history. Its content is the study of the emergence, development, and impact of scientific concepts, ideas, and approaches within the context of social processes typical of a given epoch. In the United States, this discipline developed further into a social history of ideas, that is, the study of an idea not only as an abstraction, but with consideration to its cultural context, the people involved, and the historical processes. Political, cultural, intellectual, and social factors became important variables, both in chronological and contemporary contextualization. The history of thought eventually included many disciplines.

Philosophy of Science

Philosophy of science is a subbranch of philosophy (Humphreys, 2016; Kuhn, 1970; Ladyman, 2002; Morrison, 2016; "Philosophy of Science," 2021).

It is concerned with the conceptualization and the form of knowledge acquisition in science. There are connections especially with the philosophical fields of epistemology and methodology. The central concern of this discipline is the question of correct and exact cognition and the clarification of what science is and what it is not.

The basic themes of this philosophy of science are general questions about science, such as the definition of the term science, the methodology, reliability, and validation of its results. Also belonging to this subject are fundamental questions concerning individual particular sciences.

Further important questions arise from the question of comparisons of differences and correspondences in methods, objects, material, and topics of each discipline.

History of the Philosophy of Science

(Hepburn & Andersen, 2021; "History and Philosophy of Science," 2021; Patton, 2014) A first phase in the history of the philosophy of science is seen from antiquity until the middle of the 17th century when science was regarded as absolutely certain knowledge, generated from deduction and derivation from evident axioms. In a second phase until the end of the 19th century, scientific methods in the sense of inductive procedures with strict rules are introduced. This is followed by a third phase which lasted until the late 20th century, in which the scientific methods for obtaining science are retained, but the demand for absolute certainty is abandoned. In this phase, knowledge becomes fallible (Hoyningen-Huene, 2015).

Methodologies of Science, Logic, and Philosophy

Logic (Bobzien, 2020; "History of Logic," 2021) can be described as a method of reasoning, which is considered to lead to correct conclusions. Consistency is its topic. It is also called a doctrine of thought (laws of thinking). Traditionally, logic was a subfield of philosophy. Its roots for European culture can be found in the pre-Socratics, Sophists, Stoics, and Peripatetics. On the one hand, according to an ancient and a medieval logic, a so-called classical, formal, or Aristotelian-scholastic logic can be distinguished from a modern mathematical or symbolic logic that has been developing since 1847. Today the term logic can be understood as a relatively fuzzy collective term for different logics that have developed over time.

Theory

A theory, ("Theory," 2021) generally speaking, is usually a cognition achieved by thinking. The scientific concept of theory has its origins in Pythagoras and mathematical logic. A scientific theory stands for a system of scientifically founded statements with the goal of explaining underlying laws of sections of reality and, if necessary, making prospective forecasts. From a positivistic point of view, it stands for a model of reality with descriptive and explanatory statements, which can be checked and, if necessary, verified or falsified by observation methods or methodical-systematic collection of data. Nowadays, however, all theories are understood to be ultimately provisional.

Theoretical elements are the so-called basic assumptions, the basic concepts (Freud, 1900, p. 75; 1917, p. 222; 1927, p. 30), or the underlying assumptions of theoreticians with descriptive and explanatory statements (the latter are also called hypotheses). These include measurement concepts and empirical evidence. The decisive factor is a scientific method that meets scientific criteria.

The term scientific theory ("Scientific Theory," 2021) is distinguished from both the term scientific models and the term hypotheses.

The scientific model (Hatzimanolis, 2018; "Scientific Modelling," 2021) can mean, for example, an abstract, simplified compact conceptualized construction based on scientific work for the logical explanation of complex processes or complex reality. Such models can—when experimentation and measurement are impossible—be used as an abstraction and simplified substitute (for these where theory construction is not yet possible).

Hypotheses ("Hypothesis," 2021) are generally proposed explanations for reality, based on previous observations. They are assumptions, which are formulated in a logical statement and whose validity is not yet proven. A hypothesis has to be verifiable by scientific methods in order to be considered scientific.

Theses on the other hand are considered to be assertions. Scientific theses should be confirmed or rejected with the help of scientific proof.

The Classical Axiom and the Term "Assumption"

The axiom can be seen as a principle that is accepted as true ("Axiom (Disambiguation)," 2021). It can be seen as a principle of a theory but also of a whole science. It is not substantiated or deductively derived but assumed without proof. It serves as a starting point for other statements or positions and does not require further examination.

The classical axiom is based on Euclid and Aristotle. Closely related concepts from this period are postulate and basic assumptions. From an axiom or axioms, logically compelling consequences can be deduced. The axiom is the basis of deductive knowledge (Balzer, 2009).

Assumptions as Axioms

From this point of view, what Freud called underlying assumptions in his early work can be seen as equivalent to axioms for that which is called psychoanalysis.

Psychoanalysis and Science

Now knowing the elements, or better, the basics of science and sciences, we will look at the implications of these basics for psychoanalysis as a science (Walsh et al., 2014).

The Differentiation of Sciences in Nature and Human/ Social Sciences

In the course of the history of science, the natural sciences first developed, then, for example, beginning with the scientific revolution over the course of about two centuries, new disciplines such as history, psychology, or later, sociology, which often had to emancipate themselves from philosophy. Wilhelm Dilthey (Makkreel, 2021) distinguished nature and human sciences which were later called social sciences in the development of science.

Different Methods for the Two Science Groups, Natural and Social Sciences

Natural and social sciences differ in particular in the method by which their respective subject matter is recorded. The natural sciences make use of empirical research, objects or events, data, and fact-gathering if necessary. Experiments or laboratory tests and corresponding interpretations are based on this. In social sciences the method of choice is the interpretation of data or events in the sense of a hermeneutic access to understanding. For the interpretation, both the approaches of interpretation and the meanings of interpretations are important. Friedrich Schleiermacher called the interpretation of data and context the hermeneutic circle ("Hermeneutic Circle," 2021).

Hermeneutics can be seen as a study of the interpretation of human meanings and experiences. Sometimes it is called a "philosophy of interpretation."

Now we come to the so-called hard problem of consciousness and the mind-brain problem.

The Objectivity or the Subjectivity of the Respective Observation

These two science groups were discriminated by methodological differences.

In the natural sciences, one researches objects and aims to reach objectivity in one's results. In social or human sciences one can only reach a subjective view of the subject. You can differentiate the empirical and analytic sciences from the historical and hermeneutic sciences. The main question is which type of the result of research and observation can be reached. This depends on the topic of the search for information, the so-called objectivity of an object in natural sciences or the subjectivity of the subject of the observation. Causality remains a very complex question.

Social Sciences and Psychology

History of Psychology as Science and as Profession

The history of psychology as a science and a profession then became widely discussed by Walsh et al. (2014) in their book *A Critical History and Philosophy of Psychology*.

For many centuries to millennia, the study of psychic phenomena has been the subject of philosophy. It was not until the 19th century that the discipline of psychology developed hesitantly. During the scientific revolution, natural philosophers were still concerned with psychic phenomena. Only Helmholtz's studies made early natural science psychology possible. Wundt then founded a natural science psychology with his physiological psychology and his psychological laboratory. While psychology has so far been attributed to philosophy, it has been divided into a natural science psychology or a human or social sciences psychology with a humanistic philosophical tradition. At the same time, the knowledge of psychology and the professional profile of the psychologist, the scientific discipline, and the profession slowly developed. Psychology increasingly became an independent autonomous science.

Psychology as part of philosophy was the past, scientific psychology was the future. An institutionalization of the "New Psychology" with societies and magazines followed. Binet founded test psychology and William James, along with others, American functional psychology. In addition to experimental psychology, Gestalt psychology, different versions of behaviorism and person-centered psychology developed. Natural-scientific psychology is marked by analytical and explanatory methods, the human-scientific psychology by descriptive. Habermas differentiated between empirical-analytic and historical-hermeneutical sciences.

Paradigms

Thomas Kuhn, in *The Structure of Scientific Revolutions*, which was a history of science, coined the term "paradigm" for the basics of each respective discipline. This is very helpful in a variety of ways. Competing paradigms or conceptual systems are seen within a wide range of intellectual, cultural, economic, and political developments. He is referring to a particular set of untestable essential concepts, which build the basic structure of the respective discipline and provide generally accepted examples of its methods of investigation (Kuhn, 1962, p. 137; Walsh et al., 2014).

In the context of a constantly changing scientific world with ever-new insights, Kuhn sees not an evolutionary development of science but rather a revolutionary one. Scientific changes are seen to be following what Kuhn called paradigm shifts. The concepts within a paradigm continue to change as new knowledge is added and finally the paradigm itself is discarded. According to Kuhn, science changes in five steps.

1 At first, the old science has become brittle in its explanations. This leads to considerations as to how to solve the problems identified. This can be seen as a hallmark of a pre-paradigmatic phase.
2 This is followed by a normal scientific phase of changes in scientific foundations.

3 This can be followed by a period of crisis as a result of even newer findings or problems.
4 This leads to confusion of the revolution phase, during which the respective discipline eventually integrates scientific progress.
5 This is followed by a normal phase of the now-renewed science. Scientific development can have not only a rational but also a social and an interpersonal dimension.

It can be said that followers of different paradigms can live psychologically in different worlds.

The Development of Psychoanalysis as a Discipline via Two Different Approaches, Medicine and Psychology

After Freud had established psychoanalysis as a theory and treatment method it remained for a long time as a medical subdiscipline. Its main domain was psychiatry, the discipline for severe mental illnesses. In the United States, in addition to biological psychiatry, a dynamic psychiatry based on psychoanalysis was being developed. Psychoanalysis became a subdiscipline of psychiatry and thus of medicine. The American Psychoanalytic Association was established and until the 1950s it was necessary to be an MD in order to be able to practice psychoanalysis.

On the other hand, after WWII, psychology as a discipline began to grow. During the 1920s, Floyd Allport had developed an experimental social psychology, and this discipline expanded with the recognition of social problems after WWII. Interpersonal relations and the behavior of groups became important subjects of study. Also the WWII veterans needed help. Therefore, psychologists were allowed to practice psychotherapies. However, psychologists were not allowed to offer psychoanalytic treatment until the late 1950s.

Many social conflicts within society had to be managed. The problems and conflicts became more evident, and in this situation, psychology became the discipline for the study of social problems of a particular time. Personality and intelligence tests and their operators, clinical psychologists, were needed; special treatments and trainings too. Psychology was expanding and differentiating into an applied and a professional psychology. During the 1950s and the 1960s, clinical programs and clinical specializations were developed. Psychologists wanted to practice treatment and special psychological schools were founded, while specialization and subspecialties were developed (Walsh et al., 2014). After psychologists experienced problems with the American Psychoanalytic Association (APA), the APA developed a psychoanalytical division, Division 39 (Eisold, 2018b).

What Were the Implications of these Historical Developments for the Discipline of Psychoanalysis?

Here again my questions mentioned above:

1 Can psychoanalysis be a science?
2 Have I discovered the reasons for so many psychoanalytic approaches?
3 Can there be a correct view?

1 Can Psychoanalysis Be a Science?

Nowadays, science is seen as a system of knowledge that deals with the phenomena of our world and is based on observation and experiments. Knowledge is seen as a search for truths or general rules. Science will be divided into different areas depending on the subject, such as physical, biological, or social sciences, each with its own methods.

This study for this book has led me to the conclusion that psychoanalysis is a science, however not a natural science, which it considered itself at the start, but a human/social science. The method of psychoanalysis is hermeneutics, the theory of the interpretation of texts and understanding all the questions and problems that arise from it (Walsh et al., 2014).

2 Reasons for So Many Psychoanalytic Approaches

In the beginning of my professional life I was confused by the contrast between the cohesive nature of medical thinking and the great variety of psychoanalytic schools and perspectives. Through my medical education, the standpoint of objectivity was clear to me and dear to me. So, what were the reasons for this variety in the many psychoanalytic perspectives?

2.1 Paradigm Shifts

Thinking about the development of so many psychoanalytic approaches we need a great deal of information. Like Kurt Danzinger I think we can understand the development, or better, the history of psychoanalysis as a subgroup of psychology yet not without its respective context, social (cultural, intellectual, and technological), and individual history. The development of scientific theory is always context-dependent (Danziger, 1979, 1990, 1997; Kuhn, 1962; Rieber, 2012).

When looking at the beginnings of psychoanalysis we see that it started with Freud's discovery of the unconscious. However, he was a child of his Victorian time. His social and scientific context was marked (in a history of science sense) by a mechanistic-energistic-positivistic structure of thinking. He emerged at a time when psychology was still philosophy in the context of the respective social conditions and natural-science models of thought. In the course of the historical development of psychoanalysis as described in this book, it is possible to see that the psychoanalytic models have been influenced by the respective prevailing social, intellectual, and scientific currents.

Terms and concepts are subject to change through the increase in knowledge, but the framework, the psychoanalyst-patient relationship and the notion of the unconscious remain important constants.

2.2 Paradigm Shifts in Psychoanalysis

Applying the considerations of Thomas Kuhn and Kurt Danzinger and many others (Kuhn, 1962; Walsh et al., 2014), the development can be seen to have taken place in the following way.

Because at the beginning of psychoanalysis the developers were medical doctors, the development, or better, the focus, was influenced by their thinking and the principles of medicine. Freud was very much connected with the natural scientific models and concepts of his time and the 19th-century paradigms of natural science.

When with Ferenczi and Abraham an object relation view emerged, gradually the mother-child relationship entered into the focus of the observation to add to, but sometimes replace, the Oedipal focus. The paradigm became the observation of the mother-child relationship (here medicine more as a human or applied science), later called infant research.

Here also began the shift from the one-person-psychology to a two-person psychology. The growth of social psychology before and after WWII changed the world of psychoanalysis.

Before WWII, there was some interest in the social and cultural context (for example the Neo-Freudians). However, WWII and its consequences, especially for the veterans, made the need for the disciplines such as social psychology more and more clear. Social psychologists became regarded as specialists in their own right. As clinical psychologists they became allowed to practice psychotherapeutic treatment and later to train in psychoanalysis. They needed training facilities and seem to have adapted psychoanalytic concepts to their social psychological concepts and knowledge based on their psychological and not a medical training.

This appears to have changed psychoanalysis from the inside as it were, in a direction from a natural or human or applied science (medicine) to a social science (psychology). These two areas of knowledge only sometimes have the same ideas about the world, which hopefully leads to useful tensions, conflicts, and constructive outcomes.

The latest paradigm shifts seem to be linked to new insights through improved investigation techniques and technological progress (video, fMRI).

Other local paradigm shifts seem to be caused by a philosophical Zeitgeist, such as Lacan (structuralism) and relational psychoanalysis (constructivism).

Thus there were many developments of different psychoanalytic approaches and shifts (Eisold, 2018c, 2018d) over the decade in the last century and a quarter.

People could or can hold on to them, adapt them to the respective developments or develop new, correspondingly new knowledge and perspectives. Psychoanalysis will remain an always-changing discipline, adapted to the respective knowledge and requirements of ever-new types of patients (Eisold, 2018a). Eisold describes all these developments. "Some belong to strict or strong schools: Kleinian, Lacanian, interpersonalists, ego psychologists, and so forth. Others are more eclectic, more accepting of the current pluralistic world" (Eisold, 2018b, p. 186).

2.3 Subjectivity of the Psychoanalysts

When looking at the varieties of subjectivity of psychoanalytic perspectives, remember the positions of Nietzsche about subjectivity. To understand the varieties of the schools of thought, Bion and his terms of transformations and vertices were especially helpful for me. He argued that a psychoanalyst transforms the facts he describes "by regarding them in a particular way. My description is therefore a transformation, analogous to the artist's painting that is a product of the particular artist's approach" (Bion, 1965, p. 10).

> "Transformations may be scientific, aesthetic, religious, mystical, (or) psycho-analytical."
>
> (Bion, 1965, p. 140)

Bion saw the work of a psychoanalyst lying

> between the point where a man receives sense impressions and the point where he gives expression to the transformation that has taken place. The principles of this investigation must be the same whether the medium is painting, music, mathematics, sculpture, or a relationship between two people, whether expressed verbally or by any other means. (These principles must be determined so that they remain constant whether the transformation is effected in a mind which is sane or insane.)
>
> (Bion, 1965, p. 46. or similar in Bion, 1970, p. 21)

Respective to my questions about the various schools of thought, Bion wrote that it would be "helpful to regard psycho-analytical theories as belonging to the category of groups of transformations, a technique analogous to that of a painter, by which the facts of an analytic experience (the realization) are transformed into an interpretation (the representation)" (Bion, 1965, p. 4).

3 Can There Be a Correct Way?

I believe now after editing this book that this question cannot be asked in this way. In the course of the historical development of psychoanalysis, as described before, the psychoanalytic thinking, the models, concepts, and methods seem to have been adapted to the respective prevailing social, intellectual, and scientific currents and the increasing knowledge by research. Nowadays, we can find analysts who are still working according to old models, concepts, and methods, others according to adapted ones, others eclectic or after the newer or the latest ones (for example see Chapter 9, Leon Hoffman, p. 101).

There are different ways of thinking in psychoanalysis, not one correct way. Personal subjectivity seems to be the main reason for the diverse schools of mind and the different perspectives. The personal standpoint, the subjectivity of the analyst seems to affect his choice of perspective and respective assumptions, conscious/unconscious. He is also influenced by the cultural assumptions of the major centers of the psychoanalytic movement/development.

Under the collective term or umbrella of psychoanalysis we can find the most diverse schools of psychoanalysis. However, the importance of the framework, the psychoanalyst-patient relationship and the idea of the unconscious remain the two major constants in this enterprise.

I would like to end this chapter today with the still relevant words of Freud from 1923: The goal of psychoanalysis is the accumulation "of psychological information … accumulated into a new scientific discipline" (p. 235). As we have seen, much depends on your definition of science.

References

Axiom (Disambiguation). (2021, September 2). In *Wikipedia*. https://en.wikipedia.org/w/index.php?title=Axiom_(disambiguation)&oldid=1027731275

Balzer, W. (2009). *Science and its methods, principles of philosophy of science*. Alber.

Bion, W. R. (1965). *Transformations: Change from learning to growth*. Tavistock.

Bion, W. R. (1970). *Attention and interpretation*. Tavistock.

Bobzien, S. (2020). Ancient logic. *The Stanford Encyclopedia of Philosophy* (Summer 2020 Edition). Retrieved August 22, 2021, from https://plato.stanford.edu/archives/sum2020/entries/logic-ancient/

Chessick, R. D. (1997). Perspectivism, constructivism, and empathy in psychoanalysis: Nietzsche and Kohut. *Journal of the American Academy of Psychoanalysis*, *25*(3), 373–398.

Danziger, K. (1979). The social origins of modern psychology. In A. R. Buss (Ed.), *Psychology in social context* (pp. 29–45). Irvington.

Danziger, K. (1990). *Constructing the subject: Historical origins of psychological research*. Cambridge University Press.

Danziger, K. (1997). *Naming the mind: How psychology found a language*. Sage.

Eisold, K. (2018a). Psychoanalysis and psychotherapy. A long and troubled relationship. In K. Eisold (Ed.), *The organizational life of psychoanalysis: Conflicts, dilemmas, and the future of the profession* (pp. 55–81). Routledge.

Eisold, K. (2018b). Psychoanalysis as a profession: Past failures and future possibilities. In K. Eisold (Ed.), *The organizational life of psychoanalysis: Conflicts, dilemmas, and the future of the profession* (pp. 181–209). Routledge.
Eisold, K. (2018c). The intolerance of diversity in psychoanalytic institutes. In K. Eisold (Ed.), *The organizational life of psychoanalysis: Conflicts, dilemmas, and the future of the profession* (pp. 85–110). Routledge.
Eisold, K. (2018d). The splitting of the New York Psychoanalytic Society and the construction of psychoanalytic authority. In K. Eisold (Ed.), *The organizational life of psychoanalysis: Conflicts, dilemmas, and the future of the profession* (pp. 32–54). Routledge.
Encyclopædia Britannica, Incorporated. (2020). Perspective. In *Britannica.com dictionary*. Retrieved September 4, 2020 from www.britannica.com
Freud, S. (1900). The interpretation of dreams. In J. Strachey (Ed. and Trans.), *The standard edition of the complete works of Sigmund Freud* (Vol. 4–5, pp. 1–627). Hogarth Press.
Freud, S. (1914). On the history of the psycho-analytic movement. In J. Strachey (Ed. and Trans.), *The standard edition of the complete works of Sigmund Freud* (Vol. 14, pp. 1–66). Hogarth Press.
Freud, S. (1917). A metapsychological supplement to the theory of dreams. In J. Strachey (Ed. and Trans.), *The standard edition of the complete works of Sigmund Freud* (Vol. 14, pp. 217–235). Hogarth Press.
Freud, S. (1923). Two encyclopedia articles. In J. Strachey (Ed and Trans.), *The standard edition of the complete works of Sigmund Freud* (Vol. 18, pp. 235–259). Hogarth Press.
Freud, S. (1925). An autobiographical study. In J. Strachey (Ed. and Trans.), *The standard edition of the complete works of Sigmund Freud* (Vol. 20, pp. 1–74). Hogarth Press.
Freud, S. (1927). The future of an illusion. In J. Strachey (Ed. and Trans.), *The standard edition of the complete works of Sigmund Freud* (Vol. 21, pp. 1–56). Hogarth Press.
Friedman, L. (1974). Perspectivism in psychotherapy. *Contemporary Psychoanalysis*, *10*, 125–142.
Gabbard, G. O. (1997). A reconsideration of objectivity in the analyst. *International Journal of Psycho-Analysis*, *78*, 15–26.
Giere, R. (2006). *Scientific perspectivism*. University of Chicago Press.
Hatzimanolis, D. (2018). Scientific models. *Investigating Science*. Retrieved August 23, 2021, from https://investigatingsciencehsc.com/scientific-models/
Hermeneutic Circle. (2021, August 29). In *Wikipedia*. https://en.wikipedia.org/w/index.php?title=Hermeneutic_circle&oldid=1035330914
Hepburn, B. & Andersen, H. (2021). Scientific method. The Stanford Encyclopedia of Philosophy (Summer 2021 Edition). Retrieved August 27, 2021, from https://plato.stanford.edu/archives/sum2021/entries/scientific-method/
Hinshelwood, R. (2012). On being objective about the subjective: Clinical aspects of intersubjectivity in contemporary psychoanalysis. *International Forum of Psychoanalysis*, *21*, 136–145.
History and Philosophy of Science. (2021, August 24). In *Wikipedia*. https://en.wikipedia.org/w/index.php?title=History_and_philosophy_of_science&oldid=1033551104

History of Logic. (2021, August 22). In *Wikipedia*. https://en.wikipedia.org/w/index.php?title=History_of_logic&oldid=1039156787
History of Science. (2021, July 30). In *Wikipedia*. https://en.wikipedia.org/w/index.php?title=History_of_science&oldid=1037187392
Horowitz, M. C. (Ed.). (2004). *New dictionary of the history of ideas* (6 volumes). Scribner.
Hoyningen-Huene, P. (2015). *Systematicity: The nature of science*. (2nd ed.). Oxford University Press.
Humphreys, P. (Ed.). (2016). *The Oxford handbook of philosophy of science*. Oxford University Press.
Hypothesis. (2021, August 23). In *Wikipedia*. https://en.wikipedia.org/w/index.php?title=Hypothesis&oldid=1024930586
Intellectual History. (2021, August 22). In *Wikipedia*. https://en.wikipedia.org/w/index.php?title=Intellectual_history&oldid=1026098843
Jacobson, J. I. (1973). *Perspectivism in art*. Philosophical Library.
König, G. (1989). Perspective, perspectivism, perspectival subjectivism. In J. Ritter & K. Gründer (Eds.), *Historical dictionary of philosophy* (Vol. 7, pp. 362–375). Scientific Book Society.
Kuhn, T. S. (1962). *The structure of scientific revolutions*. University of Chicago Press.
Kuhn, T. S. (1970). *The structure of scientific revolutions* (2nd ed.). University of Chicago Press.
Ladyman, J. (2002). *Understanding philosophy of science*. Routledge.
Leibniz, G. W. (1989). *Philosophical essays*. (R. Ariew & D. Garber, Trans.). Hackett Publishing.
Levenson, E. A. (1972). *The fallacy of understanding*. Basic Books.
Levenson, E. A. (1989). Whatever happened to the cat?—Interpersonal perspectives on the self. *Contemporary Psychoanalysis, 25*, 537–553.
Levenson, E. A. (1990). Reply to Hoffman. *Contemporary Psychoanalysis, 26*, 299–304.
Makkreel, R. (2021). Wilhelm Dilthey. *The Stanford Encyclopedia of Philosophy* (Spring 2021 Edition). Retrieved August 29, 2021, from https://plato.stanford.edu/archives/spr2021/entries/dilthey/
Merriam-Webster, (n.d.). Perspective. In *Merriam-Webster.com dictionary*. Retrieved from https://www.merriam-webster.com/dictionary/perspective
Merriam-Webster, (n.d.). Perspectivism. In *Merriam-Webster.com dictionary*. Retrieved from https://www.merriam-webster.com/dictionary/perspectivism
Morrison, M. (2016). Models and theories. In P. Humphreys (Ed.), *The Oxford handbook of philosophy of science* (pp. 378–396). Oxford University Press.
Nietzsche, F. (2014a). Beyond good and evil, Preface. In A. Del Caro (Trans.), *The complete works of Friedrich Nietzsche: Beyond good and evil/On the genealogy of morality* (Vol. 8, p. 2). Stanford University Press.
Nietzsche, F. (2014b). On the genealogy of morality. In A. Del Caro (Trans.), *The complete works of Friedrich Nietzsche: Beyond good and evil/On the genealogy of morality* (Vol. 8, p. 308). Stanford University Press.
Nietzsche, F. (2020). 2 (149) 218. In A. Del Caro (Trans.), *The complete works of Friedrich Nietzsche: Unpublished Fragments (Spring 1885 – Spring 1886)* (Vol. 16, p. 377). Stanford University Press.

Nietzsche, F. (in press). 6 (14). In G. H. Leiner (Trans.), *Unpublished Fragments: Summer 1886–Fall 1887, The Complete Works of Friedrich Nietzsche* (Vol. 17). Stanford University Press.

Patton, L. (2014). *Philosophy, science, and history*, pp. 27–33. Routledge.

Philosophy of Science. (2021, August 22). In *Wikipedia*. https://en.wikipedia.org/w/index.php?title=Philosophy_of_science&oldid=1035988737

Protter, B. (1988). Ways of knowing in psychoanalysis—Some epistemic considerations for an autonomous theory of psychoanalytic praxis. *Contemporary Psychoanalysis*, *24*, 498–526.

Protter, B. (1996). Classical, modern, and postmodern psychoanalysis: Epistemic transformations. *Psychoanalytic Dialogue*, *6*(4), 533–562.

Rieber, R. W. (Ed.). (2012). *Encyclopedia of the history of psychological theories*. Springer.

Science. (2021, August 27). In *Wikipedia*. https://en.wikipedia.org/w/index.php?title=Science&oldid=1040341076

Scientific Modelling. (2021, August 23) In *Wikipedia*. https://en.wikipedia.org/w/index.php?title=Scientific_modelling&oldid=1039442249

Scientific Theory. (2021, August 22). In *Wikipedia*. https://en.wikipedia.org/w/index.php?title=Scientific_theory&oldid=1039501290

Theory. (2021, September 4). In *Wikipedia*. https://en.wikipedia.org/w/index.php?title=Theory&oldid=1038058231

Walsh, R. T. G., Teo, T., & Baydala, A. (2014). *A critical history and philosophy of psychology*. Cambridge University Press.

Chapter 29

Prospectus and Perspectives

Bernd Huppertz

During my journey through the world of schools of thought, I found perspectives that were particularly interesting to me and which I suggest may permit a glimpse into the future development of psychoanalysis.

The Motivational Systems

Joseph Lichtenberg developed, starting in 1989, a new integrated experience-based vision of psychoanalysis in theory and practice. Attempting to study human experience and the concepts of identity, development, and motivation, he developed a model of what has become seven motivational systems. He connected the term human experience with a doer's experiences of doing, so-called lived experience. The subjects of the study were the changing experiences of individuals during the course of their lives in the context of internal and external events. Identity in this context means the experience of who we are and how we are shaped, shown in the analysands' narratives, particularly their narratives of identity (Lichtenberg, 1989).

Based on his study of mother-child research, he found that people could, by observing the mother and baby interacting over 24 hours and day by day, recognize how driven by motivation their interactions are for both and therefore, what motivation means. For Lichtenberg, intentions are signs of motivation. The seeking of the respective baby or later the individual for something which is suitable for his respective needs and wishes is a manifestation of a motivation. Based on mother and child research, he recognized five motivational systems at first. Later he added two further systems. He wished to provide an overview of all experiences that people undergo during their lives. Each of these systems has its typical affects, intentions, and goals. The development of these motivational systems begins at birth and lasts throughout life. Intersubjective experience, from the very first hour of mother-infant interaction, shapes the affective tone, as an affective matrix of the individual and his respective disposition and expectations. This underlying basic tone can be changed during the whole lifetime and reflects the respective adaptive successes or failures achieved. Thus intersubjective

DOI: 10.4324/9781003027768-30

experience can influence and develop the affective basic tone of the individual throughout his life.

Motivational systems are self-organizing and stabilizing. Each of these systems is marked by respective affects, intentions, and goals, which interact with the affects and intentions of the other systems. The respective affects have a wide range of intensity. Alternately, depending on the respective moment and according to the existing needs or desires, one of the motivational systems is the dominant one and in the foreground.

Motivational systems are dynamic and open systems. Affects have a wide range of intensities and can vitalize and soothe. Vitalization is the driving force.

For Lichtenberg et al. (2021), seeking, not drive or instinct, represents the starter and spark for the activating affects, the intentions, and the goals of the respective motivational system. Seeking is the motivational source for experiences and seeking can be accompanied by other functions to achieve various intentions and goals: (1) clarification of needs, (2) planning, (3) reflection, and (4) the examination of boundaries. The experience of seeking can be found at the beginning of the start of every system.

Lichtenberg had tried since the 1980s and later, together with his colleagues, Lachman and Fosshage, to integrate both the latest research results of science, especially neuroscience, epigenetics, and infant research, as well as the newer and latest concepts in psychoanalysis into this concept of motivational systems. This concept further developed over the last four decades into the seven motivational systems (Lichtenberg, 1989; Lichtenberg et al., 1992, 1996, 2002, 2011, 2021).

The first is the motivational system for the regulation of physiological requirements. This stands for the physiological regulation of the body, health, and psychophysical balance. The second is the attachment motivational system. This stands for relationship, closeness, trust, or affection. The third is the exploratory (and the assertion of preferences) motivational system. This stands for exploring, searching, and mastering the environment, and the activities of learning, working, and playing. The fourth is the aversive (aversive antagonism and withdrawal) motivational system. This stands for the ability to recognize aversive situations and to behave and regulate them accordingly. The fifth is the sensuality and sexuality motivational system. This stands for sensual vitality, together or alone, and for orgasmic experience in the sense of sexuality.

Later in 2011, a sixth and seventh motivational systems were added by Lichtenberg. The sixth is the affiliative motivational system. This stands for the connection and belonging to a group (family, tribe, peers, team, state, or country). The seventh is the caregiving motivational system. This stands for caring for the needs of others with compassion and for altruism.

Lichtenberg's theory is called the model of motivational systems (attachment, caregiving, affiliation, regulation of physiological requirements, sensuality and sexuality, exploration and assertion of preferences, and aversive antagonism and withdrawal). It is based on the newest research. Lichtenberg et al. differentiate three development pathways: (1) of human relatedness and intimacy, (2) of mastering of the environment, and (3) of physiological regulation and a healthy body, which in turn are influenced in the course of life by changes, extensions, and limitations that occur.

The infant is looking for what they want from the very beginning. Intersubjective experience in infancy is rather holistic. Later as a child or adult, reflection is used to try to achieve what is sought and not easy to achieve. In the search for intimacy, mastery, and health, the affective basic tone can change in the course of life and influence the core sense of self. Failure in seeking can result in disappointment and search for alternatives or in disillusionment and termination of the respective intention. During the first year of life, the individual starts to categorize his experiences and assign them to the respective motivational systems.

Three generalized emotional states may develop from the corresponding experiences, 1) a generalized affect tonality of positive affection, 2) a sense of the degree of power, mastery, and ability, and 3) a feeling of physical well-being. These, in turn, have a great influence on the identity and disposition of the individual.

Thus, the psychoanalytic method of therapy in Lichtenberg's sense is based on the following factors: associative and interpretative process with formation of insight and meaning, empathetic listening and formation of a relationship, as well as the changing nonverbal ambience between analyst and analysand. Treatment aims to influence the generalized implicit underlying affect tone of the analysand, which reflects his lifelong experiences. Every individual analysand, at the beginning of a treatment has an underlying affect tone that is influenced by success or failure with regard to the intentions and goals of the individual as a doer. Depending on lifelong success or failure, people can have a positive or negative tint in their underlying affect tones. Analysands often can have, because of trauma, a negative underlying affect tone. This affect tone of the analysand reflects the generalized experiences of affection, competence, and physical well-being. The aim over the time of treatment is to change the mostly negative by a "working through" of the generalized state. Important for the progress of a therapy is the interest of both the analysand and the analyst to solve problems.

Lichtenberg et al. believe that the subtle changes of the affect in the ambiance of a treatment relationship can have a significant influence on the progress of therapy.

Lichtenberg's exploratory technique aimed to clarify the intentions and objectives of the analysand. His way of working was characterized by an open friendliness and security-radiating manner. In an empathetic way, he sought to understand the analysand and his motivation and its origins. For him, the information from the analysand was important. He sought to explore the affective experience in episodic stories, statements, and thoughts at all levels and by these the past and current experiences of analysand and its context. For him, "the message contains the message" (Lichtenberg, 2013, p. 51) on a verbal and a non-verbal level, so all the information levels were important and nothing was left behind for him. He sought to fully explore the stories of the analysands and to form episodes, so-called narratives, affective clinical narratives together with the analysand. Lichtenberg called this "filling the narrative envelope" (Lichtenberg, 2013, p. 70). He paid particular attention to the way the analysand and therapist develop the on-going narrative of the analysand. Lichtenberg named the new look of managing transference and countertransference "wearing the attribution" (Lichtenberg, 2013, p. 84). This means the exploration of how both analysand and psychotherapist talk about self and self with other and the way they see, talk, and form their interaction over the whole time of the treatment.

In biographical episodes, he sought to find, together with the analysand, typical situations, so-called "model scenes" (Lichtenberg, 2013, p. 98). Model scenes were marked by typical constellations, which show interactional schemas in the sense of the typical behaviors of the analysand in dealing with the other and himself. Lichtenberg would also be looking out for aversive motives (Lichtenberg, 2013, personal communication, March 23, 2021).

Here are two typical examples of his way of interacting:

> When in the treatment the patient comes and says, "I don't sleep well at night and it's so bad," there's a puzzle to be solved. What about this sleep thing? Well, the analyst has to say, "Yeah, I'm into that puzzle with you so the two of us can puzzle about, seek an answer to the same puzzle." And if you do that, then you're working together.
>
> (Lichtenberg, personal communication, March 18, 2021)

Another example would be this.

> The patient is talking about an argument she had with her husband the night before and she stops talking. She's silent. Now, I could say, "You have thoughts, then you've defended against them by becoming silent."
>
> Well, then she's going to take out of that, "Oh I did something wrong I shouldn't have done, I was bad." That is not a joint interest. That's a shaming.
>
> Alternatively, if the analyst says, "Where did you drift to in your mind? Where did you go off to?"
>
> "Oh I was thinking about going to the store and trying to remember to pick up the things I need to pick up."
>
> "Oh, has that been a concern that you might forget it?"

> And "Yeah, I was trying to remind myself so I wouldn't have."
>
> "Was that then a part of the earlier discussion with your husband in the argument?"
>
> "Yeah, he was saying I didn't do—"
>
> And you're both playing around with the issue.
>
> (Lichtenberg, personal communication, March 18, 2021)

The late Lichtenberg saw the sense of power, the experience of power of a doer doing it, as the motivating goal of the daily life (personal communication, April 4, 2021). This means the experience of a doer doing it and as a result of the success the feeling of power, conscious or unconscious. In the case of lack of success, Lichtenberg distinguished different ways of restoring the sense of power by adaptive reactions or intentions or by switching to maladaptive reactions or intentions (by anger, fantasy, imagination, or avoidance). The result, therefore, can be constructive or destructive.

According to Lichtenberg, the experience of a sense of power is reflected in the episodes of success and failure in episodic memory and has great significance for the sense of self. A sense of power can be found in the events as well as in the respective moments of daily life. It is also evident during explorative therapy. It can be found in the context of exploration of the past and the history of success and failure as well as in the respective moment of the therapeutic session in different ways. It can be a change of power for example in the interaction or in the context of interpretations. Changes in the sense of power during the treatment can have the above-described results and influences so the therapeutic process should be observed and reflected by the analyst. Thus the sense of power, the experience of a doer doing, can be found in every experience and in every moment.

Systems Theories

Thinking in systems has gained increasing importance over the last century. This interest in the behavior of systems developed in parallel with that of the discipline of physics, where people such as Ernst Mach, Christian von Ehrenfels, Max Wertheimer, Heinz von Foerster, and Ernst von Glaserfeld aimed to extend and document a new scientific view of the world ("Systems Theory," 2021).

General Systems Theory

The biologist Ludwig von Bertalanffy described the general nature of systems, which he then called "general systems theory." It serves as an interdisciplinary approach to the foundations and principles of systems and is intended to clarify and explain different complex phenomena, structures, and dynamics (von Bertalanffy, 1969).

Open Systems Theory

Bertalanffy evolved the notion of "closed" and "open" systems; the latter was later developed as "open systems theory." This was of interest across the board for biologists and social scientists, as well as for information theorists. Open systems theory deals with systems that are related to their environment and are not isolated ("Open System (Systems Theory)," 2021).

Linear and Nonlinear Systems

Systems as such can be regarded as a set of objects that are in a holistic context, are related to each other through interrelationships and are delimited from their environment. Such systems can follow simple or complicated, constant or changeable rules. Simple and complicated, calculable and non-calculable, and linear and nonlinear systems can be distinguished. Linearity means the property of a system to react to the change of one of its parts, a so-called parameter, always known with a corresponding proportional change of another of its parts or another parameter. This refers to a simple system following rules, which is a natural or artificial whole composed of individual parts with different properties with certain ordered, one-dimensional relationships with each other. As long as linear behavior alone was known, the idea that the world could be generally calculable was valid ("Linear System," 2021; "Nonlinear System," 2021).

Chaos Theory

Chaos theory deals with the natural phenomenon of chaotic behavior of nonlinear systems with high sensitivity to the initial conditions. In particular, small changes can cause large changes in the sequence of developing processes ("Chaos Theory," 2021).

Complexity Theory

The discovery of nonlinearity, so-called nonlinear behavior as a result of the mutual influence of parts of objects, objects, systems, and system parts among themselves, opened up the possibility of capturing system states and the complexity of nonlinear behavior. The analysis of such conditions is the task of complexity theory ("Complex System," 2021; Strevens, 2016).

So-called complex systems have a multitude of elements that act dynamically and extensively on each other, nonlinearly, multilaterally, and not in a single direction. The interactions have a short range and can have a direct or indirect effect on themselves, have open borders, are constantly changing, and their information is limited. They develop and remain complex. Often, they arise through spontaneous self-organization and self-organizing order formation, so-called emergence and autonomy. There are a large number of components that have to be considered multi-dimensionally. The nonlinearity of systems can lead to large deviations or large effects, but also to stabilization. The idea of nonlinearity and complex nonlinear systems developed over two centuries (see J. C. Maxwell, H. Poincarè, E. Lorenz, R. May, or J. Yorke) and its influence increased in the last century (Higgins, 2002).

Dynamical Systems Theory

Most living and social systems are nonlinear complex systems. The human organism, for example, as a complex cellular system, is in a fluid equilibrium between order and chaos in health, in which the various elements synergistically interact with each other and nonlinearly influence each other within a complex dynamic system. The task of dynamical systems theory is the behavioral description of these systems. An attempt to investigate system behavior is possible if, as in linear thinking or in the context of linear modeling, the system is reduced to two simple individual components, whose relationship to each other and their corresponding data are recorded and which are intended to show a constant, calculable behavior. In nonlinear thinking and modeling, if the system is reduced to the investigation of its elements, the complex dynamic interactions of the various elements with each other and their variability cannot be properly grasped. The problem with these systems is variability and the resulting predictability. It is comparable to a concert performance. Listening to the respective individual instruments is a different experience than an orchestral performance with all instruments in their acoustic interaction and interactions. Presenting such complex interactions in complex systems presents us with difficult questions (Higgins, 2002).

Dynamic Systems Theory

The consideration of reality as a system or as complex system has led to various theories such as systems theory, chaos theory, complexity theory, and dynamical systems theory. The latter contains a description of the behavior of complex dynamic, nonlinear systems. These dynamic systems themselves form patterns of order, which they change continuously. The dynamic systems theory is particularly concerned with the observation and description of development processes. The developing human being can be regarded as such a system, whose pattern of order or behavior results from spontaneous, local, decentralized interactions of all internal and external components as a type of self-organization. Dynamic systems theory can be defined as theories that "conceptualize development as change within a complex system that involves interactions of multiple factors at different levels and on different timescales (e.g., Smith & Thelen, 2003)" (Alibali et al., 2019).

This new way of looking at and presenting the world has become increasingly important over the decades (Lakshmikantham, 1977; Smith & Thelen, 2003; Strogatz, 2014).

Systems Theories and Medicine and Psychoanalysis

The influence of systems theories on medicine, psychology, and psychoanalysis became increasingly evident (for example, Belair, Bendicsen, Coburn, Dodds, Galatzer-Levy, Ghent, Glass, Hopkins, Metzger, Rai, Rose, Shulman, Rustin, and Tuffin), in this instance, from dynamic systems theory. Alexandra Harrison's (2014) sandwich model is an example of the influence of thinking in systems in respect to the dynamic systems theory (Smith & Thelen, 1993). The sandwich model is based in particular on the experience of the evaluation of video recordings and the corresponding micro-processes viewed in the microanalyses. This is a powerful integrative model that captures the different levels of the psychoanalytic process that develops during therapeutic sessions. It includes, so to speak, "a 'polysemic bundle' of communicative behaviors" (Harrison & Tronick, 2011).

Harrison distinguishes three main levels of "therapeutic action or interaction," although theoretically other diverse levels would be possible. These diverse levels, in turn, constantly maintain diverse interactions with each other (see also Tronick's dyadic expansion of consciousness model (Tronick, 1998, 2005; Troncik & Beeghly, 2011)).

Making meaning of an experience can take place simultaneously on all possible levels during an interaction. According to dynamic systems theory, growth or progress and development are reflected in an increase in the complexity and coherence of the open living system. Applied to psychoanalysis, this means for the analysand, an increase in the adaptability and flexibility of the meanings the individual makes of his experience and his experiences.

In this model, the top and the bottom levels of change cannot be understood by linear models that explain causality. The unpredictability and variability of the evolution of rivers or mountain ranges requires a nonlinear model. The upper level represents the general level of occurring or developing macro-processes of change. Change can be understood here as a reorganization of a system. This level follows the nonlinear theory, the results can be diverse and unpredictable. This level is included to maintain consistency in terms of conceptualization of the change process and is best understood in the psychoanalytic framework in terms of the inability to predict exactly when and in what way a patient will change in response to a treatment. (On this level, it is about linguistic and symbolic meaning and it serves the conceptualization of therapeutic activity in the sense of change.)

The middle level includes the story of what happens in the sessions and in the treatment itself as it is formulated by the analyst in the traditional manner of case presentation. (This is called psychoanalytic theory.) It is the symbolic level. This level uses language and symbols, follows a mostly linear theory, develops a so-called coherent narrative, and wants to create sense and causality. It shows the problems of analysands that are repeated in the different stories. One story can stand for many others. The aim is to change and develop new, different, and more adaptive responses to challenges for the analysands. The lower level, the floor, contains the continuous micro-processes ("the music and dance," the vocal rhythms, and the movements of the two partners of the therapeutic action (Harrison, 2014)).

This conceptualization of change includes the somatic, the non-symbolic, and the moment-to-moment processes, whereby somatic here means the non-conscious somatic communication of the vegetative system. Overall, bodily movement, gestures, or non-verbal speech elements of both, the analysand and the analyst are meant here, which typically, but not always, take place in very short, seconds or millisecond interactive events (for example, body and voice communication, vocal rhythms). These are of such short duration that they cannot be consciously perceived. This level in turn follows nonlinear theory. According to the dynamic systems theory model, the meaning of a narrative depends on its nonverbal context. Somatic meaning, for example, represents the context for the symbolic meaning and vice versa the symbolic meaning represents the context for the somatic meaning. These three levels of the sandwich model also have different time levels: the top level can be measured in decades to centuries, the middle level in minutes to years and the lower level in seconds or milliseconds. Because of the multiple possible meanings that can be made of any human gesture (due to the nonlinearity of the therapeutic interactions and their resulting unpredictability or predictability), there can be no right or wrong interpretation, for example—way of analysis and resulting change. Important for analysand and analysts is the joint development of co-creating a process that creates something new and more adaptable than there was before, meaning understanding and therapeutic change.

The theory can be illustrated by a case of a four-year-old boy who invites the analyst into a struggle by refusing to play with her (Harrison, personal communication, May 20, 2022). Here, the top slice of bread—growth in dynamic systems—represents the child's inability to risk (does not have the energy for) an action at a higher level of organization and stays in the familiar struggle pattern that typifies his problems with his mother and other adults. The child moves toward a symbolic level—the meat of the sandwich—when he tells the analyst that he wants to "throw the girl (doll) in the dump (the fireplace)," but he accompanies his words with the threat of destructive action, which compromises the symbolic meaning. The analyst feels stressed and drawn into the struggle; she too cannot find the energy for the higher level of function—reflective function—and she makes a prohibiting remark—"No, we cannot do that" (throws the doll into the fireplace). In the bottom slice of bread, the micro-process initially shows high attunement of vocal coordination only at points of conflict. Moments later, after the boy leaves the room to enter an adjacent toy closet, the analyst recovers her reflective capacity and when the child reenters, she makes a transference interpretation linking the boy's struggles with his mother and his oppositional behavior with the analyst. She has moved to the level of the meat of the sandwich. The prosody of the analyst's voice and the rhythm of the analyst's vocalizations have become more regular. They are approaching a moment in the session when the micro-process demonstrates a mutually regulated coordination and the dyad moves into pretend play that is enjoyable to both. The micro-process forms a context for the symbolic, and the symbolic forms a context for the micro-process, the meat and the bottom slice of bread fitting together. The top slice of bread functions as a reminder of the overarching context of nonlinear processes of change.

Psychoanalysis has become over time more experimental, more subjective, more interpersonal, and more personal without giving up its search for knowledge. Psychoanalysis is and will remain a field of further explorations, perspectives, and meanings.

References

Alibali, M. W., Brown, S. A., & Menendez, D. (2019). Understanding strategic change: Contextual, individual, and metacognitive factors. In J. Benson (Ed.), *Advances in child development and behavior* (Vol. 56, pp. 227–256). Academic Press.

Chaos Theory. (2021, August 21). In *Wikipedia*. https://en.wikipedia.org/w/index.php?title=Chaos_theory&oldid=1039536507

Complex System. (2021, August 21). In *Wikipedia*, (1.2 Complexity). https://en.wikipedia.org/w/index.php?title=Complex_system&oldid=1039490908

Harrison, A. M. (2014). The sandwich model: The 'music and dance' of therapeutic action. *International Journal of Psycho-Analysis*, *95*(2), 313–340.

Harrison, A. M., & Tronick, E. (2011). "The noise monitor": A developmental perspective on verbal and nonverbal meaning-making in psychoanalysis. *Journal of the American Psychoanalytic Association*, *59*(5), 961–982.

Higgins, J. P. (2002). Nonlinear systems in medicine. *The Yale Journal of Biology and Medicine*, *75*(5–6), 247–260.

Lakshmikantham, V. (Ed.). 1977. *Nonlinear systems and applications: An international conference*. Academic Press.

Lichtenberg, J. D. (1989). *Psychoanalysis and motivation*. The Analytic Press.

Lichtenberg, J. D. (2013). *Craft and spirit: A guide to the exploratory psychotherapies*. Routledge.

Lichtenberg, J. D., Lachmann, F. M., & Fosshage, J. L. (1992). *Self and motivational systems: Toward a theory of psychoanalytic technique*. The Analytic Press.

Lichtenberg, J. D., Lachmann, F. M., & Fosshage, J. L. (1996). *The clinical exchange: Techniques derived from self and motivational systems*. The Analytic Press.

Lichtenberg, J. D., Lachmann, F. M., & Fosshage, J. L. (2002). *A spirit of inquiry: Communication in psychoanalysis*. The Analytic Press.

Lichtenberg, J. D., Lachmann, F. M., & Fosshage, J. L. (2011). *Psychoanalysis and motivational systems: A new look*. Routledge.

Lichtenberg, J. D., Lachmann, F. M., & Fosshage, J. L. (2021). *An experience-based vision of psychoanalytic theory and practice*. Routledge.

Linear System. (2021, September 9). In *Wikipedia*. https://en.wikipedia.org/w/index.php?title=Linear_system&oldid=1031714783

Nonlinear system. (2021, September 9). In *Wikipedia*. https://en.wikipedia.org/w/index.php?title=Nonlinear_system&oldid=1032173630

Open System (Systems Theory). (2021, September 6). In *Wikipedia*. https://en.wikipedia.org/w/index.php?title=Open_system_(systems_theory)&oldid=1035189846

Smith, L. B., & Thelen, E. (Eds.). (1993). *A dynamic systems approach to development: Applications*. The MIT Press.

Smith, L. B., & Thelen, E. (2003). Development as a dynamic system. *Trends in Cognitive Sciences*, *7*, 343–348. 10.1016/S1364-6613(03)00156-6

Strevens, M. (2016). Complexity theory. In P. Humphreys (Ed.), *The Oxford handbook of philosophy of science* (pp. 695 ff). The Oxford University Press.

Strogatz, S. H. (2014). *Nonlinear dynamics and chaos: With applications to physics, biology, chemistry, and engineering* (2nd ed.). Routledge.

Systems Theory. (2021, August 30). In *Wikipedia*. https://en.wikipedia.org/w/index.php?title=Systems_theory&oldid=1028933865

Tronick, E. (1998). Interventions that effect change in psychotherapy: A model based on infant research. *Infant Mental Health Journal*, *19*(3), 277–279.

Tronick, E. (2005). Why is connection with others so critical? The formation of dyadic states of consciousness and the expansion of individuals' states of consciousness: Coherence governed selection and the co-creation of meaning out of messy meaning making. In J. Nadel & D. Muir (Eds.), *Emotional development: Recent research advances* (pp. 293–315). Oxford University Press.

Tronick, E., & Beeghly, M. (2011). Infants' meaning making and the development of mental health problems. *American Psychologist*, *66*(2), 107–119.

von Bertalanffy, L. (1969). *General system theory: Foundations, development, applications* (Revised ed.). George Braziller.

Index

For Product Safety Concerns and Information please contact our EU representative GPSR@taylorandfrancis.com
Taylor & Francis Verlag GmbH, Kaufingerstraße 24, 80331 München, Germany

www.ingramcontent.com/pod-product-compliance
Ingram Content Group UK Ltd.
Pitfield, Milton Keynes, MK11 3LW, UK
UKHW020145200926
475702UK00005B/937

* 9 7 8 0 3 6 7 4 6 2 5 5 0 *

